MRCGP
Applied Knowledge Test
1001 Questions and Answers

Rob Daniels

MA (Cantab), MB BChir, MRCGP
General Practitioner

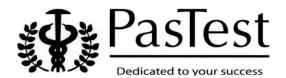

PasTest

Dedicated to your success

© 2013 PASTEST LTD
Egerton Court
Parkgate Estate
Knutsford
Cheshire
WA16 8DX

Telephone: 01565 752000

A percentage of the material in this book was previously published in *MRCGP Practice Questions: Applied Knowledge Test, Second Edition* (ISBN 9781905635665) and *nMRCGP Practice Papers: Applied Knowledge Test, Second Edition* (ISBN 9781905635597).

First Published 2013. Reprinted July 2014.

ISBN: 1905635869
9781905635863

A catalogue record for this book is available from the British Library.

PasTest Revision Books and Intensive Courses

PasTest has been established in the field of undergraduate and postgraduate medical education since 1972, providing revision books and intensive study courses for doctors preparing for their professional examinations.

Books, courses and online revision available for:
Medical undergraduates, MRCGP, MRCP Parts 1 and 2, MRCPCH Parts 1 and 2, MRCS, MRCOG, DRCOG, DCH, FRCA, Dentistry.

For further details contact:

PasTest, Freepost, Knutsford, Cheshire WA16 7BR

Tel: 01565 752000 Fax: 01565 650264

www.pastest.co.uk enquiries@pastest.co.uk

Text prepared in the UK by Keytec Typesetting Ltd, Bridport, Dorset
Printed and bound in the UK by Page Bros Ltd, Norwich

Contents

Acknowledgements

I would like to thank the patients of Townsend House Medical Centre, whose images appear in this book. I would also like to acknowledge, with thanks, the following people who have contributed additional clinical images:

Mr Peter Simcock, Consultant Ophthalmologist, Royal Devon & Exeter Hospital

Dr Chris Bower, Consultant Dermatologist, Royal Devon & Exeter Hospital

Mr Malcolm Hilton, Consultant Surgeon, Royal Devon & Exeter Hospital

Mr Ian Daniels, Consultant Surgeon, Royal Devon & Exeter Hospital

Dr Chris Cates, Senior Research Fellow, St Georges University London (www.nntonline.net)

Townsend House Medical Partnership

Thanks also to Lisa Daniels.

Dedicated to Grant Neumegen,
a great friend and colleague
who contributed both to this book and others,
and who sadly passed away in August 2013

Contributors to the previous editions

Julius Bourke MBBS, MRCPsych
Specialist Registrar, General Adult Psychiatry and Neuropsychiatry
The Maudsley Hospital
London

Erika Damato MA (Cantab) MBBS MRCP
Medical Ophthalmology Registrar
Bristol Eye Hospital

Rob Daniels MA (Cantab) MB BChir MRCGP
General Practitioner
Devon

Alison Johnstone MBChB MRC GP DFFP
General Practitioner
Hampshire

Priya Joshi MB ChB DRCOG MRCGP
General Practitioner
Cambridge

Grant Neumegen MBChB (Otago) MRCGP
General Practitioner
Devon

Seamus Phillips MA BM MRCS DOHNS MSc
Otolaryngology SpR
South Thames Rotation

Suzanne Renshaw BM DRCOG MRCGP
General Practitioner
Hampshire

Andrew Rosewarne MBBS MRCS DFPP DCH MRCGP
General Practitioner
Exeter

Pinki Singh MBBS DGO DNB MRCOG
Specialist Registrar Obs & Gynae
Worcester (West Midlands Deanery)

Ramanathan Visvanathan BM BCh, FRCS (Irel, Eng, Ed), ILTM
Consultant Surgeon, Bronglais General Hospital, Wales
Honorary Senior Lecturer, Cardiff University

Amy Wilson MBChB MRCPCH
Paediatric Registrar
Manchester

Kurt Wilson BSc MBChB MRCGP
General Practitioner
Manchester

Introduction

This book is intended predominantly to help candidates prepare for the Membership examination of the Royal College of General Practitioners, which is the qualifying exam for a career in general practice. It is also hoped that this book will be useful for established GPs to identify learning needs as part of their appraisal process and perhaps prepare them for any future knowledge-based test introduced as part of revalidation.

In line with changes in other specialty exams, the MRCGP now consists of a written exam, a formal clinical skills assessment and workplace-based assessment. The written paper encompasses clinical scenarios, hot topics and critical reading, and is in the form of a 200 question MCQ exam known as the Applied Knowledge Test (AKT). The subject matter is divided between critical appraisal and evidence-based clinical practice components, which make up approximately 10% of the questions; 10% will comprise health informatics and administrative questions, with the remaining 80% clinical questions. Questions are of the single best answer, extended matching questions and free text forms, and may require interpretation of pictures, results, and experimental or statistical data. The exam aims to test higher problem-solving rather than simple fact recall. A wealth of information about the curriculum and exam format is available on the Royal College of General Practitioners' website (www.rcgp.org.uk).

The Applied Knowledge Tests take place at the end of January, May and October each year, via computer terminals at 152 Pearson Vue professional testing centres around the UK (www.pearsonvue.co.uk). Detailed feedback will be provided for candidates who are unsuccessful, allowing them to take remedial action where necessary before the next sitting. Candidates may take the exam at any point in their general practice specialty training, but it is expected that most will do so during their third year of specialty training, when they will be working in primary care. All questions will address important issues relating to general practice in the UK, and international applicants should note that the answers will relate to standard clinical practice in the UK, which may differ from their own country.

The key to successful preparation is twofold. Exam technique is vital in many medical exams and the AKT is no exception. Two hundred questions have to be completed in 3 hours at a rate of just over one question a minute. The questions are of the single best answer, extending matching question and algorithm completion format, and there are many examples of each type in this book. The second component of successful exam performance is an adequate knowledge base. The content of the questions in this book is based on the GP curriculum, which is available on the RCGP's website, and the questions are loosely based on my clinical experience. This GP curriculum (www.rcgp-curriculum.org.uk) is an excellent resource in planning your revision, especially in less clinical areas of the curriculum such as practice management and information technology.

The RCGP website gives the pass mark and exam feedback for each sitting. In 2012 the pass mark was 68% and the pass rate was 75%. It is well worth reading the examiners' reports on previous sittings as these describe areas of weak performance, which the examiners may concentrate on in future exams. Candidates usually perform well in clinical medicine, less well in critical appraisal and worst in administration questions.

The best way to prepare for clinical questions is to read up on problems that you see in general practice, ideally keeping a list of PUNs and DENs (patient's unmet needs and doctor's educational needs) encountered during each surgery. Try to do as many practice multiple choice questions as you can; the old-style MRCGP exam questions are still mostly valid and there are a number of excellent practice MCQ books still available in shops and medical libraries. PasTest also offer an online revision package specifically for the AKT, which gives instant progress feedback (www. pastest.co.uk). It should be possible to pick up on hot topics just through working in general practice and reading the *British Medical Journal* and *British Journal of General Practice*, but a 'Hot topics' course just before the exam is usually money well spent. In the previous incarnation of the MRCGP exam, editorials from the *British Journal of General Practice* had an uncanny habit of turning up as hot topic questions in the next paper. Exam questions are likely to be drawn from several well-known journals, including those listed above. The RCGP's website gives useful information on this, so keep your eyes peeled.

Information on management issues is best picked up by spending a session or two with a practice manager, attending practice meetings and doing multiple-choice questions to identify specific learning needs. It often helps to revise this area with a textbook, such as *Notes for the MRCGP*, although this is now somewhat out of date. Practising critical appraisal of journal articles with a group from your GP training scheme is a useful way of learning this skill, and a lot more enjoyable than trying to read a statistics textbook. The Bandolier website (www.jr2.ox.ac.uk/bandolier) is an excellent source of information about critical appraisal. I have included several statistics questions to illustrate various concepts, but all of the data and graphs are made up, so please do not take the results too seriously.

I have done my best to ensure that all the questions and answers are accurate and current. If you find any discrepancies or have any other comments please let me know and I will make the necessary changes.

Good luck!

Rob Daniels

Abbreviations

A&E	accident and emergency
ABPI	ankle–brachial pressure index
ACE	angiotensin-converting enzyme
ACL	anterior cruciate ligament
ACTH	adrenocorticotrophic hormone
ADH	antidiuretic hormone
ADHD	attention deficit hyperactivity disorder
AF	atrial fibrillation
AG	anion gap
AIDS	acquired immune deficiency syndrome
ALL	acute lymphoblastic leukaemia
ALP	alkaline phosphatase
ALT	alanine transaminase
AML	acute myeloid leukaemia
ARB	angiotension receptor antagonist
ARDS	acute respiratory distress syndrome
ARI	absolute risk increase
ARR	absolute risk reduction
APTT	activated partial thromboplastin time
AST	aspartate transaminase
AV	atrioventricular
BCC	basal cell carcinoma
BCG	bacille Calmette–Guérin
BIPP	bismuth iodoform paraffin paste
BMI	body mass index
BNP	brain natriuretic peptide
BP	blood pressure
BTS	British Thoracic Society
CBT	cognitive–behavioural therapy
CC	case–control (study)
CER	control event rate
CF	cystic fibrosis
CHADS$_2$	**C**CF, **h**ypertension, **a**ge >75, **d**iabetes and **s**troke
CHD	coronary heart disease
CI	confidence interval
CIN	cervical intraepithelial neoplasia
CK	creatine kinase
CKD	chronic kidney disease
CLL	chronic lymphoblastic leukaemia
CML	chronic myeloid leukaemia
CMV	cytomegalovirus
CNS	central nervous system

COC(P)	combined oral contraceptive (pill)
COPD	chronic obstructive pulmonary disease
COX	cyclooxygenase
CPAP	continuous positive airway pressure
CPR	cardiopulmonary resuscitation
CREST	calcinosis, Raynaud's disease, (o)esophageal dysmotility, sclerodactyly and telangiectasia
CRP	C-reactive protein
CSF	cerebrospinal fluid
CT	computed tomography
CTG	cardiotocography
CVD	cardiovascular disease
CVS	chorionic villous sampling
DCIS	ductal carcinoma *in situ*
DES	direct enhanced service
DIC	disseminated intravascular coagulation/coagulopathy
DIP	distal interphalangeal
DKA	diabetic ketoacidosis
DMARD	disease-modifying anti-rheumatic drug
DNA	deoxyribonucleic acid
DSM-IV	*Diagnostic and Statistical Manual of Mental Disorders*, 4th edition
DVLA	Driver and Vehicle Licensing Agency
DVT	deep vein thrombosis
DXA	dual-energy X-ray absorptiometry
EBV	Epstein–Barr virus
ECG	electrocardiogram
EEG	electroencephalogram
EER	experimental event rate
eGFR	estimated glomerular filtration rate
ENT	ear, nose and throat
EPA	enduring power of attorney
ERCP	endoscopic retrograde cholangiopancreatography
ESR	erythrocyte sedimentation rate
FBC	full blood count
FEV_1	forced expiratory volume in 1 second
FFP	fresh frozen plasma
FRC	functional residual capacity
FSH	follicle-stimulating hormone
FT_4	free thyroxine
FVC	forced vital capacity
G6PDH	glucose-6-phosphate dehydrogenase
GFR	glomerular filtration rate
GGT	γ-glutamyltransferase
GI	gastrointestinal
GMS	General Medical Services
GPPAQ	General Practice Physical Activity Questionnaire
GPwSI	general practitioner with a special interest
GnRH	gonadotrophin-releasing hormone
GTN	glyceryl trinitrate
GUM	genitourinary medicine

HbA1c	glycated haemoglobin
βhCG	β-human chorionic gonadotrophin
HDL	high-density lipoprotein
HELLP	haemolysis, elevated liver enzymes, low platelets
HIV	human immunodeficiency virus
HPV	human papillomavirus
HR	heart rate
HRT	hormone replacement therapy
HSP	Henoch–Schönlein purpura
IBS	irritable bowel syndrome
ICD-10	*International Classification of Disease*, 10th revision
ICP	intracranial pressure
ICU	intensive care unit
INR	international normalised ratio
IOP	intraocular pressure
IQ	intelligence quotient
IUCD	intrauterine contraceptive device
KUB	kidneys, ureters and bladder
LDH	lactate dehydrogenase
LDL	low-density lipoprotein
LES	local enhanced service
LFTs	liver function tests
LH	luteinising hormone
LHRH	luteinising hormone-releasing hormone
LMWH	low-molecular-weight heparin
LPA	lasting power of attorney
LTOT	long-term oxygen therapy
LVF	left ventricular failure
MALT	mucosa-associated lymphoid tissue
MAOI	monoamine oxidase inhibitor
MCH	mean corpuscular haemoglobin
MCV	mean corpuscular volume
MI	myocardial infarction
MMR	measles, mumps and rubella
MRI	magnetic resonance imaging
MRSA	methicillin-resistant *Staphylococcus aureus*
MSU	midstream urine
NCAA	National Clinical Assessment Authority
NICE	National Institute for Health and Care Excellence
NNH	number needed to harm
NNT	number needed to treat
NSAID	non-steroidal anti-inflammatory drug
NSTEMI	non-ST-elevation myocardial infarction
NYHA	New York Heart Association
OCD	obsessive–compulsive disorder
OSA	obstructive sleep apnoea
PCL	posterior cruciate ligament
PCOS	polycystic ovarian syndrome
PCR	polymerase chain reaction
PCT	primary care trust

PEFR	peak expiratory flow rate
PE	pulmonary embolus
PICA	posterior inferior cerebellar artery
PID	pelvic inflammatory disease
PIP	proximal interphalangeal
PMR	polymyalgia rheumatica
POP	progestogen-only pill
PPI	proton pump inhibitor
PSA	prostate-specific antigen
PT	prothrombin time
PTH	parathyroid hormone
PUVA	psoralen + UVA
RCT	randomised controlled trial
QALY	quality-adjusted life-year
QOF	Quality and Outcomes Framework
RA	rheumatoid arthritis
RICE	rest, ice, compression and elevation
RR	relative risk
RSV	respiratory syncytial virus
SCC	squamous cell carcinoma
SIGN	Scottish Intercollegiate Guidelines Network
SIR	standardised incidence ratio
SLE	systemic lupus erythematosus
SNRI	serotonin and noradrenaline reuptake inhibitor
SSRI	selective serotonin release inhibitor
STEMI	ST-elevation myocardial infarction
STI	sexually transmitted infection
SVC	superior vena cava
T_3	triiodothyronine
T_4	thyroxine
TB	tuberculosis
TED	thromboembolic deterrent
TIA	transient ischaemic attack
TNF	tumour necrosis factor
TSH	thyroid-stimulating hormone
TFT	thyroid function test
U&Es	urea and electrolytes
UTI	urinary tract infection
UTRI	upper respiratory tract infection
UVA	long-wavelength ultraviolet (light)
UVPP	uvulopalatoplasty
VEGF	vascular endothelial growth factor
VIN	vulval intraepithelial neoplasia
VRE	vancomycin-resistant enterococci
WCC	white cell count
WOMAC	Western Ontario and McMaster Universities Index of Osteoarthritis

Chapter 1
Cardiovascular

SINGLE BEST ANSWER QUESTIONS

1.1 Blood pressure
At a routine blood pressure check your practice nurse discovers a
20 mmHg difference in systolic blood pressure between the right and left
arms of a patient. She asks him to return and see you and, when he does,
you note the same findings. What would be the single most appropriate
next step in his management?

○ A   Ambulatory blood pressure monitoring

◉ B   Ankle–brachial pressure measurement   ✗

○ C   Chest X-ray

○ D   Refer for tilt-table tests

○ E   Urinary catecholamines

1.2 Cholesterol
A 29-year-old man asks for a cholesterol test. His father, aged 53, has just
had a heart attack, although he was a heavy smoker. On checking his
blood pressure you notice pale nodules on the tendons of his wrists. He
tells you that he also has them on the back of his ankles, and that these
are a family trait. His cholesterol is 7.8 mmol/l and his blood pressure is
134/80 mmHg. Which one of the following would be appropriate
management for this patient?

○ A   Advise on a low-fat diet and repeat his blood test in 6 months

○ B   Calculate his Framingham risk score and treat him with statins if his
10-year risk is >20%

○ C   Start atorvastatin 10 mg once daily

○ D   Start simvastatin 20 mg once daily

○ E   Start simvastatin 80 mg once daily

? Atorvastatin

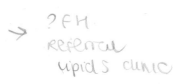
*→ ?FH.
Referral
lipids clinic*

1.3 Atrial fibrillation

Your practice is asked by your local commissioning group to conduct an audit of all patients with atrial fibrillation using the CHADS$_2$ score to optimise anticoagulation. Which one of the following statements is true regarding this tool?

- A CHADS$_2$ calculates the risk of atrial fibrillation developing in the next 12 months *10 yr stroke risk in those with AF*
- B Net benefit from anticoagulation is seen when the score is ⩾2
- C Patients with a score of 1 should be anticoagulated *men score 1 femaur sce 2*
- D Patients with a score of <4 should have aspirin, while those with a score of >4 should be anticoagulated *No role aspirin*
- E The CHADS$_2$-VASc score is included in the Quality and Outcomes Framework from 2012

1.4 Fainting

A 21-year-old student rower who is training for national trials complains that he has had a few episodes of palpitations and fainted during a heavy training session. On examination he is in sinus rhythm with a resting pulse of 54, his heart sounds reveal a soft systolic murmur and his blood pressure is 112/66. An ECG shows slightly enlarged R waves. Which one of the following is the single most likely diagnosis?

- A Hypertrophic obstructive cardiomyopathy
- B Overexertion
- C Paroxysmal atrial fibrillation
- D Recurrent supraventricular tachycardia
- E Wolff–Parkinson–White syndrome

1.5 Leg pain

A 72-year-old man who underwent coronary artery bypass surgery 5 years ago presents with intermittent cramp-like pain in the buttock, thigh and calf. The symptoms are worse on walking and relieved by rest. On examination, both legs are of normal colour, but the pedal pulses are difficult to palpate. Sensation is mildly reduced in the left foot. Which of the following is the single most appropriate action?

- A Advise him to reduce walking distance to prevent pain
- B Doppler ultrasound
- C Measure ankle–brachial systolic pressure index
- D Magnetic resonance imaging (MRI) of the lumbar spine
- E Referral for angiography

1.6 Hypertension

You see a newly diagnosed hypertensive patient for review after his baseline investigations. According to the Quality and Outcomes Framework (QOF), which one of the following statements is correct regarding assessment of new hypertensives?

- A Cardiovascular risk assessment must be carried out within 6 months of the date of diagnosis
- B Lifestyle advice must be given in the 3 months before or after diagnosis of hypertension
- C Risk assessment must use the Framingham assessment tool
- D The QRISK assessment tool should be used for patients with pre-existing ischaemic heart disease
- E There must be an assessment of physical activity

1.7 Ablation therapy

A 52-year-old man with paroxysmal atrial fibrillation comes to see you requesting referral for ablation therapy, which he has read about on the internet. He is currently taking flecainide but finds that he is having to take increasing amounts of time off work and has been cardioverted three times. Which one of the following statements is correct about ablation for paroxysmal atrial fibrillation?

- A Of patients 76% are successfully treated with this procedure
- B It is a first-line treatment for younger patients with paroxysmal atrial fibrillation
- C Serious side effects are extremely rare
- D The procedure is usually carried out as an outpatient
- E Usually requires insertion of a pacemaker as part of the procedure

1.8 Cholesterol wrong guidance

The following results show the fasting lipid profile of a 35-year-old man who underwent routine testing as part of a general health check: total cholesterol 7.9 mmol/l, low-density lipoprotein (LDL) 4.9 mmol/l, high-density lipoprotein (HDL) 0.83 mmol/l and triglyceride 5.2 mmol/l. His father died of myocardial infarction (MI) at the age of 52. Which one of the following would be the most appropriate initial management?

- A Initiate dietary modification and monitor response by re-testing in 3 months
- B Initiate treatment with a fibrate
- C Initiate treatment with simvastatin 10 mg once daily
- D Initiate treatment with simvastatin 80 mg once daily; further testing is not required
- E Refer for specialist opinion

1.9 Driving after myocardial infarction

A 65-year-old man has recently been discharged from hospital having suffered an ST-elevation MI. Coronary artery stenting was performed and he is now pain free. He enquires whether he can drive his own car. Which one of the following is the most appropriate advice?

○ A After an MI patients should not drive until they have undergone exercise or functional testing

○ B Driving must cease for 6 months

✓ C Driving must cease for at least 4 weeks

1 week

○ D The patient must notify the DVLA

○ E The patient should be informed that the GP is obliged to inform the DVLA of this event

1.10 Antibiotic prophylaxis

A 64-year-old man who underwent mitral valve replacement 5 years ago has forgotten the advice that he was given regarding the use of prophylactic antibiotics to prevent endocarditis when he undergoes dental treatment or other procedures. Which one of the following is the most appropriate advice?

○ A Antibiotic prophylaxis is not recommended for routine procedures, but he should be advised about the importance of maintaining good oral health

○ B He should receive antibiotic prophylaxis for any future dental or surgical procedures

○ C He should receive antibiotic prophylaxis for any procedures on the gastrointestinal or genitourinary tracts

○ D He should receive antibiotic prophylaxis for dental procedures only

○ E He should use chlorhexidine mouthwash before dental treatment

1.11 Hypertension

A 42-year-old man of Asian origin attends for a general health check. He is a non-smoker, drinks 21 units of alcohol per week, is physically well and active, and enjoys regular moderate exercise and a healthy diet. His body mass index (BMI) is 27.2 kg/m^2. His BP, measured on three occasions, was 162/100, 165/100 and 168/102 mmHg. Which one of the following would be the most appropriate initial management?

○ A Advise about lifestyle modification and review in 6 months

○ B Refer for investigation of a secondary cause of hypertension

○ C Start a calcium-channel blocker

○ D Start a thiazide diuretic

○ E Start an ACE inhibitor

1.12 Calf pain

A 42-year-old woman has varicose veins that are normally asymptomatic. She presents with a 3-day history of moderately severe pain and erythema surrounding a superficial vein, below and medial to the right knee. On palpation, the varicose vein is hardened and tender; the rest of the calf is unremarkable. Which one of the following is the most appropriate management?

- A   Refer for surgical assessment
- B   Request a Doppler ultrasound scan of the leg
- C   Start oral flucloxacillin
- D   Treat with an NSAID and crepe bandage
- E   Treat with topical corticosteroid

1.13 Collapse

A 21-year-old female student with no significant medical history consults you 24 hours after collapsing in a shop. The event was witnessed by a friend, who reports that she suddenly became pale and clammy, lost consciousness and fell to the floor. There was a short episode of twitching of all four limbs. She regained consciousness after less than 1 minute, rapidly became oriented and has felt well since the event. Neurological and cardiovascular examinations are normal, with a heart rate (HR) of 76/min and BP of 120/65 mmHg. Which of the following is the single most likely diagnosis?

- A   Epilepsy
- B   Hyperglycaemia
- C   Neurocardiogenic syncope
- D   Paroxysmal arrhythmia
- E   Pseudoseizure

1.14 Syncope

A 78-year-old man with a history of atrial fibrillation treated with sotalol complains of recurrent syncopal episodes. Examination reveals atrial fibrillation with a rate of 84/min and normal blood pressure. You ask your practice nurse to do an electrocardiogram (ECG) and while this is taking place he has another syncopal episode. A rhythm strip is obtained, which is shown below.

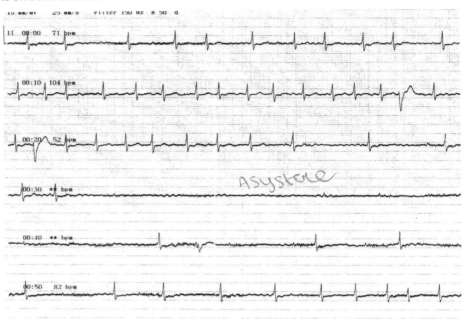

What would be the most appropriate action in this situation?

- A Admit for pacemaker
- B Check bloods to exclude myocardial infarction
- C Give intravenous adrenaline and commence cardiopulmonary resuscitation (CPR)
- D Start amiodarone
- E Stop his β blocker

1.15 ECG abnormalities

A 35-year-old man presents with chest pain. The ECG below is carried out. Select the one feature from A to E shown that is most consistent with a diagnosis of pericarditis.

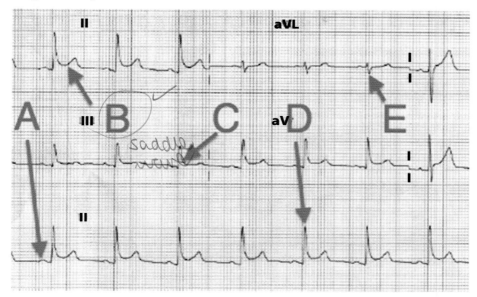

1.16 Raised blood pressure

A 56-year-old woman who looks after her daughter's three young children attends for a flu jab and is found to have raised blood pressure by the nurse. You see her and find that her blood pressure is elevated, but not as much as when the nurse saw her. There is no difference between her arms. You arrange a 24-hour blood pressure recording, the results of which are shown below.

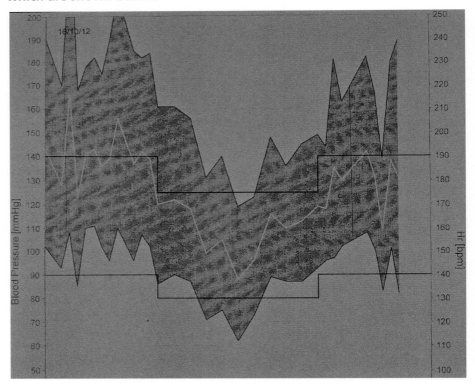

Which one of the following would be appropriate management in this situation?

○ A Advice her about healthy lifestyle and review in 3 months

○ B Ask her to purchase her own blood pressure monitor and keep a diary of regular recordings for 2 weeks

○ C Encourage her to attend relaxation classes

○ D Reassure her that she has white coat hypertension and no treatment is needed

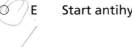 E Start antihypertensives

1.17 Data interpretation

A study looking at risk factors for a disease is carried out. The data shown below relate to the association between alcohol consumption and risk of disease.

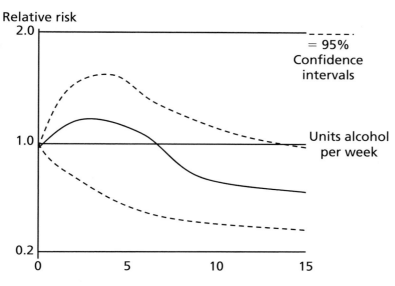

Which one of the following statements is a correct interpretation of the data? Select one option only.

A   Increased consumption of alcohol is associated with an increased risk of disease

B   Increased consumption of alcohol is protective against disease

C   Increased risk of disease is correlated with number of years drinking

D   Non-drinkers are at higher risk than all drinkers

E   The data do not reach statistical significance

1.18 Shortness of breath

A 79-year-old man presents with a 1-month history of mild shortness of breath on exertion. On examination, his pulse is irregular with a rate of 90 beats/min at rest. A systolic murmur is heard on auscultation. His ECG is shown below.

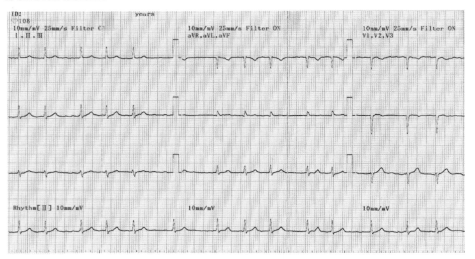

Which one of the following would be most appropriate in his management?

○ A   Amiodarone 200 mg once daily

○ B   Aspirin 300 mg once daily

○ C   Bendroflumethiazide 2.5 mg once daily

✓ D   Diltiazem hydrochloride 60 mg twice daily

○ E   Furosemide 40 mg once daily

1.19 Management of essential hypertension in patients under 55 years of age

Select the rank order of the options (1–4) that best fulfils the requirements given in the question.

The following is a list of treatments for essential hypertension for white people aged <55:
1   ACE inhibitor or β blocker
2   α Blocker
3   Calcium-channel blocker
4   Thiazide diuretic

The responses (A–E) rank the treatments for essential hypertension in various orders. Select the response that places the options (1–4) in the order of **initial** treatment first to **final** step last. Select one rank order only.

- ○   A: 1, 3, 2, 4
- ○   B: 1, 3, 4, 2
- ○   C: 1, 4, 3, 2
- ○   D: 3, 1, 4, 2
- ○   E: 4, 3, 1, 2

EXTENDED MATCHING QUESTIONS

Antiplatelet therapy

Options

A   Aspirin 75 mg daily
B   Aspirin 150 mg daily
C   Aspirin 300 mg daily
D   Aspirin 75 mg daily and dipyridamole 200 mg twice daily
E   Clopidogrel 75 mg daily
F   Dipyridamole modified-release 200 mg twice daily
G   Ticagrelor 75 mg daily
H   Warfarin
I   None of the above

For each of the situations below, select the single most appropriate option from the list above. Each option may be used once, more than once or not at all.

1.20   A 76-year-old man develops a facial palsy and slurred speech that resolve after 4 hours. *C*

1.21   A 57-year-old man attends for a review 3 months after a successful coronary artery bypass graft. He had a myocardial infarction *A* 12 months ago but was not suitable for angioplasty.

1.22   A 78-year-old woman develops a left-sided hemiplegia. This does not resolve and she is left with residual disability. CT confirms an ischaemic event, but an ECG and echocardiogram are normal. *E*

1.23   A 48-year-old man is seen for a routine review 3 months after having a second ischaemic stroke, despite taking clopidogrel. On examination you note that he is in atrial fibrillation, although this has not been previously noted. *H*

1.24   A 42-year-old woman with a history of hypertension and diabetes develops a severe headache, diplopia when looking laterally and has a seizure. On admission to hospital she has a CT scan that shows an intracerebral haemorrhage. *I*

Heart failure

Options

A   Amlodipine
B   Atenolol
C   Carvedilol
D   Digoxin
E   Diltiazem
F   Furosemide
G   Ramipril
H   Spironolactone
I   Valsartan
J   None of the above

For each of the scenarios below, select the most appropriate option from the list above. Each option may be used once, more than once or not at all.

1.25   A 67-year-old man had a heart attack last year. An echocardiogram 6 months after the heart attack showed left ventricular dysfunction for which he was started on an ACE inhibitor. He is still symptomatic and on examination he has a sinus tachycardia with a rate of 100. His previous medical history includes hypertension and hypercholesterolaemia, and he is taking aspirin, simvastatin and ramipril.   *B .*

1.26   An 86-year-old man with heart failure has been started on lisinopril 8 weeks ago but complains of a persistent cough. His *I* previous medical history includes chronic obstructive pulmonary disease for which he takes tiotropium and salmeterol.

1.27   A 73-year-old woman with left ventricular dysfunction after a myocardial infarction is taking valsartan and nebivolol at maximum doses. She was previously treated with ramipril but *H* developed a cough. She is keen to improve her exercise capacity so that she can play with her grandchildren.

1.28   A 92-year-old woman who has been treated for many years for heart failure is taking digoxin for atrial fibrillation, ramipril and spironolactone. She has previously tried β blockers but developed cold feet. She is particularly bothered by her oedematous legs which make it very hard to find shoes that fit.   *F*

Treatment of hypertension

Options

A   Amlodipine
B   Atenolol
C   Bendroflumethiazide
D   Candesartan
E   Doxazosin
F   Furosemide
G   Hydralazine
H   No change indicated
I   Ramipril
J   Specialist referral

Select from the options above the most appropriate treatment for each of the following scenarios. Each option can be used once, more than once or not at all.

1.29   A white 49-year-old man takes ramipril and amlodipine at their maximum doses for essential hypertension. His BP over the last 3 months has persistently been found to be between 148/92 and 154/96 mmHg.

1.30   A 56-year-old man of African–Caribbean origin takes bendroflumethiazide 2.5 mg once daily. His BP is persistently found to lie between 148/94 and 156/96 mmHg. He has a healthy diet and takes regular exercise.

1.31   A white 69-year-old man, who is otherwise well, takes atenolol and bendroflumethiazide for essential hypertension. His BP is 136/88 mmHg.

1.32   A 39-year-old businessman complains of daily headaches and stress at work. His BP is 186/116 mmHg and his urine is positive for protein on dipstick testing.

1.33   A previously well 42-year-old man has recently started taking an ACE inhibitor for essential hypertension. He complains of a dry cough, and has decided to stop his medication. On examination, his BP is 148/98 mmHg and auscultation of the chest is normal.

Angina

Options

A   Amlodipine
B   Anticoagulation
C   Atenolol
D   Clopidogrel
E   Emergency hospital admission
F   Glyceryl trinitrate (GTN)
G   Isosorbide mononitrate
H   Lisinopril
I   Nicorandil

For each of the scenarios below, select the most appropriate treatment from the list above. Each option can be used once, more than once or not at all.

1.34 A 48-year-old man is seen at the end of the morning surgery, having experienced four episodes of chest pain that morning. Each episode lasted for 15–20 minutes and radiated to the left arm. He smokes 20 cigarettes a day and has a family history of MI. He takes no regular medication. He is now pain free, with a BP of 155/95 mmHg. Examination of the chest is normal.

1.35 A 72-year-old woman with angina experiences chest pain three to four times a week. Episodes usually occur on exertion and are relieved by sublingual GTN. She takes no other medication.

1.36 A 79-year-old man with known left ventricular dysfunction requires further control of his angina despite the use of a long-acting nitrate. He takes no other medication.

1.37 A 59-year-old man with angina, for whom standard treatment with calcium antagonists, β blockers and long-acting nitrates has been unsuccessful.

Stroke risk

1.38 –1.42

Options

A Anticoagulation
B Antiplatelet
C Antiplatelet or warfarin
D Dipyridamole
E Heparin
F No treatment
G Patient aged >75 years
H Patient aged <75 years

Complete the algorithm below for the management of stroke risk in atrial fibrillation, using the CHADS$_2$ (**C**CF, **h**ypertension, **a**ge >75, **d**iabetes and **s**troke) scoring system, from the list of options above. Each option may be used once, more than once or not at all.

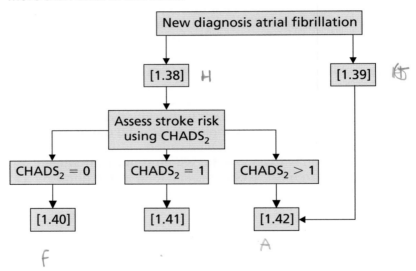

Pharmacological treatment of symptomatic heart failure due to left ventricular systolic dysfunction

1.43–1.48

Options

A   ACE inhibitor
B   Angiotensin II receptor antagonist
C   β Blocker
D   Digoxin
E   Diuretic therapy
F   Spironolactone

Complete the following algorithm, selecting options from the list above. Each option can be used once, more than once or not at all.

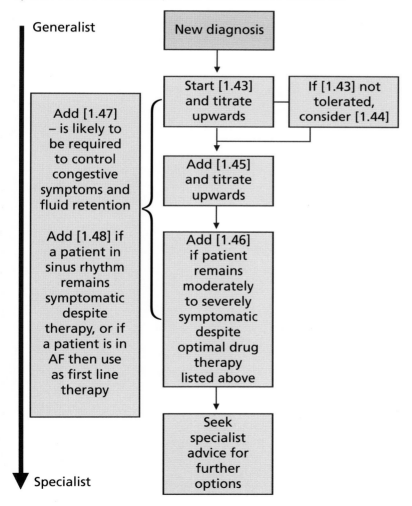

Generalist

New diagnosis

Start [1.43] and titrate upwards

If [1.43] not tolerated, consider [1.44]

Add [1.47] – is likely to be required to control congestive symptoms and fluid retention

Add [1.45] and titrate upwards

Add [1.48] if a patient in sinus rhythm remains symptomatic despite therapy, or if a patient is in AF then use as first line therapy

Add [1.46] if patient remains moderately to severely symptomatic despite optimal drug therapy listed above

Seek specialist advice for further options

Specialist

FREE TEXT QUESTION

1.49 **Shortness of breath**

A 32-year-old woman with no previous medical history is seen 3 weeks after an uneventful delivery of her second baby. She complains that she has swollen ankles, is short of breath and has been waking up at night unable to breathe. Examination confirms pitting oedema of the ankles, a resting tachycardia of 120, with a regular heartbeat and bilateral basal crepitations on auscultation. In the box below, write the most likely diagnosis in this case.

Preserved Ejection Fraction HF

SINGLE BEST ANSWER

1.1   **B:**   **Ankle–brachial pressure measurement**

A difference in systolic blood pressure between the arms of >10 mmHg is a risk factor for cardiovascular disease; systematic reviews suggest that a 15 mmHg difference is associated with a 70% increase in risk of occult peripheral arterial disease. Sustained differences should prompt ankle–brachial pressure index (ABPI) testing, particularly in patients with other cardiovascular risk factors. Ambulatory blood pressure monitoring should be used in patients with suspected white coat hypertension, whereas urinary catecholamines are used to exclude phaeochromocytoma in patients with fluctuating resistant hypertension.

1.2   **E:**   **Start simvastatin 80 mg once daily**

Tendon xanthomas are diagnostic of familial hypercholesterolaemia. He is at very high risk of ischaemic heart disease and should be treated with simvastatin 80 mg once daily or equivalent regardless of his Framingham score. Diagnostic criteria for familial hypercholesterolaemia are a total cholesterol >7.5 with tendon xanthomas. Prevalence in the UK is 1:500 but it is higher in certain ethnic groups such as Afrikaners. Familial hypercholesterolaemia accounts for 10% of cases of heart disease in the under 60 group.

1.3   **B:**   **Net benefit from anticoagulation is seen when the score is ⩾2**

$CHADS_2$ assigns 1 point each for the presence of CCF, hypertension, age >75 years and diabetes. A score of 1 should be treated with antiplatelet or anticoagulation whereas a score >1 should be treated with anticoagulation. The $CHADS_2$ score is a part of the QOF. An extended formula, the $CHA2DS_2$-VASc score uses additional risk factors such as previous cerebrovascular disease and gender, and has been shown to be a more accurate predictor of risk.

1.4   **A:**   **Hypertrophic obstructive cardiomyopathy**

HOCM has a prevalence of 1:500 and is a common cause of sudden cardiac death in young people. Early symptoms include angina, dyspnoea and syncope. ECG changes include left ventricular hypertrophy and examination may show a systolic murmur, which characteristically diminishes on squatting and increases on Valsalva's manoeuvre. Echocardiography is the examination of choice.

1.5   C: Measure ankle–brachial systolic pressure index

These symptoms are typical of intermittent claudication. The history and an ABPI of <0.9 support the diagnosis. Walking distance can be improved by exercise and patients should be encouraged to continue walking beyond the distance at which pain occurs. Referral to a vascular surgeon is indicated if symptoms are lifestyle limiting. If there are bilateral symptoms, spinal stenosis should be considered.

1.6   E: There must be an assessment of physical activity

The cardiovascular disease primary prevention indicators require that, for patients with hypertension, there should be an assessment using the General Practice Physical Activity Questionnaire (GPPAQ). Lifestyle advice needs to be given in the previous 15 months, but does not need to be given face to face. Previously the QOF required newly diagnosed patients to have a face to face CVS risk assessment, but this has been dropped from April 2013.

1.7   A: Of patients 76% are successfully treated with this procedure

Radiofrequency ablation via the femoral vein is carried out in patients who have refractory symptoms despite medical therapy or where medical therapy is contraindicated. It is combined with electrophysiological mapping of the heart to identify aberrant pathways and is usually carried out under sedation. Meta-analysis suggests success rates of 76% but the complication rate is 6%, with cardiac tamponade, transient ischaemic attack (TIA), oesophageal perforation and pulmonary vein stenosis all being reported.

1.8   A: Initiate dietary modification and monitor response by re-testing in 3 months

The premature death (at 52 years) of this patient's father and his abnormal lipid profile suggest a diagnosis of familial hyperlipidaemia, of which there are several types. Combined elevation of cholesterol and triglycerides suggests familial combined hyperlipidaemia, which affects 0.5–1% of the population and approximately 15% of patients who have an MI before the age of 60. In the absence of other risk factors (smoking, diabetes, hypertension) he can safely be managed by diet and, if there is no response, with statins. Should other risk factors be present, these should also be addressed.

1.9   C: Driving must cease for at least 4 weeks

DVLA medical standards of fitness to drive state that driving of a private car (a group 1 vehicle) must cease for 4 weeks after an ST-elevation MI. All acute coronary syndromes, including MI, result in disqualification from driving group 2 vehicles (eg a heavy goods vehicle or bus) for 6 months before re-licensing.

1.10   A: Antibiotic prophylaxis is not recommended for routine procedures, but he should be advised about the importance of maintaining good oral health

The use of prophylactic antibiotics to prevent endocarditis for patients with structural cardiac abnormalities and replacement valves has been longstanding, accepted medical practice, but there is little evidence of its effectiveness. Recommendations have been changed, based on the best available published evidence and multidisciplinary and expert consensus (NICE, March 2008).

1.11   E: Start an ACE inhibitor

This patient has a diagnosis of hypertension. With a BP >160/100 mmHg, he should be offered drug therapy. An ACE inhibitor is recommended as first-line treatment for patients aged <55 years. Patients aged >55, and black patients of any age, should initially be treated with a calcium-channel blocker or a thiazide diuretic.

1.12   D: Treat with an NSAID and crepe bandage

These features are typical of superficial thrombophlebitis, which can usually be adequately treated with NSAIDs. A crepe bandage will compress the vein and help prevent propagation of the thrombus. If phlebitis extends upwards in the medial thigh, towards the saphenofemoral junction, refer for Doppler ultrasound because there is potential for extension into the femoral vein.

1.13   C: Neurocardiogenic syncope

These features are typical of neurocardiogenic (vasovagal) syncope. The condition is benign and can be triggered by the following factors: emotion, pain, fear and anxiety, micturition, defecation, dehydration, a warm environment and prolonged standing. Advice to patients should include avoidance of precipitating factors. Other methods of prevention include compression hosiery or voluntary forceful contraction of the limb muscles at the onset of symptoms.

1.14   A: Admit for pacemaker

This ECG shows a 12-second episode of asystole. Atropine can be used if the episode is prolonged but a permanent pacemaker is needed. Amiodarone is used for atrial fibrillation, whereas adrenaline would be used in an arrest situation. If the patient collapses, basic life support should be instituted until he reaches hospital. Where pacing is not available, short-term treatment with isoprenaline might be helpful until definitive treatment is possible.

1.15   B

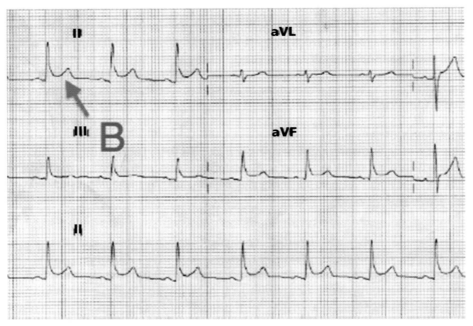

B indicates a saddle wave typical of acute pericarditis. This condition may cause ST elevation and also initially depression between the P wave and the start of the QRS complex. In later stages T-wave inversion may be seen.

1.16   E: Start antihypertensives

This graph shows that she has sustained hypertension with systolic readings consistently >140 mmHg. There are peaks, suggesting a stress response, but her average readings will be well above treatment targets. She should have lifestyle advice, start treatment and be assessed for end-organ damage and causes of hypertension, as well as having her 10-year cardiovascular risk calculated.

1.17   B: Increased consumption of alcohol is protective against disease

The data show that drinkers drinking more than 7 units a week have a reduced risk of disease, and that this reaches statistical significance at around 11 units a week (95% confidence interval <1.0). Moderate drinkers (<7 units a week) have increased risk relative to non-drinkers although the confidence intervals are wide. Longevity of drinking is not shown on this graph.

1.18   D: Diltiazem hydrochloride 60 mg twice daily

The ECG reveals AF with a rapid ventricular response. NICE clinical guidance on AF (2006) recommends that the most appropriate management strategy for this patient would be rate control with a rate-limiting calcium antagonist (or β blocker). Stroke risk stratification and anticoagulation are important, and it is likely that this patient would be a candidate for warfarin therapy (aged >75 with clinical evidence of valve disease).

1.19   **B:**   **1 3 4 2**

               1 ACE inhibitor or β blocker; 3 Calcium-channel blocker; 4 Thiazide diuretic; 2 α Blocker

NICE guidance for the management of essential hypertension in adults aged >55 is to start with an ACE/ARB or if this is contraindicated with a β blocker. Poor control should prompt addition of a calcium-channel blocker. If control is still not gained a thiazide diuretic should be tried next. Spironolactone, although unlicensed for this indication, is recommended at stage 4 in the BNF. Failure to respond should prompt either an α blocker or specialist referral. Those aged >55 or of African–Caribbean origin should start with a calcium-channel blocker at stage 1.

EXTENDED MATCHING ANSWERS

Antiplatelet therapy

1.20   **D:**   **Aspirin 75 mg daily and dipyridamole 200 mg twice daily**

Aspirin and dipyridamole are recommended as first-line treatment after a TIA. Clopidogrel is not licensed for this indication. If dipyridamole is not tolerated aspirin alone should be used.

1.21   **A:**   **Aspirin 75 mg daily**

Aspirin 75 mg should be used for secondary prevention after myocardial infarction.

1.22   **E:**   **Clopidogrel 75 mg daily**

Clopidogrel is the first choice after an ischaemic stroke. If there is evidence of underlying atrial fibrillation warfarin should be considered.

1.23   **H:**   **Warfarin**

Patients with sustained or paroxysmal atrial fibrillation should be treated with warfarin. In the acute phase after the stroke aspirin 300 mg once daily and dipyridamole MR 200 mg twice daily are used, but after 2 weeks they should be warfarinised.

1.24   **I:**   **None of the above**

Patients with subarachnoid haemorrhage should be treated surgically, not with antiplatelets or anticoagulants.

Heart failure

1.25   **C:**   **Carvedilol**

First-line treatment for heart failure with left ventricular dysfunction consists of ACE inhibitor and a cardioselective β blocker such as carvedilol, bisoprolol or atenolol.

1.26   I: Valsartan

If ACE inhibitors are not tolerated, patients should be treated with an angiotensin receptor blocker. An alternative would be a β blocker, but in this patient there is COPD with reversibility, so caution should be exercised with β blockers.

1.27   H: Spironolactone

Patients symptomatic despite a β blocker and ACE inhibitor/ARB should be considered for an aldosterone antagonist.

1.28   F: Furosemide

Diuretics are useful for symptom relief but do not affect prognosis. They can cause postural hypotension so should be used with caution.

Treatment of hypertension

1.29   C: Bendroflumethiazide

1.30   I: Ramipril

1.31   H: No change indicated

1.32   J: Specialist referral

1.33   D: Candesartan

The guidance produced by NICE suggests a stepwise protocol for the treatment of hypertension, as follows:

Step	Patients aged <55 years	Patients aged ⩾55 years or black patients of any age
1	A	C or D
2	A + C or D	C or D + A
3	A + C + D	A + C + D

A = ACE inhibitor (AIIRA if intolerant),
C = calcium-channel blocker,
D = thiazide diuretic.

Drug therapy should be offered to the following patients:

- Those with a persistent high blood pressure of ⩾160/100 mmHg
- Those with a 10-year risk of CVD of >20%, and persistent high blood pressure of ⩾140/90 mmHg.

Patients should be referred immediately if there are signs of accelerated hypertension or if phaeochromocytoma is suspected.

Angina

1.34	E:	Emergency hospital admission
1.35	C:	Atenolol
1.36	A:	Amlodipine
1.37	I:	Nicorandil

For patients with mild angina with fewer than two attacks per week, 'as required' treatment with GTN is appropriate. Introduction of further treatments should be stepwise in the following order: (1) β blocker, (2) long-acting dihydropyridine calcium-channel blocker (eg amlodipine) and (3) long-acting nitrate.

In the presence of left ventricular dysfunction, long-acting nitrates are used first line, with the addition of a long-acting dihydropyridine calcium-channel blocker if necessary. Nicorandil is recommended if standard treatment is unsuccessful but is contraindicated in left ventricular failure (LVF) and hypotension.

Stroke risk

1.38	H:	Patient aged <75 years
1.39	G:	Patient aged >75 years
1.40	F:	No treatment
1.41	C:	Antiplatelet or warfarin
1.42	A:	Anticoagulation

Pharmacological treatment of symptomatic heart failure due to left ventricular systolic dysfunction

1.43	A:	ACE inhibitor
1.44	B:	Angiotensin II receptor antagonist
1.45	C:	β Blocker
1.46	F:	Spironolactone
1.47	E:	Diuretic therapy
1.48	D:	Digoxin

Based on NICE clinical guidance, *Management of adults in chronic heart failure in primary and secondary care*, July 2003.

FREE TEXT ANSWER

1.49   Peripartum cardiomyopathy

Peripartum cardiomyopathy occurs in the final 4 weeks of pregnancy or the first 6 months of delivery, and is characterised by impaired LVF. Most patients are managed medically but cardiac transplantation may be needed. The mortality rate is 20–50% although 30–50% recover without long-term complications. Recurrence rates are high and patients should be counselled about future pregnancies.

Chapter 2
Dermatology

SINGLE BEST ANSWER QUESTIONS

2.1 Urticaria
A 17-year-old boy comes to see you about his recurrent attacks of urticaria. Over the years he has tried excluding possible triggers but is now getting regular attacks. These involve itch and rash but he has no signs of angioedema. He has not tried any prescription medications yet. Which one of the following would be appropriate as the next step in his treatment?

○ A   Issue an EpiPen with advice on how to use it

○ B   Loratadine tablets

○ C   Montelukast tablets

○ D   Prednisolone to use orally when he develops attacks

○ E   Topical steroids to use for short periods

2.2 Sweaty palms
A 36-year-old businessman complains that he has suffered from sweaty palms for many years, but is now finding this increasingly embarrassing in business meetings. He has a friend who has had successful treatment for this but is not sure what this was. He asks your advice. Which one of the following treatments is most effective for this condition?

○ A   Botox injections

○ B   Cervical sympathectomy

○ C   Excision of sweat glands

○ D   Topical aluminium hydroxide

○ E   Topical hydrocortisone

2.3 Psoriasis
Which one of the following is the most appropriate initial treatment for a patient presenting with palmar psoriasis?

○ A   Betamethasone valerate ointment

○ B   Hydrocortisone 1% ointment

○ C   Oral prednisolone

○ D   Regular emollients

○ E   Tacrolimus cream

2.4 Prurigo
A medical student has seen a 40-year-old man with prurigo nodularis. The medical student asks you to explain more about this condition. Which one of the following pieces of information is correct?

○ A   Hydrocortisone cream often worsens the condition

○ B   Patients with the condition often suffer with intense itch that lasts for about 1 day

○ C   The majority of patients have a personal or family history of atopy

○ D   The trunk is often the most affected area of the patient's body

○ E   Young children are more likely to be affected by prurigo nodularis than adults

2.5 Finger lump
A 56-year-old man attends having knocked his finger while working in the garage. He reports having had a small lump on his finger for some months and, since knocking his finger, this has been leaking, as shown below.

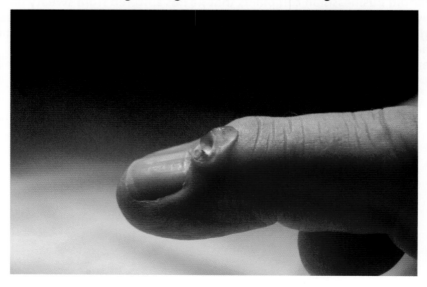

What is the single most likely diagnosis?

- ○ A Keratoacanthoma
- ○ B Myxoid cyst
- ○ C Pyogenic granuloma
- ○ D Sebaceous cyst
- ○ E Wart

2.6 Arm lesion
A 78-year-old retired farmer shows you the lesion below, which he has noticed on his arm.

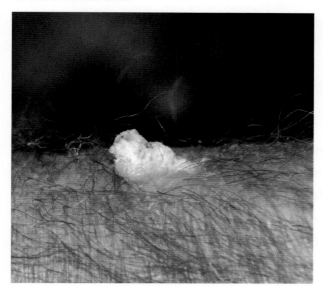

What would be the most appropriate management of this lesion?

- ○ A Cryotherapy
- ○ B Curettage
- ○ C Excision biopsy
- ○ D Shave biopsy
- ○ E Watchful waiting

2.7 Skin lesion

A 93-year-old man complains that for the last few weeks he has had a bleeding lesion on his chest that seems to be growing rapidly. The lesion is shown below.

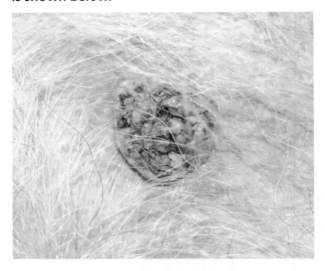

What is the single most likely diagnosis?

○ A Basal cell carcinoma

○ B Malignant melanoma

○ C Seborrheic keratosis

○ D Squamous cell carcinoma

○ E Wart

2.8   Skin disease

A 59-year-old woman complains that the skin lesion shown below catches on her clothing. It has been present for several years and is not associated with any other symptoms.

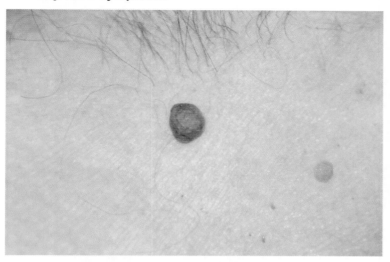

What is the single most likely diagnosis? Select one option only.

○   A   Dermatofibroma

○   B   Fibroepithelial polyp

○   C   Keratoacanthoma

○   D   Nodular basal cell carcinoma

○   E   Seborrhoeic keratosis

2.9 Skin lesion

A 63-year-old man asks if you can get rid of a wart from his back that catches on his clothes and bleeds on occasion. He thinks it has been there for only a couple of months. The lesion is shown below.

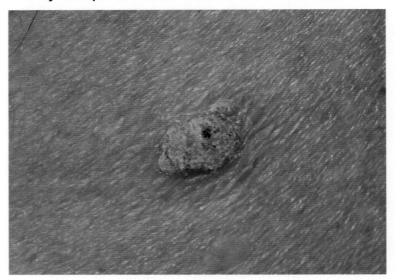

Which one of the following would be the single most appropriate treatment for this lesion?

○   A   Cryotherapy

○   B   Excision biopsy

○   C   Salicylic acid

○   D   Silver nitrate cautery

○   E   No treatment necessary

2.10 Rash affecting the hand

A 23-year-old man complains of an intensely itchy rash on the palms of his hands. This came on without any obvious cause about 2 weeks ago and was initially painful. It is now very itchy and keeping him awake at night. His hand is shown below.

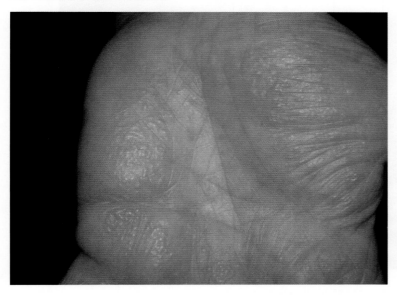

What is the most likely diagnosis?

○ A   Contact dermatitis

○ B   Eczema

○ C   Hand, foot and mouth disease

○ D   Pompholyx

○ E   Scabies

2.11 Rashes

An 87-year-old man complains of a rash on his chest, back and stomach. He has tried emollients and antihistamines without any luck. The rash is shown below.

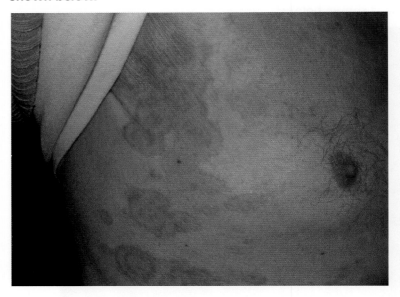

What is the most likely diagnosis?

○ A   Contact dermatitis

○ B   Erythema annulare

○ C   Erythema chronicum migrans

○ D   Erythema nodosum

○ E   Urticaria

2.12 Rash

A 14-year-old girl presented with erythematous patches affecting the dorsal aspect of both feet (shown below). The rest of her skin was clear. The rash was itchy. She had recently bought some new shoes and the rash appeared shortly after she had worn them.

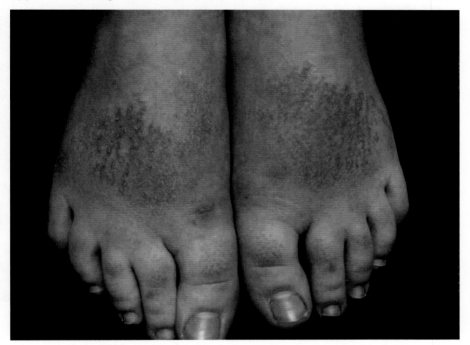

Select the single most likely diagnosis from the following list:

○ A Allergic contact dermatitis

○ B Eczema

○ C Irritant contact dermatitis

○ D Perniosis (chilblains)

○ E Tinea pedis

2.13 Skin lesions

A senior citizen asks you whether you can arrange to have this lesion on his back treated (shown below). He is not sure how long it has been there but he complains that it is now catching on his clothes.

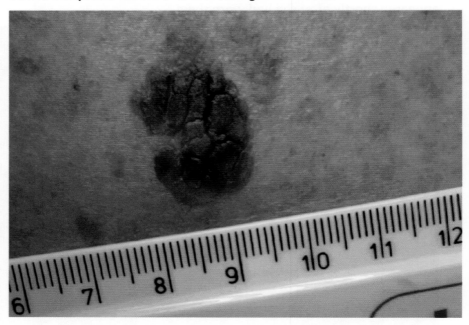

What is the single most appropriate course of action?

○ A   Refer to a local minor surgery service for complete excision with 2-mm borders

○ B   Refer to dermatology for a routine opinion

○ C   Refer to dermatology for an urgent outpatient opinion

○ D   Treat with 5-fluorouracil cream

○ E   None of the above

2.14 Rashes

A 54-year-old man took paracetamol after a minor injury 3 months ago. He developed a pruritic, oval skin lesion on his right shoulder. The lesion gradually resolved after he stopped the paracetamol. He recently restarted paracetamol for a headache. He quickly developed a recurrent skin lesion affecting his right shoulder (shown below).

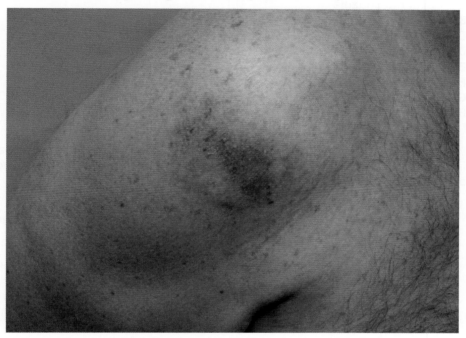

Which one of the following options is the most likely skin diagnosis? Select one option only.

○ A Drug hypersensitivity syndrome

○ B Drug-induced photosensitivity

○ C Fixed drug eruption

○ D Gout

○ E Mycetoma

EXTENDED MATCHING QUESTIONS

Fungal infections

Options

A   Oral fluconazole
B   Oral nystatin
C   Oral terbinafine
D   Refer for specialist opinion
E   Topical amorolfine
F   Topical clotrimazole
G   Topical hydrocortisone
H   Topical terbinafine
I   None of the above

For each of the statements below about the management of common fungal infections, select the most appropriate management from the list above. Each option may be used once, more than once or not at all.

2.15   **A 23-year-old woman who has recently had a course of co-amoxiclav now complains of vaginal soreness and discharge. She has not improved with a course of over-the-counter clotrimazole.**

2.16   **A 34-year-old man with no previous history of note has had a red itchy rash in both sides of his groin for 4 weeks.**

2.17   **A 3-year-old girl who has been treated for a small patch of suspected ringworm on her scalp has developed a tender, inflamed, cystic lesion on her scalp**

2.18   **A 39-year-old woman has a discoloured thickened fingernail on her right index finger; her other finger and toenails are normal.**

2.19   **A 24-year-old amateur footballer has been self-treating his athlete's foot for 2 weeks with topical miconazole. His feet are still intensely itchy and erythematous.**

Management of psoriasis

2.20 –2.23

Options

A   Betamethasone cream
B   Coal tar
C   Hydrocortisone cream
D   Oral steroids
E   Refer for phototherapy
F   Vitamin D once daily
G   Vitamin D plus betamethasone cream
H   Vitamin D twice daily

The algorithm below has been designed to standardize the management of psoriasis on the trunk and limbs.

For each of the numbered gaps, select one option from the list to complete the algorithm. Each option may be used once, more than once or not at all.

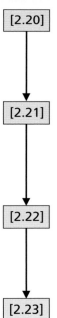

Moles

2.24 –2.27

Options

A   Basal cell carcinoma
B   Dermatofibroma
C   Dysplastic naevi
D   Keratoacanthoma
E   Lentigo maligna
F   Malignant melanoma
G   Pyogenic granuloma
H   Seborrhoeic wart
I   Squamous cell carcinoma

Complete the table below describing characteristics of skin lesions, from the list of options above. Each option may be used once, more than once or not at all.

Appearance	Usually multiple, irregular outline and pigment	Raised, red, round and bleeds easily; grows rapidly after trauma	Smooth, flesh-coloured, raised lesions on arms and legs	Rapidly growing, raised with a central plug surrounded by a collar
Size (cm)	>1	1	1	>1
Age at onset (years)	<40	Any	<40	40s
Diagnosis	**2.24**	**2.25**	**2.26**	**2.27**

Acne

2.28–2.32

Options

A   Benzoyl peroxide
B   Benzoyl peroxide plus topical clindamycin
C   Combined oral contraceptive pill
D   Isotretinoin
E   Lymecycline
F   Minocyline
G   Oxytetracycline
H   Secondary care referral
I   Topical clindamycin
J   Topical erythromycin
K   None of the above

Complete the table below detailing the stepwise approach to managing acne, using the list of options above. Each option may be used once, more than once, or not at all.

	Mild	Moderate	Severe
Description	Comedones	Comedones with inflammatory papules and pustules	Comedone, papules, pustules, nodules and cysts with scarring
First line	**2.28**	Benzoyl peroxide Consider **2.29** in females	**2.30** Consider COCP in females
Second line	**2.31**	Benzoyl peroxide plus **2.32**	

FREE TEXT QUESTIONS

2.33 Skin conditions

A 45-year-old man complains of an intensely itchy rash on both wrists. On examination he has flat-topped violaceous papules on each wrist and forearms. What is the most likely diagnosis? Write your answer in the box below.

2.34 A 72-year-old man with a history of diet-controlled diabetes comes to see you for a routine check. You notice the lesion below on his forehead, which he tells you has been there for some months, but does not cause him any trouble and does not bleed.

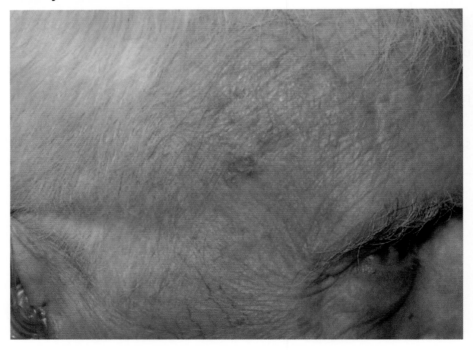

In the box below write the single most likely diagnosis

2.35 **What would be the most appropriate initial treatment? Write your answer in the box below.**

SINGLE BEST ANSWER

2.1   B: Loratadine tablets

Urticaria has multiple causes and avoidance can be difficult if an obvious precipitant cannot be identified. Symptomatic treatment with oral antihistamines is usually sufficient to control symptoms of simple urticaria but where there is associated angioedema parenteral adrenaline might be needed. Montelukast in association with antihistamines can be useful in refractory cases but is ineffective as monotherapy. In severe cases not responding to oral antihistamines, short courses of steroids orally might be needed but topical steroids are not effective.

2.2   A: Botox injections

Botulinum toxin injections are effective treatment for this condition but require repeated treatment every 4–6 months. They are effective for axillary, palmar and facial sweating. With prolonged use they can cause the production of antibodies, which reduce their efficacy. An alternative treatment is iontophoresis. Aluminium hydrochloride is useful for axillary hyperhidrosis but is less so for sweating of the hands and often leaves a residue.

2.3   A: Betamethasone valerate ointment

The British Association of Dermatology recommends using potent topical steroids as part of the initial treatment of palmar psoriasis. Keratolytic agents, such as salicylic acid in Lassar's paste, might be required to remove scale from hyperkeratotic skin. Tars and vitamin D analogues can also help. Palms and soles can be difficult areas to treat, and the patient should be referred to a dermatologist if initial treatments fail after 2–3 months or if there is diagnostic uncertainty. Specialists may recommend treatments including clobetasol propionate under occlusion or PUVA.

2.4   C: The majority of patients have a personal or family history of atopy

Prurigo nodularis is an intensely itchy skin condition of unknown aetiology. Adults are affected more frequently than children and the condition is equally distributed between males and females. Affected individuals are likely to have a personal or family history of atopy; up to 80% have a positive history compared with 25% of the normal population. Nodular, itchy lesions, 1–2 cm in diameter, are symmetrically distributed, particularly on the extensor limb surfaces. Itching is often difficult to treat and is commonly a long-standing problem. High-potency corticosteroids can be tried to treat itchy lesions, under occlusive dressings to increase absorption. Many topical and systemic treatments have been tried in the past with limited success.

2.5   B: Myxoid cyst

Myxoid cysts are ganglions of the distal interphalangeal joint. They grow slowly and often cause grooving of the nail as they grow. They are benign, but can become painful. Treatment is by aspiration of the thick jelly inside or injection with steroid, or surgical excision if they recur. A keratoacanthoma has a plug of keratin in the centre whereas a pyogenic granuloma usually grows rapidly at the site of trauma. Sebaceous cysts are not typically seen on digits.

2.6   C: Excision biopsy

Keratin horns should be excised fully including the base to allow histological exclusion of an underlying squamous cell carcinoma. Cryotherapy will not provide a tissue for histology and curettage or shave biopsy may yield insufficient depth for diagnosis.

2.7   D: Squamous cell carcinoma

This is a squamous cell carcinoma. The bleeding, rapid growth and irregular surface differentiate from a seborrhoeic keratosis or wart. A basal cell carcinoma usually has a rolled edge.

2.8   B: Fibroepithelial polyp

Fibroepithelial polyps are frequently seen at sites of chafing such as the groin, axilla or neck. They are benign and typically have a narrow stalk. They are occasionally associated with insulin resistance but in most cases are idiopathic. Dermatofibromas are usually seen on the legs or arms and are within the skin. Keratoacanthomas have a central plug of keratin.

2.9   B: Excision biopsy

Although most likely a wart, the irregular appearance, rapid growth and history of bleeding raise a possible diagnosis of squamous cell carcinoma (SCC). Excision biopsy with histology would be the most appropriate treatment. Cryotherapy or cautery does not provide tissue for histology. Curettage is an option with tissue sent for histology but a further excision would be necessary if SCC is confirmed.

2.10   D: Pompholyx

This is a typical appearance for pompholyx, with painful, itchy vesicles on the palms (and sometimes soles). It is difficult to treat without potent topical steroids but usually subsides over 2–3 weeks. Potassium permanganate can be used for treatment if vesicles break down and, in refractory cases, topical calcineurin inhibitors, Botox or PUVA (psoralen plus UVA) can be effective.

2.11　B:　Erythema annulare

This annular and erythematous rash is erythema annulare. It affects all ages and usually starts as a small papule, which slowly enlarges to form a ring while the central area clears. The rash is not usually very itchy but does persist. It is often idiopathic but can be associated with underlying malignancy (particularly where there are multiple, concentric, whirling rings), tuberculosis, liver disease and Graves' disease. Patients should have blood tests, ultrasound of the liver and a chest X-ray if there is suspicion of underlying disease. The rash usually settles spontaneously, but this can take up to 12 months. Topical steroids might be helpful in speeding resolution.

2.12　C:　Irritant contact dermatitis

Allergy and irritants can both trigger contact dermatitis. Irritant contact dermatitis is usually well demarcated and itchy and often has a glazed appearance; there can be some surface scaling. Causes include exposure to detergents and damage due to repeated friction and sweating. On further questioning the patient admitted that her new shoes felt too tight and had been rubbing.

2.13　E:　None of the above

This is seborrhoeic keratosis, a benign epidermal tumour common in elderly people. Note the characteristic stuck-on appearance and rough, warty surface. Treatment is not necessary unless there is diagnostic certainty. Troublesome lesions can be removed by shave excision or curettage; smaller lesions can by treated with cryotherapy. Most commissioners will not authorise removal.

2.14　C:　Fixed drug eruption

Fixed drug eruptions manifest as painful oval or round lesions. They characteristically occur at the same site 30 minutes to 8 hours after taking the medication responsible. The lesions sometimes blister and occur most commonly on the hands, feet, glans penis and lips. Many drugs have been implicated.

EXTENDED MATCHING ANSWERS

Fungal infections

2.15　A:　Oral fluconazole

Failure to respond to topical antifungals should prompt a review of the diagnosis and if no alternative is suspected a stat dose of fluconazole 150 mg is usually effective.

2.16　H:　Topical terbinafine

Topical terbinafine for 2–4 weeks will usually treat tinea cruris. If it fails to respond alternative diagnoses such as erythrasma should be considered.

2.17   D: Refer for specialist opinion

Cases of suspected kerion should be referred for urgent specialist opinion. They are usually caused by zoonotic fungal infections, eg from family pets.

2.18   E: Topical amorolfine

Topical amorolfine can be used for tinea unguium where it is confined to one nail. More widespread disease should be treated with oral antifungals.

2.19   G: Topical hydrocortisone

Addition of topical hydrocortisone to antifungals may help where there is significant inflammation

Management of psoriasis

2.20   G: Vitamin D plus betamethasone cream
2.21   H: Vitamin D twice daily
2.22   B: Coal tar
2.23   E: Refer for phototherapy

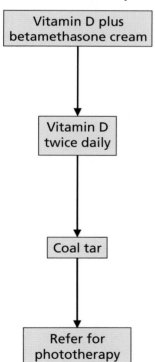

Moles

2.24	C:	Dysplastic naevus
2.25	G:	Pyogenic granuloma
2.26	B:	Dermatofibroma
2.27	D:	Keratoacanthoma

Appearance	Usually multiple, irregular outline and pigment	Raised, red, round and bleeds easily; grows rapidly after trauma	Smooth, flesh-coloured, raised lesions on arms and legs	Rapidly growing, raised with a central plug surrounded by a collar
Size (cm)	>1	1	1	>1
Age at onset (years)	<40	Any	<40	40s
Diagnosis	C Dysplastic naevus	G Pyogenic granuloma	B Dermato-fibroma	D Keratoacanthoma

Acne

2.28	A:	Benzyl peroxide
2.29	C:	Combined oral contraceptive pill
2.30	H:	Secondary care referral
2.31	B:	Benzoyl peroxide plus topical clindamycin
2.32	E:	Lymecyline

	Mild	Moderate	Severe
Description	Comedones	Comedones with inflammatory papules and pustules	Comedone, papules, pustules, nodules and cysts with scarring
First line	Benzoyl peroxide	Benzoyl peroxide Consider COCP in females	Secondary care referral Consider COCP in females
Second line	Benzoyl peroxide plus topical clindamycin	Benzoyl peroxide plus oral lymecycline	

FREE TEXT ANSWERS

2.33   Lichen planus

Cutaneous lichen planus affects men three times more frequently than women, with a mean age of onset of 40–45. It is intensely itchy and may be widespread. It may also be a sign at sites of previous scarring. It may be associated with hepatitis C infection. Management is with topical steroids. Cases affecting the genital area should be referred for specialist review.

2.34   Solar keratosis (or actinic keratosis)

Bleeding or rapid growth would suggest the alternative diagnosis of squamous cell carcinoma.

2.35   Topical 5-fluorouracil treatment

Topical 5-fluorouracil treatment, usually with pulsed hydrocortisone for the resultant inflammation. Alternatives include cryotherapy or topical 3% diclofenac.

Chapter 3
Ear, nose and throat

SINGLE BEST ANSWER QUESTIONS

3.1 Reduced hearing
A 67-year-old woman complains of 3 weeks of reduced hearing in one ear after an upper respiratory tract infection. She says that her head feels as if it is in a bucket. On examination she has no evidence of acute infection in her middle or outer ear but does have clinical evidence of a middle-ear effusion. She is otherwise well, and 2 months before this she had a full ENT assessment for reduced smell, which was normal. Which one of the following management strategies is effective in this situation?

○   A   Nasal steroids

○   B   Oral decongestant

○   C   Otovent device

○   D   Reassurance that her symptoms should resolve within 1–2 weeks

○   E   Refer for grommets

3.2 Sore throat
A 19-year-old student is diagnosed with tonsillitis and starts antibiotic therapy. Twenty-four hours later she presents to the out-of-hours service with fever, ear pain, dysphagia and trismus. On examination her uvula is displaced away from the midline and her tonsils appear asymmetrically enlarged. What is the most likely diagnosis?

○   A   Epiglottitis

○   B   Glandular fever

○   C   Lemierre syndrome

○   D   Quinsy

○   E   Tonsillar lymphoma

3.3 Sore throat

A 16-year-old schoolboy complains of flu-like symptoms, sore throat and enlarged glands in his neck. On examination he has a temperature of 38.5°C, significantly enlarged lymph nodes in his neck, enlarged tonsils with white exudate and a yellowish tinge to his skin. Abdominal examination reveals some tenderness in the right upper quadrant. What is the most likely diagnosis?

○ A   Epstein–Barr virus infection

○ B   Hepatitis A

○ C   Quinsy

○ D   Streptococcal tonsillitis

○ E   Viral sore throat

3.4 Enlarged tonsils

Asymmetrical tonsil enlargement in a 40-year-old man is best treated with which of the following options?

○ A   Antifungals

○ B   Antibiotics

○ C   Referral for biopsy

○ D   Steroids

○ E   Watch and wait

3.5 Neck swelling

A child presents with a 3-cm swelling to the left of the midline in the lower part of the anterior triangle of the neck. It moves with swallowing and tongue protrusion. What is it most likely to be?

○ A   Branchial cyst

○ B   Lymph node

○ C   Thyroglossal cyst

○ D   Thyroid cyst

○ E   Sebaceous cyst

3.6 Snoring

A 54-year-old man with a BMI of 22 kg/m² complains of snoring and waking up at night. He is tired during the daytime, and his partner says that he seems to stop breathing for up to a minute every night. What is the most appropriate first-line treatment?

○ A   Advice on lifestyle changes and weight loss

○ B   Advise the use of earplugs

○ C   Refer for a sleep study

○ D   Refer for surgery

○ E   Refer to a dentist for a mandibular advancement device

3.7 Hearing loss

A 6-year-old girl has a 1-year history of 30 dB conductive hearing loss, flat tympanograms and poor school performance. What is the single most appropriate next-stage treatment?

○ A   Adenoidectomy

○ B   Bilateral grommet insertion

○ C   Conservative treatment

○ D   Nasal decongestants

○ E   Tonsillectomy

3.8 Facial swelling

An 86-year-old man is seen for a new patient check. While talking to him you notice a swelling in front of and inferior to the right ear. He tells you that this has been slowly growing for 10 years. On examination the swelling is firm but non-tender and mobile. He has no other findings of note. The swelling is shown below.

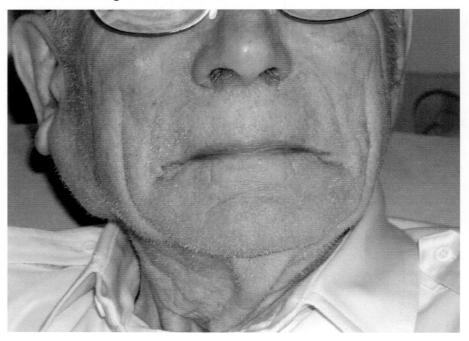

What is the most likely diagnosis?

○ A   Acute bacterial parotitis

○ B   Adenocarcinoma

○ C   Lymphoma

○ D   Mumps

○ E   Parotid adenoma

3.9 Earache

A 10-year-old girl complains of earache and a discharge from her ear and she has a fever. On examination you note the appearance below.

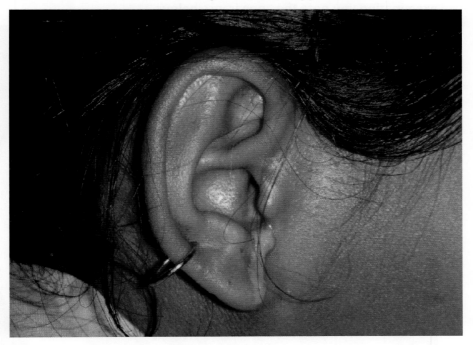

What is the single most likely diagnosis?

○   A   Acute otitis externa

○   B   Acute tympanic membrane perforation

○   C   Chronic otitis externa

○   D   Chronic tympanic membrane perforation

○   E   Glue ear

3.10 Itchy ears

A 27-year-old man with itchy ears has had several courses of eardrops over the last 3 months. He now complains of recurrent itchiness. On examination you note the appearance below.

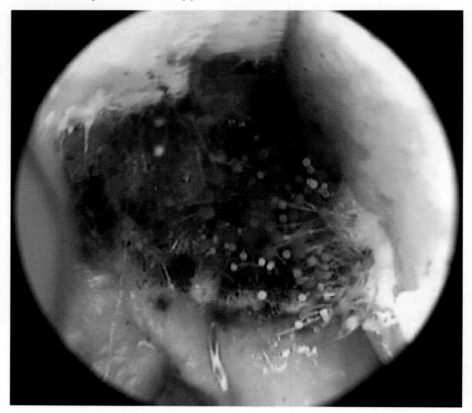

What is the most appropriate medical treatment?

○ A   Betnesol drops

○ B   Ciprofloxacin drops

○ C   Clotrimazole drops

○ D   Locorten-Vioform drops

○ E   Sofradex eardrops

3.11 Painful ear

A 21-year-old girl has just returned from a holiday in Greece, where she developed a very painful ear. She has been taking regular ibuprofen, paracetamol and codeine from a local pharmacy, but to no effect. On examination her ear has the appearance shown below.

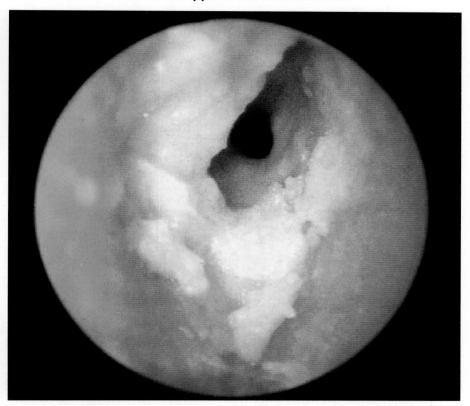

What is the diagnosis?

- ○ A   Acute otitis externa
- ○ B   Chronic suppurative otitis media
- ○ C   Fungal otitis externa
- ○ D   Otitis media with effusion
- ○ E   Otitis media with perforation

3.12 Loss of hearing

This picture shows the right tympanic membrane of a patient who presented with reduced hearing and discharge 2 days after the onset of earache and fever. The patient reports that the pain has eased somewhat since the onset of the discharge.

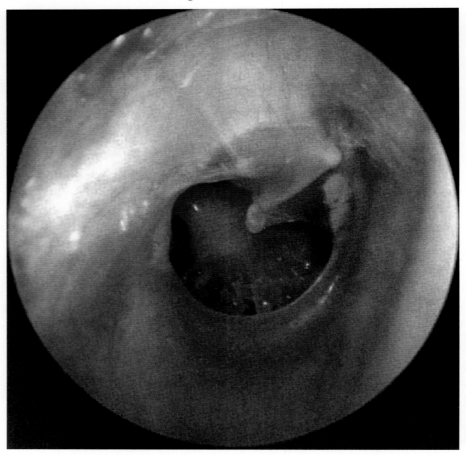

What is the most likely diagnosis?

- ○ A Cholesteatoma
- ○ B Otitis externa
- ○ C Otitis media
- ○ D Otosclerosis
- ○ E Tympanosclerosis

3.13 Audiograms

A patient with hearing problems has an audiogram carried out. Which one of the options A–E would be most likely to be seen in a patient with presbyacusis?

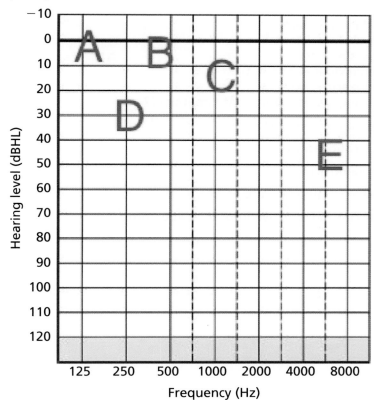

3.14 Ear discharge

A 45-year-old man presents with left ear discharge after swimming. The swab from this discharge shows the following results:

Organism: *Pseudomonas aeruginosa*

Sensitivity:

- Penicillin – resistant
- Neomycin – resistant
- Framycetin – resistant
- Metronidazole – resistant
- Ciprofloxacin – sensitive

What is the single most appropriate treatment?

- ○ A   Intravenous co-amoxiclav
- ○ B   Oral ciprofloxacin
- ○ C   Oral co-amoxiclav
- ○ D   Topical aluminium acetate eardrops
- ○ E   Topical ciprofloxacin eyedrops used as eardrops

3.15 Management of glue ear

A   4 weeks
B   6 weeks
C   3 months
D   6 months
E   12 months

Your local audiology department have produced a flowchart for the management of suspected glue ear in children. Complete the algorithm from the list of options above.

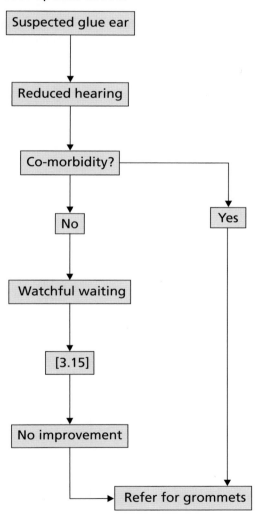

3.16 Medical management of chronic rhinosinusitis

Select the rank order of the options (1–4) that best fulfils the requirements given in the question.

The following is a list of treatment options for chronic rhinosinusitis:

1   1–2 weeks of oral antibiotics
2   4–6 weeks of oral antibiotics
3   Nasal steroid drops
4   Nasal steroid spray

The responses (A–E) rank the treatment options in various orders. Select the response that places the treatment options (1–4) in the order in which they should be used, with the **initial treatment** first to the **maximal medical therapy** last.

Select one rank order only.

   ○   A: 4, 2, 3, 1

   ○   B: 4, 3, 2, 1

   ○   C: 1, 3, 4, 2

   ○   D: 4, 1, 3, 2

   ○   E: 3, 4, 1, 2

EXTENDED MATCHING QUESTIONS

Investigations in ENT

Options

A   Audiogram
B   Caloric testing
C   CT scanning
D   MRI
E   Plain X-ray
F   None of the above

For each of the scenarios described below, select the most appropriate investigation from the list of options above. Each option may be used once, more than once or not at all.

3.17   **A 27-year-old man with acute sinusitis.**

3.18   **A 57-year-old woman with a history of neurofibromatosis who has developed unilateral tinnitus.**

3.19   **A 72-year-old man who struggles to follow conversations in church.**

3.20   **A 47-year-old man with a history of nasal polypectomy who complains of recurrent symptoms.**

Drug management of ENT disease

Options

A   Amoxicillin
B   Betnesol
C   Ciprofloxacin drops
D   Doxycycline
E   Erythromycin
F   Mometasone nasal spray
G   Montelukast
H   Phenxymethylpenicillin
I   Sofradex
J   Sterimar

For each of the scenarios described below, select the most appropriate treatment option from the list above. Each option may be used once, more than once or not at all.

3.21   A 4-year-old boy complains of earache on one side. Examination shows a red, dull, bulging eardrum on that side. He has a temperature of 39.2°C and looks unwell.

3.22   A 24-year-old woman with long-standing perennial rhinitis not helped by antihistamines.

3.23   A 19-year-old man with a history of a chronically discharging ear. A swab is sent which shows *Pseudomonas* species.

3.24   A 51-year-old woman who is on a long-term nasal steroid spray complains of a blocked nose, and reduced smell and taste. Examination reveals bilateral nasal polyps.

FREE TEXT QUESTION

3.25 Hot topics

How many attacks of tonsillitis in a 12-month period are considered sufficient to justify tonsillectomy in an otherwise healthy patient? Write your answer in the box below.

SINGLE BEST ANSWER

3.1   C: Otovent device

Middle-ear effusions are often seen on a background of acute upper respiratory tract infection and are typically unilateral. They can take several months to clear, but this can be improved with an Otovent device. Grommets might be necessary for refractory cases. Nasal decongestants and steroids are ineffective. Patients presenting with acute middle-ear effusions in adulthood should have nasendoscopy performed to exclude postnasal space lesions.

3.2   D: Quinsy

This presentation is typical of quinsy, or peritonsillar abscess. Treatment usually involves intravenous antibiotics and fluids, and incision of the abscess if it does not settle. Interval tonsillectomy is offered in most centres. Epiglottitis affects the epiglottis rather than the uvula and a lymphoma would not normally present over such a short period. Glandular fever does not usually cause significant asymmetry, whereas Lemierre syndrome causes more widespread disease throughout the mediastinum and patients are usually much more unwell.

3.3   A: Epstein–Barr virus infection

Epstein–Barr virus causes glandular fever. Most patients develop a sore throat, fever, malaise and cervical lymphadenopathy. Hepatosplenomegaly is not uncommon and most patients develop transient abnormalities of liver function. Treatment is supportive and most patients make a full recovery. Complications include cranial nerve palsies, encephalitis and splenic rupture, but these are rare. The symptoms usually last 2–4 weeks but up to 50% of patients report ongoing fatigue, which can take months to resolve.

3.4   C: Referral for biopsy

Asymmetrical tonsil enlargement in adults is suspicious of neoplasia, and biopsy is needed, as well as imaging of the head and neck.

3.5   C: Thyroglossal cyst

The thyroglossal cyst is a remnant of the thyroglossal duct, which descends from the tongue via the hyoid and neck to the thyroid during development. There can be a connection to the hyoid bone which explains its pattern of movement. Treatment is with surgical excision via Sistrunk's procedure.

3.6   C: Refer for a sleep study

Surgery for snoring is controversial, and evidence on its effectiveness is conflicting – some surgery might provide short-term help with snoring, but problems tend to recur. Any surgery should be carefully targeted at the source of the snoring. Lifestyle changes and earplugs will be ineffective with this patient. A mandibular advancement device might help, depending on the site of snoring, but, with a clear history of daytime somnolence and apnoea, a sleep study should be performed first – night-time continuous positive airway pressure (CPAP) might be all that is necessary to improve the patient's quality of life.

3.7   B: Bilateral grommet insertion

Typically, glue ear produces a 20–40 dB conductive loss with flat tympanograms – it is most common in children aged between about 3 years and 8 years, and tends to improve with time, although if it starts to affect development intervention is indicated. For cases of recurrent glue ear adenoidectomy has been shown, in the TARGET trial, to reduce the rate of recurrence.

3.8   E: Parotid adenoma

The most likely diagnosis in this case is a parotid adenoma. Parotid adenomas account for 90% of benign parotid tumours and are typically in the lower pole of the parotid. They are benign but can cause local damage to the facial nerve. They grow slowly and elderly patients might not require treatment. The diagnosis should be confirmed by fine-needle aspiration. Malignant tumours of the parotid tend to present more acutely due to rapid growth. Lymphomas tend to be more aggressive and often have a rubbery feel.

3.9   B: Acute tympanic membrane perforation

The history of fever and otalgia followed by otorrhoea suggests an acute otitis media followed by perforation. The discharge is thin and mucoid, which suggests middle-ear involvement rather than otitis externa, which causes a much thicker discharge which seldom runs from the ear. Chronic perforations can behave in this way but usually follow water exposure or coryza rather than an acute febrile illness. The tympanic membrane usually heals in 4–6 weeks.

3.10   C: Clotrimazole drops

This is a fungal otitis externa. Treatment is with 2 weeks of antifungal therapy and management of underlying risk factors, such as diabetes and excessive use of antibiotic or steroid preparations. Microsuction might be necessary where there is a lot of exudate.

3.11   A: Acute otitis externa

The presence of pain, particularly when moving the tragus, with creamy, thick exudate and meatal oedema is typical of otitis externa. The discharge in a tympanic membrane perforation tends to be more mucoid whereas in otitis media with effusion there is no exudate in the canal. Fungal otitis externa shows typical spores and hyphae.

3.12   C: Otitis media

This patient has most probably suffered from an acute middle-ear infection, resulting in a perforation and discharge, and later resolution of symptoms. Cholesteatoma usually causes a painless perforation that tends to be peripheral. Otitis externa rarely causes a perforation. Otosclerosis is a disease of the ossicles and causes a slowly progressive conductive hearing loss, and tympanosclerosis causes a conductive loss that is usually stable.

3.13   E

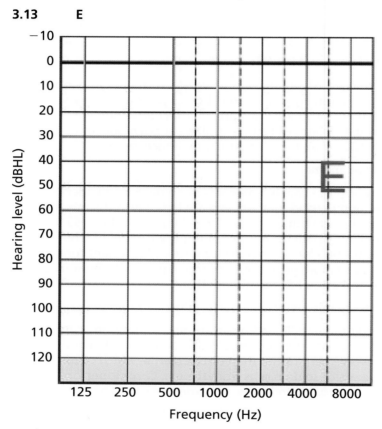

Presbyacusis is characterised by high frequency sensorineural hearing loss. Low-frequency loss is usually seen in Ménière's disease or conductive loss, whereas mid-frequency loss is often congenital. Severe hearing loss of any aetiology may affect any frequency.

3.14   E: Topical ciprofloxacin eyedrops used as eardrops

The presence of discharge after swimming suggests otitis externa. This is best treated with topical drops. Ciprofloxacin eye drops used topically in the ear, although off license, are effective in this situation. The patient should also be asked to keep his ears dry, and oral ciprofloxacin can be considered as a second-line treatment.

3.15   C: 3 months

Of cases of glue ear 90% settle within 3 months, so intervention before this period is indicated only if there is significant co-morbidity, eg blindness or Down syndrome.

3.16   D: 4, 1, 3, 2

Rank ordering: 4 Nasal steroid spray; 1 1–2 weeks of oral antibiotics; 3 Nasal steroid drops; 2 4–6 weeks of oral antibiotics

Initial management of chronic rhinosinusitis should be saline douching, which has a good evidence base for maintenance treatment of chronic rhinosinusitis. If this is not tolerated or is ineffective a nasal steroid spray is indicated. Failure to improve with regular nasal spray in the presence of signs of infection should prompt oral antibiotics. If there is still no improvement, 2–4 weeks of nasal steroid drops may prove effective. Continuing purulent discharge despite this is an indication for a 4- to 6-week course of antibiotics.

EXTENDED MATCHING ANSWERS

Investigations in ENT

3.17   F: None of the above

Plain X-rays are of limited value in sinusitis. Patients with chronic sinusitis where surgery is being considered should have a CT scan, or where recurrent polyps are found.

3.18   D: MRI

Unilateral tinnitus can be a sign of an acoustic neuroma and MRI is indicated in this situation.

3.19   A: Audiogram

Simple deafness should be investigated initially with an audiogram.

3.20   C: CT scanning

Drug management of ENT disease

3.21   A: Amoxicillin

Acute otitis media in a child who is unwell should be treated with antibiotics. If the child is not unwell a symptomatic approach might be appropriate, with the option of returning for antibiotics should the patient worsen.

3.22   F: Mometasone nasal spray

Second-line treatment in patients with rhinitis who have tried oral antihistamines is a nasal steroid. This can also help with ocular symptoms.

3.23   C: Ciprofloxacin drops

Pseudomonas sp. is often seen in patients with discharging ears and topical ciprofloxacin will often cure this. An alternative is Sofradex, but there are theoretical arguments against using this in patients without an intact tympanic membrane.

3.24   B: Betnesol

A short course of nasal steroid drops will often shrink nasal polyps, affording symptomatic relief in patients who are not fit for or who do not wish to have surgery. Mometasone nasal spray is licensed for the treatment of nasal polyps and is often effective in patients with smaller polyps and useful for preventing recurrence.

FREE TEXT ANSWER

3.25   6

The Paradise criteria are widely used by commissioning organisations to determine the cut-off for intervention in recurrent tonsillitis. Patients who have six attacks in 1 year, five a year for 2 years or four a year for 3 years are likely to have improved quality of life if they have tonsillectomy compared with medical treatment.

Chapter 4
Endocrinology

SINGLE BEST ANSWER QUESTIONS

4.1   Breast symptoms
A 52-year-old man complains of pain in the area of his nipples. He is otherwise fit and well, and his only medication is ranitidine for dyspepsia. Examination reveals tenderness in both breasts and slightly enlarged breast tissue. There is no lymphadenopathy. What is the single most likely cause of his symptoms?

○   A   Breast cancer

○   B   Hormonal changes with age

○   C   Over-the-counter drug use

○   D   Ranitidine

○   E   Recreational drug use

4.2   Weight gain
A 66-year-old woman who is being treated for polymyalgia rheumatica complains that she has gained 15 kg weight in the last 6 months. She is particularly bothered by weight gain in her face and says that she has developed a hump on her back. Her skin is thin and her face flushed. What is the single most likely diagnosis?

○   A   Addison's disease

○   B   Cushing's disease

○   C   Cushing syndrome

○   D   Diabetes mellitus

○   E   Hypothyroidism

4.3 Infertility

A 32-year-old man attends with his partner for fertility advice. She has two children by a previous partner but they would like children of their own. On closer questioning he admits to poor sex drive and difficulty maintaining erections, and that he has always needed to shave less than his peers. He has no previous history of note and takes no regular medications. He is otherwise well. You check his bloods and these show a raised FSH level with a low testosterone and a normal prolactin level. What is the most likely diagnosis?

○ A   Cushing's disease

○ B   Drug use

○ C   Primary hypogonadism

○ D   Prolactinoma

○ E   Secondary hypogonadism

4.4 Pregnancy

A 35-year-old woman with a history of hypothyroidism comes to see you having found out that she is pregnant. She is currently taking 75 µg levothyroxine a day. What advice would you give her?

○ A   Aim for a treatment TSH <0.01

○ B   Continue taking her current dose of levothyroxine

○ C   Increase her levothyroxine dose by 25 µg immediately

○ D   Monitor her TSH levels at the beginning of each trimester and treat accordingly

○ E   Reduce her levothyroxine dose by 25 µg immediately

4.5 Bone health

You see a 57-year-old postmenopausal woman who has just had a DXA scan carried out at a local private hospital as part of a well woman check. The results show that she has a T score of −1.8. She has a normal diet, normal BMI, exercises most days and does not smoke. You review her medical records and these show that she has no major previous medical history. Routine blood tests are carried out, which are normal. She would like to be treated. Which one of the following is the most appropriate management?

○ A   Calcium and vitamin D supplements

○ B   No treatment required

○ C   Oral bisphosphonate

○ D   Teriparatide

○ E   Three-monthly intravenous bisphosphonate

4.6 Erectile dysfunction

A 46-year-old man complains of problems with erections. He has been through a divorce after a long and unhappy marriage and has now started a new relationship. His new partner is frustrated by his erectile problems and would like him to try Viagra. His previous medical history is unremarkable, he takes no regular medications and he has no children. He is a new patient so you undertake a physical examination, which is normal. Which of the following would be the most appropriate next step in his management?

- ○ A Check FSH and testosterone levels
- ○ B Prescribe sildenafil at 25 mg initially and review in 2 weeks
- ○ C Prescribe testosterone supplements
- ○ D Refer for psychosexual counselling
- ○ E Start treatment with LHRH analogues

4.7 Skin changes

A 39-year-old woman joins your practice after relocating to the area. She comes to see you for a new patient check and to ask about fertility treatment. She is nulliparous, has diabetes mellitus for which she takes metformin. You note that she has acne and is obese, and that she has hirsutism with dark skin in her axillae. Which one of the following is the most likely cause of her symptoms?

- ○ A Addison's disease
- ○ B Cushing's disease
- ○ C Cushing syndrome
- ○ D Hypopituitarism
- ○ E Polycystic ovary syndrome

4.8 Leg pain
A 27-year-old woman of south Asian origin is brought to see you complaining of chronic pain in her legs. This seems to have started insidiously and there is no history of trauma. She lives according to strict cultural rules and wears full Muslim dress. You arrange for an X-ray and blood tests. These both show evidence of osteomalacia. What would be the most appropriate next step in her management?

○ A   Arrange for DEXA scan

○ B   Investigate for causes of vitamin D deficiency

○ C   Prescribe bisphosphonates

○ D   Prescribe calcium and vitamin D supplements

○ E   Refer to social services

4.9 Lump in neck
A healthy 16-year-old girl became concerned about a prominence in her neck, which was found to be a smooth, diffuse, non-tender enlargement of the thyroid gland. Which one of the following is the most likely diagnosis?

○ A   Colloid goitre

○ B   Endemic goitre

○ C   Physiological goitre

○ D   Thyroglossal cyst

○ E   Thyroid nodule

4.10 Breast symptoms
A 21-year-old woman presents with a non-tender, firm, mobile, 2-cm lump in the upper inner quadrant of the right breast. She has been on oral contraception for 5 years. Select the single most likely cause of her symptoms from the following options.

○ A   Breast carcinoma

○ B   Breast cyst

○ C   Fibroadenoma

○ D   Galactocele

○ E   Gynaecomastia

4.11 Lump in breast

A 79-year-old woman in a residential home was found by her carers to have a painless lump in the lower inner quadrant of the left breast. Clinically, there is a 4-cm lump adherent to the overlying skin, with nipple retraction on extending the arm. Select the single most likely diagnosis from the list below.

○ A Breast carcinoma

○ B Breast cyst

○ C Fat necrosis

○ D Fibroadenoma

○ E Mastitis

4.12 Neck lump

A 34-year-old woman who has recently arrived from India attends for a new patient check. You note an asymmetric goitre, shown below.

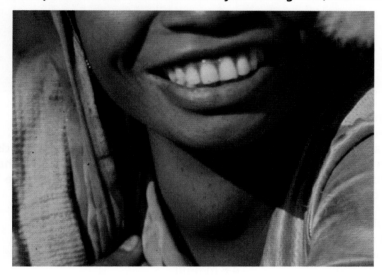

Which one of the following statements with regard to this situation is correct?

○ A If she is asymptomatic, no treatment or investigation is needed

○ B She is probably suffering from endemic goitre and should receive iodine supplementation

○ C She should be referred for surgical assessment

○ D She should be started on carbimazole

○ E She should have thyroid function tests carried out and if these are normal she can be reassured

4.13 Neck lumps

Indicate at which one of the options A–E would be the most likely location for a thyroglossal cyst, on the picture below.

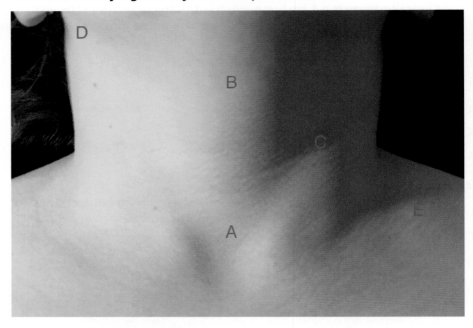

4.14 Interpreting blood test results

A 46-year-old woman presents with a 3-month history of weight gain, tiredness and irritability with night sweats. She reports that her periods have been rather irregular for the last 6 months but that she had not had any missed periods. She says that she is not depressed. Blood tests are taken which give the following results:

Haemoglobin	13.2 g/dl
White cell count	$5.2 \times 10^9/l$
Platelet count	$232 \times 10^9/l$
Glucose	4.8 mmol/l
TSH	6.4 mU/l (normal range 0.5–4.5 mU/l)
FT$_4$	11 pmol/l (normal range 10–24 pmol/l)
FSH	2.5 U/l
βhCG	<1 U/l

FT$_4$, free thyroxine; FSH, follicle-stimulating hormone; βhCG, β human chorionic gonadotrophin.

Normal range for FSH: follicular phase = 3.5–12.5 U/l; ovulatory phase = 4.7–21.5 U/l; luteal phase = 1.7–7.7 U/l; postmenopausal range = 25.8–134.8 U/l.

What is the single most likely diagnosis?

○ A   Clinical hypothyroidism

○ B   Depression

○ C   Hyperthyroidism

○ D   Perimenopause

○ E   Pregnancy

4.15 Management of diabetes in pregnancy
Which one of the following statements is true with regard to recent developments in the management of diabetes in pregnancy?

○ A   Mild gestational diabetes should be monitored initially rather than treated aggressively

○ B   Pregnancy outcomes are similar in diabetic and non-diabetic women

○ C   Screening for gestational diabetes based on clinical risk factors is more effective than universal screening

○ D   The rates of caesarean section in diabetic women are approximately twice the rate in non-diabetic women

○ E   Two-thirds of pregnant women with diabetes have an HbA1c >7% in the first trimester

4.16 Stepwise management of type 2 diabetes mellitus

Select the rank order of the options (1–4) that best fulfils the requirements given in the question.

The following is a list of treatments used in the management of a patient newly diagnosed with type 2 diabetes mellitus:

○ 1   Exenatide

○ 2   Gliclazide

○ 3   Insulin

○ 4   Metformin

The responses (A–E) rank the treatments in the management of type 2 diabetes mellitus in various orders. Select the response that places the options (1–4) in the order of the **first** treatment to **last**.

Select one rank order only.

○   A: 2, 4, 1, 3

○   B: 4, 2, 1, 3

○   C: 2, 1, 3, 4

○   D: 4, 1, 2, 3

○   E: 1, 4, 2, 3

EXTENDED MATCHING QUESTIONS

Diabetes trials

Options

A ADDITION-Cambridge study
B Cardiff UK GPRD Study
C DCCT (Diabetes Complications and Control Study)
D Diabetes Prevention Study
E DURATION trial
F UKPDS (United Kingdom Prospective Diabetes Study)
G VADT (Veterans Affairs Diabetes Trial)
H None of the above

For each of the statements below, select the most appropriate option from the list above. Each option may be used once, more than once or not at all.

4.17 **For patients with poorly controlled long-standing diabetes found no benefit for intensive over standard treatment.**

4.18 **Showed that aggressive lifestyle interventions in patients with impaired glucose tolerance can reduce the risk of developing diabetes.**

4.19 **Found the optimal HbA1c for reducing mortality to be 7.5%.**

4.20 **Showed no benefit from population screening.**

4.21 **Found that exenatide once weekly has better glycaemic control and fewer side effects than twice-daily exenatide.**

Breast pain

Options

A Benign breast change
B Blunt injury
C Breast abscess
D Breast carcinoma
E Breast engorgement
F Breast hypertrophy
G Gynaecomastia
H Haematoma
I Mondor's disease
J Shingles (herpes zoster)

For each of the scenarios described below, select the most appropriate diagnosis from the list above. Each option can be used once, more than once or not at all.

4.22 **A 19-year-old man complains of a diffuse swelling and discomfort of the right breast over a 9-month period. Clinically and on ultrasound scanning there is no discrete lesion.**

4.23   A 22-year-old woman presents in the immediate postpartum period with moderately severe bilateral breast pain and swelling; she is unable to initiate lactation.

4.24   A 53-year-old woman presents with a 4-day history of severe left-sided breast pain and the appearance of a red rash and blisters over the breast.

4.25   A 38-year-old woman who underwent excision of a large fibroadenoma of the left breast 10 days ago complains of pain, swelling and bruising at the operation site.

Blood tests in endocrinology

Options

A   Addison's disease
B   Clinical hypothyroidism
C   Cushing's disease
D   Hypercalcaemia
E   Hyperparathyroidism
F   Hyperthyroidism
G   Hypocalcaemia
H   Hypopituitarism
I   Menopausal
J   Subclinical hypothyroidism

For each of the blood result profiles below, select the most likely diagnosis from the list above. Each option may be used once, more than once or not at all.

4.26   Raised TSH, normal T_4.
4.27   Low sodium, raised potassium, raised ACTH with low cortisol.
4.28   Raised follicle-stimulating hormone (FSH), low estrogen.
4.29   Low levels of T_4, T_3, TSH, prolactin, sodium and potassium.
4.30   Low TSH, raised T_4.

Breast pain

4.31–4.35

Options

A	Combined oral contraceptive
B	Fluoxetine
C	GnRH analogue
D	NSAID
E	Reassure, lifestyle advice and supportive bra
F	Routine referral
G	Urgent referral
H	Vitamin B complex

Complete the algorithm below describing the management of patients presenting with breast pain in primary care, using the list of options above. Each option may be used once, more than once, or not at all.

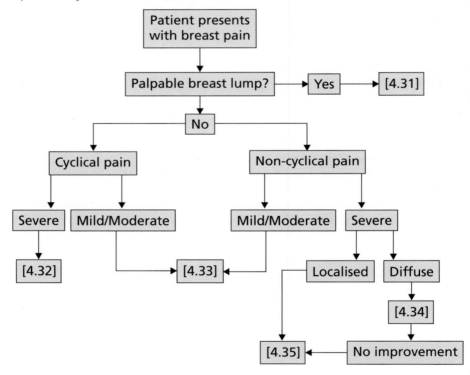

SINGLE BEST ANSWER

4.1   D: Ranitidine

Gynaecomastia can be caused by a number of medications, the most common being antacids such as PPIs and H_2-receptor antagonists. Other causes include hormone manipulation for benign and malignant prostatic conditions, recreational drug use such as marijuana or anabolic steroids. Gynaecomastia is common at puberty. Breast cancer tends to cause non-tender enlargement.

4.2   C: Cushing syndrome

This patient has symptoms of Cushing syndrome, which is usually iatrogenic due to long-term steroid use. There is characteristic 'orange on a stick' appearance of central obesity and a buffalo hump with muscle weakness, striae and thinning of skin. Cushing's disease is caused by excessive production of cortisol from the adrenals due in most cases to excessive pituitary ACTH secretion. Addison's disease is due to adrenal insufficiency and cortisol levels are low. Hypothyroidism may cause some of the symptoms of Cushing syndrome but can be differentiated on testing thyroid function, whereas elevated blood glucose in patients on steroids is often secondary to steroid therapy and resolves when doses are reduced.

4.3   C: Primary hypogonadism

This man has symptoms of hypogonadism. In the absence of obvious causes such as mumps orchitis, chemotherapy or other medication, or testicular surgery in his previous medical history, it is likely to be primary rather than secondary. Primary hypogonadism is suggested by raised FSH and LH with low testosterone, whereas secondary hypogonadism would be associated with low FSH/LH with low testosterone. He should have a karyotype to exclude Klinefelter syndrome (prevalence 1:700) and be assessed for osteoporosis. Any signs of pituitary disease should prompt referral for CT scan.

4.4   C: Increase her levothyroxine dose by 25 µg immediately

Patients with treated hypothyroidism have increased requirements for levothyroxine when pregnant. Their dose should be increased on confirmation of pregnancy by 25 µg (50 µg if they are on a low dose) and monitored to aim for a TSH in the 0.4–2.0 range. Patients with subclinical hypothyroidism who are trying to conceive should be started on thyroxine.

4.5   A: Calcium and vitamin D supplements

This patient has osteopenia rather than osteoporosis. Treatment should be aimed at lifestyle measures, calcium supplementation and reassurance. Where there are underlying risk factors such as coeliac disease these should be treated. Bisphosphonates are indicated only in otherwise healthy patients where osteoporosis is confirmed, or for prophylaxis in patients on steroids. Teriparatide is useful only in patients who do not respond to bisphosphonates.

4.6   B: Prescribe sildenafil at 25 mg initially and review in 2 weeks

If there are symptoms or signs of hypogonadism, checking FSH levels will differentiate between primary or secondary causes. A drug history should be taken to exclude reversible causes such as steroids, β-blockers, spironolactone or drugs of abuse such as marijuana. In the absence of contraindications, a trial of sildenafil starting at 25 mg may be appropriate.

4.7   E: Polycystic ovary syndrome

This patient has symptoms of PCOS. The diagnosis can be confirmed with blood tests during the first week of her period. PCOS is associated with raised free testosterone, raised LH and normal FSH. Primary Cushing's disease is rare and is caused by pituitary-dependent adrenal hyperplasia. Treatment of Cushing syndrome should be by gradual reduction of steroids and replacement where possible with steroid-sparing agents. Addison's disease is caused by a deficiency of steroids and causes low blood pressure, lassitude and depression.

4.8   B: Investigate for causes of vitamin D deficiency

Osteomalacia is characterised by abnormal mineralisation of bone and is usually caused by vitamin D deficiency in adults. It can be difficult to differentiate from osteopenia and osteoporosis, but there are typically Looser's zones evident on X-ray, and blood tests reveal reduced calcium, phosphate and vitamin D levels with raised alkaline phosphatase. It is often caused by low sunlight or poor diet, but investigation should aim to exclude secondary causes such as coeliac disease or inherited disorders of vitamin D metabolism. Treatment is usually with dietary supplements once other causes have been excluded.

4.9   C: Physiological goitre

Asymptomatic enlargement of the thyroid gland can occur at puberty or during pregnancy, when there is an increased physiological stimulation of the thyroid gland.

4.10   C: Fibroadenoma

Fibroadenomas are not uncommon in premenopausal women and are usually transient. They are small mobile lumps with a smooth surface. However, once they exceed 3 cm in size they rarely regress; rarely, they may grow into a giant fibroadenoma or a phyllodes tumour.

4.11   A: Breast carcinoma

A solid lump with overlying skin tethering or nipple retraction is clinically diagnostic of an infiltrating ductal carcinoma. In elderly people these tumours are usually slow growing and slow to metastasise. They are usually hormone receptor sensitive and respond well to tamoxifen, letrozole or anastrozole therapy.

4.12   C: She should be referred for surgical assessment

All patients with goitre should have their thyroid function tested. Where there is asymmetry, referral is indicated to exclude cancer. Hyperthyroidism is treated with carbimazole initially, although levothyroxine supplementation is often required later under a 'block-and-replace' regimen. Diffuse enlargement with normal thyroid function is usually due to endemic goitre.

4.13   B

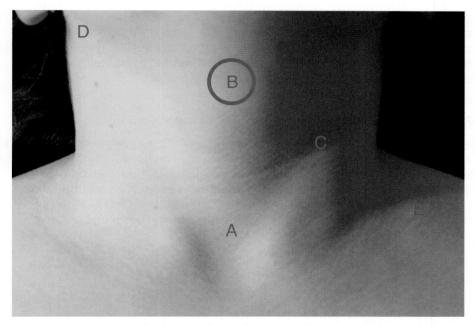

Thyroglossal cysts are usually found along the tract of the thyroglossal duct, from the thyroid to the tongue base. A lump at A is likely to be thyroid, whereas at C it is likely to be a branchial cyst or lymph node. Lumps at D are likely to be either lymph nodes or enlarged parotid gland.

4.14   D: Perimenopause

Blood tests are unreliable in diagnosing the perimenopause and clinicians should rely on a menstrual history and exclusion of other possible causes. Overt hypothyroidism is unlikely with a T_4 in the normal range. Hyperthyroidism would generally cause a raised T_4 and suppressed TSH, whereas pregnancy would cause a raised βhCG. Estradiol levels are unhelpful for diagnosing and monitoring the menopause.

4.15   E: Two-thirds of pregnant women with diabetes have an HbA1c >7% in the first trimester

Pregnancy care for diabetic women should start before conception, with joined-up care involving primary care, obstetricians and endocrinologists. Close control of diabetes is associated with lowered perinatal mortality and lowered risk of congenital malformation. The ACHOIS trial (the Australian Carbohydrate Intolerance Study) demonstrated the benefits of treating mild gestational diabetes, and therefore supports the argument for universal screening, particularly because relying on clinical risk factors alone has been shown to miss up to 50% of cases of gestational diabetes in some groups. The caesarean section rate is 60–70% in diabetic women and current NICE guidelines suggest that women should be offered delivery at 38 weeks to reduce the risk of shoulder dystocia and subsequent emergency section.

4.16   B: 4, 2, 1, 3
Rank ordering: 4 Metformin; 2 Gliclazide; 1 Exenatide; 3 Insulin

All patients with type 2 diabetes should receive lifestyle advice with regard to exercise, diet and weight loss. Metformin should be used if diet fails to control sugar levels, unless contraindicated. Second-line oral treatment is usually a sulphonylurea. Failure to respond to this should prompt an additional oral treatment such as a glitazone or gliptin. If these are ineffective, injectable treatment with exenatide may be used as an alternative to insulin.

EXTENDED MATCHING ANSWERS

Diabetes trials

4.17   G: VADT

The Veterans Affairs Diabetes Trial looked at patients with longstanding poorly controlled diabetes (mean 11 years), and found no difference between intensive and normal treatment.

4.18   D: Diabetes Prevention Study

The Diabetes Prevention Study found that aggressive lifestyle interventions could delay the onset of type 2 diabetes in patients with impaired glucose tolerance, with a 56% relative risk reduction

4.19   B: Cardiff UK GPRD Study

Mortality with HbA1c is U shaped, with lowest mortality rate seen at 7.5%, hence the thresholds seen in the Quality and Outcomes Framework.

4.20   A: ADDITION-Cambridge study

ADDITION-Cambridge found no benefit from screening high-risk patients for type 2 diabetes over a 10-year follow-up period

4.21   E: DURATION trial

DURATION trial has shown that the weekly exenatide preparation is superior in efficacy and side effects to twice-daily exenatide.

Breast pain

4.22   G: Gynaecomastia

Gynaecomastia in adolescence is due to unopposed estrogenic activity; it is usually self-limiting and resolves after puberty. Occasionally the swelling persists and when it is cosmetically unacceptable it is treated by subcutaneous mastectomy.

4.23   E: Breast engorgement

Breast engorgement in the early postpartum period is not uncommon in primips; it is also associated with a poor suckling reflex or inverted nipples.

4.24   J: Shingles (herpes zoster)

Herpes zoster infection presents as a linear subcutaneous rash with overlying blisters along intercostal dermatomes; the breast is not affected. However, the diagnosis can be difficult before the appearance of the rash and if there is no history of the infection.

4.25   H: Haematoma

Postoperative haematoma or a seroma after surgery on the breast usually resolves, provided that the collection is small and uninfected; large collections can require repeated aspiration.

Blood tests in endocrinology

4.26   J: Subclinical hypothyroidism

Subclinical hypothyroidism is associated with raised TSH with normal T_4 and T_3 levels. These patients should be monitored over time because a significant number will become overtly hypothyroid in time.

4.27   A: Addison's disease

Addison's disease is due to adrenal failure, so ACTH is elevated with a normal or low serum cortisol. A short Synacthen test will often confirm hypoadrenalism.

4.28   I: Menopausal

Luteinising hormone (LH) and follicle-stimulating hormone (FSH) levels are raised in testicular and ovarian failure, in association with low levels of estrogen or testosterone.

4.29   H: Hypopituitarism

Hypopituitarism should be suspected in patients with signs of hypothyroidism, hypogonadism or growth hormone deficiency; these patients often also have diabetes insipidus. The diagnosis can be confirmed by a combined pituitary test.

4.30   F: Hyperthyroidism

Raised T_4 with suppressed TSH is diagnostic of primary hyperthyroidism. Low TSH with normal T_4 and T_3 is usually caused by excess thyroxine replacement or high-dose steroids.

Breast pain

4.31   G: Urgent referral

4.32   F: Routine referral

4.33   E: Reassure, lifestyle advice and supportive bra

4.34   D: NSAID

4.35   F: Routine referral

Breast pain alone is seldom a symptom of breast cancer; however, persistent pain not responding to NSAIDs is an indication for routine referral. Lifestyle changes such as a low-fat diet, evening primrose oil and phytoestrogens may help. Where pain is severe and underlying pathology has been excluded, danazol or tamoxifen may help. Some women also find antidepressants helpful.

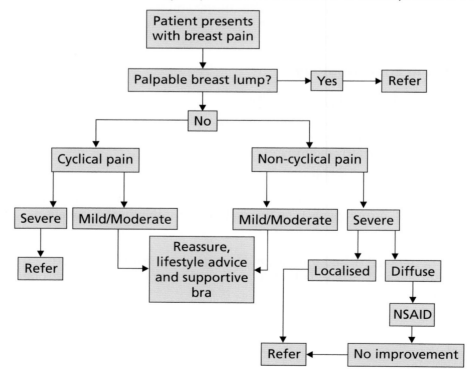

Chapter 5
Gastroenterology

SINGLE BEST ANSWER QUESTIONS

5.1 Epigastric pain
You are called to visit a 46-year-old man who complains of acute onset of severe upper abdominal pain, radiating to his back. He feels sweaty and nauseous and also reports pain in his shoulder. When you arrive he is sitting up, leaning over the back of a chair, and examination reveals marked epigastric tenderness. What is the most likely diagnosis?

- ○ A Acute cholecystitis
- ○ B Acute pancreatitis
- ○ C Oesophageal varices
- ○ D Pancreatic cancer
- ○ E Perforated duodenal ulcer

5.2 Diarrhoea
A 67-year-old man has been discharged from hospital after being treated for pneumonia. He has now developed a profuse watery diarrhoea, but has had no vomiting. There is no blood in the stool but he is febrile, tachycardic and hypotensive. What is the most likely cause?

- ○ A *Campylobacter* sp.
- ○ B *Clostridium difficile*
- ○ C *Escherichia coli*
- ○ D Norovirus
- ○ E Rotavirus

5.3 Change in bowel habit

You are updating the practice protocol for the investigation of change in bowel habit and want to base this on the NICE guidance. Which one of the following scenarios should prompt a referral under the 2-week rule?

○ A   A 28-year-old man with 6 weeks of loose stools; examination and blood tests are normal

○ B   A 34-year-old woman with 3 months of discomfort in her right iliac fossa; examination is normal, as are blood tests

○ C   A 36-year-old woman noted on routine blood testing to have a haemoglobin of 10.6 g/dl

○ D   A 45-year-old man who has routine blood tests showing a haemoglobin of 10.5 g/dl with a reduced MCV. He is otherwise well and examination is unremarkable

○ E   A 66-year-old man with 3 weeks of loose stools, but no bleeding or anal symptoms; blood tests and examination are normal

5.4 Abdominal pain

An 85-year-old woman with a previous history of peripheral vascular disease and hypertension presents with acute severe abdominal pain and loose bowels. The pain is colicky but examination findings are unremarkable apart from some tenderness in her abdomen, and an irregular pulse that has not been noted before. A rectal examination reveals blood-stained mucus. Which one of the following statements is correct with regard to this presentation?

○ A   Blood-stained mucus is likely to be due to haemorrhoids

○ B   Mesenteric ischaemia should be considered

○ C   The absence of any significant examination findings suggests that serious disease is unlikely

○ D   The most likely diagnosis is diverticulitis

○ E   The most likely diagnosis is irritable bowel syndrome (IBS) and the patient should be given mebeverine

5.5 Coeliac disease

One of your patients has been diagnosed with coeliac disease. Which one of the following can she eat normally?

○ A   Barley

○ B   Porridge oats

○ C   Rice

○ D   Rye

○ E   Wheat

5.6 Crohn's disease
Which of the following statements about Crohn's disease is true? Select one option only.

○ A Active disease should be treated initially with mesalazine

○ B Anti-mycobacterial therapies are an effective treatment if used early

○ C Anti-TNFα therapy is associated with remission rates of 80%

○ D Crohn's disease affects only the colon

○ E Patients should be referred early for surgery

5.7 Ulcerative colitis
Which one of the following statements about ulcerative colitis is true? Select one option only.

○ A Ulcerative colitis is always associated with perianal fistulas

○ B Mesalazine should always be prescribed generically

○ C Oral steroids are the mainstay of maintenance therapy

○ D Patients with ulcerative colitis should have regular colonoscopic follow-up to identify malignant change

○ E Ulcerative colitis can affect any part of the gastrointestinal tract

5.8 Abdominal pain
A 9-year-old child gives a 2-day history of intermittent abdominal pain that shifts to the right lower quadrant, preceded by nausea. She is mildly pyrexial with a tachycardia. Select the single most likely diagnosis from the list below.

○ A Appendicitis

○ B Incarcerated hernia

○ C Intussusception

○ D Malrotation

○ E Mesenteric thrombosis

5.9 Poor appetite

A 39-year-old woman who works in a dairy presents with a 9-month history of poor appetite, malaise and weight loss. Abdominal radiography reveals mesenteric nodal calcifications. There is a history of unpasteurised cheese consumption. Select the single most likely diagnosis from the list below.

○ A   Abdominal tuberculosis

○ B   Actinomycosis

○ C   Enteric *Staphylococcus aureus* infection

○ D   Hydatid disease

○ E   Trypanosomiasis

5.10 Abdominal pain

A 35-year-old woman presents with a 3-day history of upper abdominal pain that radiates to the right side, associated with nausea and bloating. She is febrile and has upper abdominal tenderness and guarding. Select the single most likely diagnosis from the list below.

○ A   Appendicitis

○ B   Cholecystitis

○ C   Ectopic pregnancy

○ D   Mesenteric thrombosis

○ E   Visceral perforation

5.11 Abdominal pain

A 74-year-old woman on long-term diclofenac for rheumatoid arthritis presents with abdominal pain. She is hypotensive with a rapid pulse and epigastric tenderness. Select the single most likely diagnosis from the list below.

○ A   Acute pancreatitis

○ B   Appendicitis

○ C   Cholecystitis

○ D   Intussusception

○ E   Perforated ulcer

5.12 Dyspepsia

Which one of the following statements about the initial management of dyspepsia in primary care is correct?

○ A   Of the UK population 20% take long-term prescription drugs for dyspepsia

○ B   Costs are greater at 1 year for test and treat compared with empirical treatment due to the relatively high cost of antibiotics compared with generic proton pump inhibitors

○ C   Endoscopy is more cost-effective than empirical treatment in the long term

○ D   Eradication of *Helicobacter pylori* might reduce the long-term incidence of cancer

○ E   Test and treat at initial consultation is more effective at 1 year than acid suppression alone

5.13 Abdominal rash

A 33-year-old woman has a violent coughing fit and shortly afterwards notices an unusual rash over her lower abdomen. Her abdomen is shown below:

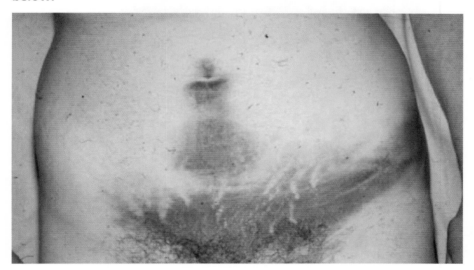

Which one of the following is the single most likely underlying diagnosis?

○ A   Disseminated intravascular coagulation (DIC)

○ B   Haemophilia

○ C   Psoas abscess

○ D   Rectus sheath haematoma

○ E   Von Willebrand's disease

5.14 Rectal bleeding

A 42-year-old man complains of fresh bleeding after defecation, discomfort, itching and intermittent soiling of his underwear with mucus. On examination of his anus you note the appearance below:

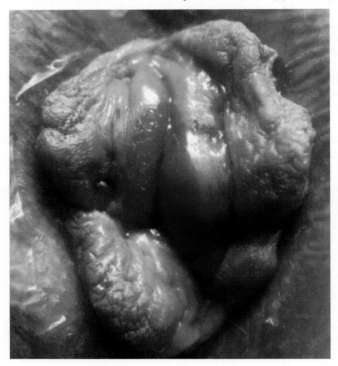

Which one of the following is the most likely diagnosis?

- ○   A   Anal fissure
- ○   B   Condyloma acuminata
- ○   C   Crohn's disease
- ○   D   Haemorrhoids
- ○   E   Squamous cell carcinoma of the anus

5.15 Bowel cancer trial

A new test has been developed to pick up asymptomatic bowel cancer. This involves patients sending specimens of stool for analysis for dyskaryotic epithelial cells. It is reported by its inventors to be non-invasive and therefore safe and accurate. Initial trial data are shown below:

Total number of samples submitted	1000
Number suitable for analysis	500
Number of samples that tested positive	50
Number of true positives (confirmed by colonoscopy)	25
Total number of diagnoses in patients who submitted suitable sample	30
Number of false negatives	5
Number of diagnoses in all patients participating in trial	60

Which one of the following statements is true with regard to this data?

- A   For patients submitting a suitable sample, the sensitivity of the test is 25/30, ie 83%

- B   For patients submitting a suitable sample, the sensitivity of the test is 25/50, ie 50%

- C   For patients submitting a suitable sample, the sensitivity of the test is 50/500, ie 10%

- D   For patients submitting a suitable sample, the specificity of the test is 25/30, ie 83%

- E   The data suggest that this test will make a significant impact on early diagnosis of bowel cancer

EXTENDED MATCHING QUESTIONS

Diarrhoea

Options

A   *Campylobacter* sp.
B   *Clostridium difficile*
C   *Cryptosporidium* sp.
D   Norovirus
E   Rotavirus
F   *Salmonella* sp.
G   *Shigella* sp.

For each of the descriptions below, select the most appropriate causative agent from the list above. Each option may be used once, more than once or not at all.

5.16   **Causes diarrhoea by contamination of drinking water with agricultural waste, usually cow slurry.**

5.17   **Causes epidemics of gastroenteritis in children.**

5.18   **Causes watery diarrhoea and abdominal cramps, progressing to bloody diarrhoea.**

5.19   **Highly infectious, with aerosol transmission; causes projectile vomiting.**

Acute abdomen

Options

A   Appendicitis
B   Cholecystitis
C   Incarcerated hernia
D   Intussusception
E   Malrotation
F   Meconium ileus
G   Mesenteric thrombosis
H   Ruptured ectopic pregnancy
I   Septic abortion
J   Urinary tract infection
K   Visceral perforation

For each of the descriptions below, select the most appropriate diagnosis from the list of options above. Each option may be used once, more than once or not at all.

5.20   **A 6-year-old girl complains of 24 hours of generalised abdominal pain. On examination she is diffusely tender with some guarding. Urine dipstick testing is positive for nitrites.**

5.21   **A 28-year-old woman is admitted with a 14-hour history of sudden onset of severe lower abdominal pain with nausea and**

retching. Her last normal period was 10 weeks ago. Her pulse is 120 beats/min and her BP is 90/70 mmHg.

5.22 A 4-year-old boy is seen with an 8-hour history of colicky central abdominal pain and vomiting. He presents with an irreducible lump in the left groin, extending into the scrotum.

5.23 An 18-month-old toddler who has been on a weaning diet becomes fretful, clutches his abdomen and cries out. He refuses feeds and passes loose motions containing blood-stained mucus.

5.24 A 7-day-old male neonate has not opened his bowels since birth. Symptoms of bowel obstruction develop, with bile-stained vomiting. Respiratory investigations suggest cystic fibrosis.

Liver disease

Options

A   Acute cholecystitis
B   Acute cholangitis
C   Acute liver failure
D   Biliary atresia
E   Biliary stricture
F   Cirrhosis
G   Gallstone ileus
H   Wilson's disease
I   Hepatocellular carcinoma
J   Liver abscess

For each of the scenarios described below, select the most appropriate diagnosis from the list above. Each option can be used once, more than once or not at all.

5.25 A 39-year-old man with a history of alcoholism complains of malaise, anorexia and weight loss. Clinically, he has a firm, enlarged liver, a palpable spleen and moderate ascites.

5.26 A 44-year-old northern European man with a dusky complexion presents with painful arthritic swelling of both knees and a 3-month history of polyuria and polydypsia. He has a 15-cm, firm hepatomegaly with cutaneous signs of chronic liver disease.

5.27 A 42-year-old woman is admitted with severe right-sided abdominal pain that is radiating to the back, with nausea and retching some hours after a meal. She is tender in the right upper quadrant and inflammatory markers in her peripheral blood are raised.

5.28 A 46-year-old woman with known gallstones is admitted acutely ill with progressive jaundice, upper abdominal pain and rigors. She has been confined to bed for the past 4 days.

Management of childhood constipation

5.29–5.35

Options

A High-dose osmotic laxative
B Impaction not present
C Impaction present
D Maintenance-dose osmotic laxative
E No red flags
F Routine referral
G Red flags present
H Urgent referral

Complete the algorithm below describing the management of childhood constipation. Each option may be used once, more than once or not at all.

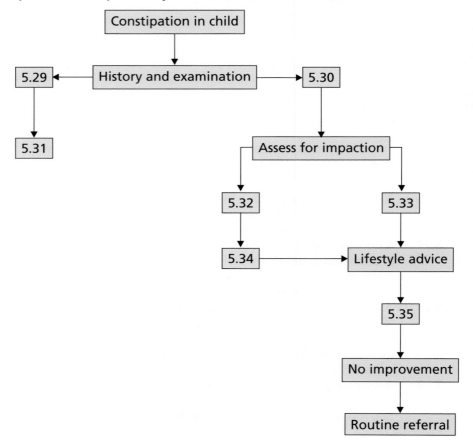

SINGLE BEST ANSWER

5.1   B: Acute pancreatitis

This is a typical presentation of acute pancreatitis. He should be admitted for investigation and management. Raised amylase will usually confirm the diagnosis. Oesophageal varices tend to cause haematemesis, whereas a perforated duodenal ulcer, although causing similar symptoms, is not usually relieved by sitting leaning forward.

5.2   B: *Clostridium difficile*

Watery diarrhoea starting after recent antibiotic therapy is usually caused by *Clostridium difficile*. The most common implicated antibiotics are amoxicillin, ampicillin, clindamycin and cephalosporins. Treatment consists of stopping the offending antibiotics, metronidazole or oral vancomycin, fluid replacement and barrier nursing. Toxic megacolon can occur and this should be managed surgically. *Campylobacter* sp. causes a diarrhoeal illness that is usually associated with eating chicken, whereas norovirus causes a transient diarrhoeal and vomiting illness. Rotavirus usually affects children.

5.3   D: A 45-year-old man who has routine blood tests showing a haemoglobin of 10.5 g/dl with a reduced MCV. He is otherwise well and examination is unremarkable

NICE guidance suggests referral in the following situations:

- People aged ⩾40 years, reporting rectal bleeding with a change of bowel habit for 6 weeks
- People aged ⩾60 years, with rectal bleeding persisting for 6 weeks without anal symptoms
- People aged ⩾60 years, with a change in bowel habit to looser stools for 6 weeks or more without rectal bleeding
- People of any age with a right lower abdominal or rectal mass
- Men with iron-deficiency anaemia and a haemoglobin ⩽11 g/dl
- Non-menstruating women with a haemoglobin ⩽10 g/dl.

5.4   B: Mesenteric ischaemia should be considered

The presentation of acute severe abdominal pain in someone with arteriopathy, out of keeping with clinical findings, should suggest the possibility of ischaemic bowel. Initially there are few signs but, later on, blood-stained mucus, signs of bowel obstruction and shock are common. The prognosis is poor due to late diagnosis. Diverticulitis generally causes milder pain with more of a change in bowel habit whereas IBS would not normally cause severe pain.

5.5   C: Rice

Patients with coeliac disease should avoid wheat, rye and barley, but can eat rice and maize. Some coeliac disease patients are sensitive to pure oats but many patients can take these without any problem, although commercially available oats such as porridge oats are usually contaminated with wheat during the milling process, so patients should try to obtain pure oats.

5.6   C: Anti-TNFα therapy is associated with remission rates of 80%

Mesalazine is no better than placebo in the management of active disease. Its main use is in prevention of relapse after surgery. Infliximab is an effective anti-TNFα therapy in up to 80% of cases, but only 24% are steroid free. Surgery should be reserved for patients who do not respond to steroids, methotrexate or infliximab. Antibiotics should be used only for septic complications and perianal disease. Crohn's disease can affect any part of the gastrointestinal tract from the mouth to the anus.

5.7   D: Patients with ulcerative colitis should have regular colonoscopic follow-up to identify malignant change

Ulcerative colitis affects only the large bowel, whereas Crohn's disease can affect any part of the gastrointestinal tract. Mesalazine should be prescribed by brand. Ulcerative colitis is associated with bowel cancer and so patients should be regularly screened with colonoscopy. In most patients the disease can be controlled with mesalazine and where steroids are needed topical steroids such as Predfoam enemas should be used to reduce systemic effects. Perianal fistulas are associated with Crohn's disease.

5.8   A: Appendicitis

Acute appendicitis in children must be distinguished from acute mesenteric adenitis caused by systemic viral infections and urinary tract infections. In adolescent girls, mid-cycle pain, twisted ovarian cysts or ruptured ovarian follicles can mimic acute appendicitis.

5.9   A: Abdominal tuberculosis

Abdominal TB is acquired through the consumption of infected milk or milk products and leads to caseation in mesenteric, portal or splenic lymphatic tissue; these lesions can eventually heal with calcification.

5.10   B: Cholecystitis

Tenderness in the gallbladder area, a tender, palpable gallbladder and a positive Murphy's sign are all suggestive of acute calculous cholecystitis. An ultrasound scan would exclude empyema of the gallbladder, confirm stones in the gallbladder, and exclude duct stones and pancreatitis.

5.11 E: Perforated ulcer

Peptic perforation is a complication of peptic ulcer disease and is associated with anti-ulcer therapy non-compliance, alcohol abuse, long-term steroids and NSAIDs. A rare cause is gastrinoma (an islet-cell tumour), which stimulates gastric hypersecretion, causing multiple ulcers.

5.12 D: Eradication of *Helicobacter pylori* might reduce the long-term incidence of cancer

Three per cent of the population take long-term drugs for dyspepsia at an estimated annual cost of £500 million. Endoscopy is the least cost-effective option when compared with test and treat or empirical treatment. Eradication of *H. pylori* in high-risk patients has reduced the incidence of gastric cancer. The MRC-CU BE trial (Multicentre Randomised Controlled Trial of ^{13}C Urea Breath Testing and *H. pylori* Eradication for Dyspepsia in Primary Care) demonstrated equivalent cost-effectiveness for test and treat and empirical treatment, and therefore supported initial empirical treatment. The researchers concluded that the decision to test for *H. pylori* should be made with the patient.

5.13 D: Rectus sheath haematoma

This is the typical appearance of a rectus sheath haematoma, which usually occurs spontaneously after coughing or vomiting. It is usually caused by blood leaking from the inferior epigastric artery, and commonly settles spontaneously.

5.14 D: Haemorrhoids

This is a typical appearance of third-degree piles. Typical symptoms are itching and irritation, dull ache, bleeding, sensation of a lump and soiling. They are classified as 'first degree' if they are within the anal canal, 'second degree' if they come down with bowel motions but return afterwards and 'third degree' if they are down all the time.

5.15 A: For patients submitting a suitable sample, the sensitivity of the test is 25/30, ie 83%

Sensitivity = 100 × true positive/(true positive + false negative)
Specificity = 100 × true negative/(true negative + false positive)

The fact that half of all samples were unsuitable suggests that this test is unlikely to be useful on a population basis, because this resulted in 30 diagnoses being missed.

EXTENDED MATCHING ANSWERS

Diarrhoea

5.16   C: *Cryptosporidium* sp.

Cryptosporidium sp. causes a self-limiting diarrhoeal illness in children and immunocompromised individuals. Treatment with spiramycin might be needed in patients with reduced immunity.

5.17   E: Rotavirus

Rotavirus is the most common cause of gastroenteritis in children in the UK. Epidemics tend to occur in winter and spring, with fewer cases in the summer. Treatment is supportive.

5.18   G: *Shigella* sp.

Shigella sp. causes dysentery and in the UK outbreaks have been seen in nurseries, psychiatric facilities and care homes. It causes bloody diarrhoea after an incubation period of 48 hours. Treatment is supportive; ciprofloxacin is useful in those who are immunocompromised or severely affected.

5.19   D: Norovirus

Norovirus causes epidemics of gastroenteritis and often causes epidemics on cruise ships, in schools and in hospitals. Symptoms usually settle with conservative treatment in 48 hours.

Acute abdomen

5.20   A: Appendicitis

Appendicitis typically starts with vague abdominal pain that tends to localise to the right iliac fossa over 12–24 hours. Nitrites have low specificity for urinary tract infection. A pelvic appendix can mimic a urinary tract infection.

5.21   H: Ruptured ectopic pregnancy

Sudden onset of severe, persistent abdominal pain with hypotension and peritonism in a woman of childbearing age strongly suggests a ruptured ectopic pregnancy. A pelvic ultrasound scan will confirm the diagnosis.

5.22   C: Incarcerated hernia

Inguinal hernia in early childhood is caused by the virtual apposition of the internal and external rings during the development of the inguinal canal. The processus vaginalis is also patent, providing access of abdominal contents to the scrotum.

5.23   D: Intussusception

Intussusception in childhood is usually caused by hyperplasia of submucosal lymphoid tissue due to changes in bowel flora during weaning. The intussusception is initially intermittent but bowel obstruction rapidly supervenes which leads to ischaemia of the intussuscepted loop.

5.24   F: Meconium ileus

Meconium ileus is caused by inspissated meconium impacting in the terminal ileum and results from changes in bowel mucus associated with cystic fibrosis. If colonic washouts fail to restore patency, surgical evacuation is required.

Liver disease

5.25   F: Cirrhosis

In cirrhosis, cutaneous signs are spider naevi, caput medusae, skin bruising, pigmentation and purpuric rash. The uncongugated plasma bilirubin can be raised, with raised liver enzymes and a low albumin.

5.26   H: Wilson's disease

Wilson's disease (hepatolenticular degeneration) is an autosomal recessive disorder of defective copper metabolism in the liver, resulting in copper deposition in tissues. Chelating agents (eg penicillamine) control disease progression and liver transplantation is indicated for advanced disease.

5.27   A: Acute cholecystitis

Ultrasound of the gallbladder would confirm the presence of gallstones in an inflamed, thick-walled gallbladder. Liver function is usually unaffected if the biliary tree is free of stones or inflammation.

5.28   B: Acute cholangitis

Cholangiohepatitis is an ascending infection of the biliary tree caused by calculus obstruction and would lead to inflammation of the liver parenchyma and microabscess formation. Urgent decompression of the biliary tree by percutaneous catheterisation, endoscopic drainage or surgical drainage is required.

Management of constipation in children

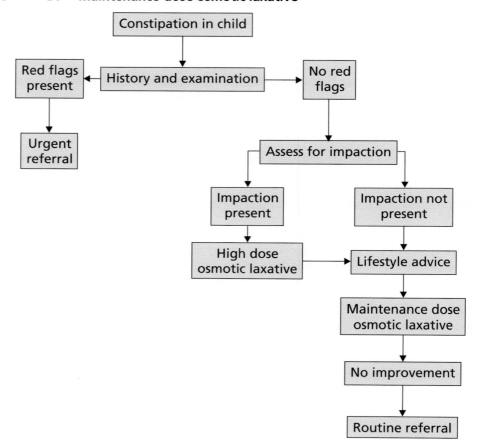

Chapter 6
Genetics

SINGLE BEST ANSWER QUESTIONS

6.1 Evidence-based practice
Which one of the following statements is correct with regard to the findings of the report *Familial cancer risk in people from ethnic minorities, 2012?*

○ A Cultural influences are a significant barrier to effective healthcare in genetic disease

○ B Risk assessment should not take into account ethnicity

○ C Standardised referral and treatment pathways across the UK ensure equality of access to specialist services

○ D The incidence of genetic disease is independent of ethnicity

○ E The report recommended that counselling on cancer risk should be undertaken by specialist genetic counsellors only

6.2 Developmental concerns
You see the parents of a 30-month-old boy who are concerned about his development. He was born at term after a normal delivery and initially seemed to be developing normally, but they have now become concerned that he is not walking as well as he should. He falls frequently and when he stands he has to push himself up with his hands. Examination shows some wasting of his quadriceps and hypertrophy of his calves. What is the single most likely diagnosis?

○ A Cerebral palsy

○ B Down syndrome

○ C Duchenne muscular dystrophy

○ D Motor neuron disease

○ E Myotonic muscular dystrophy

6.3 Causes of emphysema
A 49-year-old smoker has just been diagnosed with emphysema, and has been found to have α_1-antitrypsin deficiency. Which one of the following is a correct description of the aetiology of the emphysema?

○   A   Environmental

○   B   Multifactorial

○   C   New mutation

○   D   Single gene effect

○   E   Sporadic

6.4 Cystic fibrosis
Which one of the following statements about cystic fibrosis is true?

○   A   98% of male patients are infertile

○   B   It is transmitted as an X-linked recessive trait

○   C   The disease is common in Asian and African–Caribbean individuals

○   D   The incidence of cystic fibrosis in the UK is 1 in 10 000 live births

○   E   The prevalence of carriers is 1 in 200 in the UK

6.5 Risk of Down syndrome
A 39-year-old woman with two children by her first marriage comes to see you to discuss pre-conception counselling now that she is to remarry. She is particularly concerned about the risk of Down syndrome. Which one of the following statements is true about this situation?

○   A   All women with a risk >1 in 400 should be offered chorionic villous sampling (CVS)

○   B   Nuchal translucency testing has 98% sensitivity and specificity for Down syndrome

○   C   The risk at age 40 is 1 in 30

○   D   The risk of Down syndrome is negligible below the age of 30

○   E   The risk of having a baby with Down syndrome is significantly greater in parents who have already had a Down syndrome pregnancy

6.6 Huntington's disease

A 46-year-old man comes to see you to discuss his recent diagnosis of Huntington's disease. He was adopted and has no knowledge of his genetic family. He has two teenage sons and lost his wife 3 years ago to breast cancer. Which of the following statements is true about this situation? Select one option only.

○ A   If his teenage sons show no signs of chorea, they can be reassured

○ B   Testing the children to see if they will develop the condition is not possible

○ C   The average life expectancy from diagnosis is 25 years

○ D   The condition is inherited as an autosomal dominant trait and the risk of his sons developing the condition is 1 in 2

○ E   This condition usually presents in the late teens

6.7 Turner syndrome

Which of the following statements is true about Turner syndrome? Select one option only.

○ A   Affected individuals tend to be tall with hyperextensible joints

○ B   Affected patients have the karyotype 47XXX

○ C   The external genitalia are characteristically abnormal

○ D   The incidence is 1:2500 live births

○ E   Turner syndrome is invariably associated with learning disability

6.8 Genetic counselling

Which one of the following statements about genetic counselling in primary care is true? Select one option only.

○ A   Family trees are not helpful in counselling families affected by Down syndrome

○ B   Families with conditions with variable penetrance, eg tuberous sclerosis, can be successfully counselled in primary care

○ C   Genetic counselling is a complex field and there is no place for genetic counselling in primary care

○ D   Risk is best expressed as percentages (eg 0.1%), rather than as proportions (eg 1 in 1000)

○ E   Two generations of a family tree are sufficient to identify a genetic predisposition

6.9 Phenylketonuria

A family who have recently joined your list come to see you to discuss phenylketonuria. The parents are unaffected but have had a son who has been diagnosed on the basis of a neonatal heel-prick test. They wish to discuss the risks relating to further pregnancies.

Which one of the following statements about this situation is true?

○ A   As the parents are unaffected, the affected son is the result of a new mutation and the recurrence risks are very rare

○ B   Phenylketonuria is an autosomal dominant trait so the lack of the disease in either parent suggests that the stated father is not the biological father

○ C   Phenylketonuria is an autosomal recessive trait, so both parents must be carriers

○ D   The risk of a future child being a carrier is 1 in 4

○ E   The risk of another child having phenylketonuria is 1 in 2

6.10 Skin lesions

A patient has had the lesions shown in the photograph below all over his body since childhood. He does not know anything about his family history because he was adopted at the age of 3 months. His wife is not affected. He is planning a family and consults you for advice as to whether their children are likely to be affected.

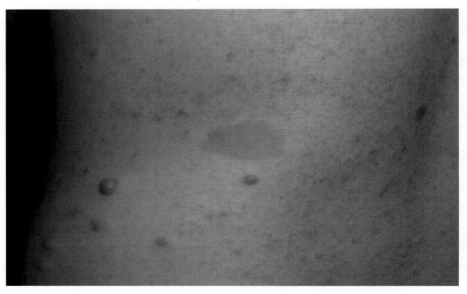

Which one of the following statements is true regarding the risk of passing the condition to any children?

○ A The condition is a spontaneous condition rather than genetic, so there is no risk of transmission to offspring

○ B The risk to affected offspring is 50%

○ C The risk to affected offspring is 100%

○ D The risk of children being carriers is 25%

○ E The risk of male children being carriers is 100%

6.11 Genetic counselling

A couple attend for pre-conception counselling after having two children affected by a genetic disease. They would like to have a third child but are concerned about the risk of recurrence. Their family pedigree is shown below:

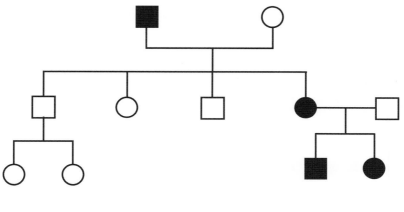

▌ Heterozygote male   □ Unaffected homozygotic male

○ Unaffected homozygotic female   ● Affected homozygotic female

■ Affected male

Which one of the following statements about the pattern of inheritance is true?

○ A The condition is inherited as an autosomal dominant trait

○ B The condition is inherited as an autosomal recessive trait

○ C The condition is inherited as an X-linked recessive trait

○ D The condition is inherited as a Y-linked trait

○ E The condition is sporadic rather than an inherited trait

6.12 Causes of learning disability

Select the rank order of the options (1–4) that best fulfil the requirements given in the question.

The following is a list of genetic syndromes causing learning disabilities:

1   Down syndrome
2   Fragile X syndrome
3   Klinefelter syndrome
4   Turner syndrome

The responses (A–E) rank the genetic syndromes causing learning disabilities in various orders. Select the response that places the options (1–4) in the order of most common syndrome to **least** common.

Select one rank order only.

A: 1, 3, 4, 2
B: 1, 3, 2, 4
C: 3, 1, 2, 4
D: 3, 1, 4, 2
E: 3, 4, 1, 2

EXTENDED MATCHING QUESTIONS

Prevalence of genetic disease

Options

A   0.05 per 1000 births
B   0.1 per 1000 births
C   0.5 per 1000 births
D   2 per 1000 births
E   5 per 1000 births
F   None of the above

For each of the disease listed below, select the option from this list above that reflects most accurately the prevalence of the condition in the UK. Each option may be used once, more than once or not at all.

6.13   Familial combined hyperlipidaemia
6.14   β-Thalassaemia
6.15   Cystic fibrosis
6.16   Haemophilia A
6.17   Sickle cell anaemia
6.18   Neurofibromatosis

Modes of inheritance

Options

A   Autosomal dominant
B   Autosomal recessive
C   Chromosomal translocation
D   Non-dysjunction
E   X-linked dominant
F   X-linked recessive

For each of the conditions below, select the most appropriate inheritance pattern from the list above. Each option may be used once, more than once or not at all.

6.19   Cystic fibrosis
6.20   Duchenne muscular dystrophy
6.21   Klinefelter syndrome
6.22   Huntington's disease

Diagnostic tests in genetics

Options

A   Amniocentesis
B   Carrier testing
C   Chorionic villous sampling (CVS)
D   Fetoscopy
E   Fluorescent *in situ* hybridisation
F   Guthrie test
G   Heel-prick test
H   Karyotyping
I   Triple test
J   Ultrasound

For each of the conditions affecting babies described below, select the most appropriate diagnostic or screening test from the list above. Each option can be used once, more than once or not at all.

    6.23   **Hypothyroidism**
    6.24   **Tay–Sachs disease**
    6.25   **Phenylketonuria**
    6.26   **Congenital cardiac disease**
    6.27   **Thalassaemia major**

Cancer genetics

Options

A   Acoustic neuroma
B   Acute lymphoblastic leukaemia
C   Colonic cancer
D   Gastrointestinal MALToma
E   Glioma
F   Kaposi's sarcoma
G   Meningioma
H   Non-Hodgkin's lymphoma
I   Oesophageal cancer
J   Retinoblastoma
K   Small-cell lung cancer
L   Thyroid cancer

For each of the genetic conditions described below, select the tumour that is most commonly associated with that condition from the list above. Each option can be used once, more than once or not at all.

    6.28   **Neurofibromatosis**
    6.29   **Tuberous sclerosis**
    6.30   **Down syndrome**
    6.31   **Familial adenomatous polypsosis**
    6.32   **Multiple endocrine neoplasia**

Antenatal testing

6.33–6.37

Options

A	0%
B	0.01%
C	0.25–0.5%
D	0.5–1%
E	5%
F	10–12 weeks
G	10–13 weeks
H	15–18 weeks
I	15–20 weeks
J	18–20 weeks
K	Diagnostic
L	Screening

The local midwives have constructed an information pack about antenatal testing to include in their booking information packs. Complete the table below from the list of options given. Each option may be used once, more than once or not at all.

Investigation	Screening or diagnostic test?	Gestation	Risk of adverse effects
Nuchal translucency	6.33		
Chorionic villous sampling		6.34	6.35
Amniocentesis			6.36
Triple test	6.37		
Anomaly scan			

SINGLE BEST ANSWER

6.1   A: Cultural influences are a significant barrier to effective healthcare in genetic disease

The report *Familial cancer risk in people from ethnic minorities* found that populations at increased risk of genetic disease face cultural and professional barriers to the delivery of effective treatment. Many patients favoured input from professionals from their own background, and the threshold for assessment should be tailored to both cultural beliefs and risk in that population.

6.2   C: Duchenne muscular dystrophy

Duchenne muscular dystrophy is an X-lined trait that usually manifests from 18 months of age but is typically not diagnosed until the age of 4–5 years. It causes progressive weakness, starting in the legs, and most patients are wheelchair bound by the age of 20. Myotonic dystrophy has an onset from late teens onwards and is characterised by hypogonadism, cataracts, weakening and wasting of sternocleidomastoid in particular. Motor neuron disease affects adults whereas cerebral palsy is non-progressive and usually present from birth.

6.3   B: Multifactorial

Patients with α_1-antitrypsin deficiency are at increased risk of heart and lung problems. The condition is inherited as a co-dominant trait, ie heterozygotes have 50% of normal enzyme activity, whereas homozygotes have only 10% normal activity. The development of emphysema depends on the enzyme activity and environmental insult, so development of pulmonary complications frequently occurs in the third and fourth decades in smokers, later in non-smokers. Homozygotes are also prone to cirrhosis and hepatocellular carcinoma. Treatment is aimed at avoiding smoking and in some centres recombinant α_1-antitrypsin is used.

6.4   A: 98% of male patients are infertile

Cystic fibrosis is the most common inherited condition in the UK and is transmitted as an autosomal recessive trait. The gene is carried by 1 in 25 people in the UK, but is rare in non-white individuals. The incidence is 1 in 2000 live births. Ninety-eight per cent of male patients are infertile and, now that the life expectancy is well into the 30s, fertility counselling plays an increasingly important role in the management of patients.

6.5   E: The risk of having a baby with Down syndrome is significantly greater in parents who have already had a Down syndrome pregnancy

Most cases of Down syndrome are due to non-dysjunction during meiosis, although some parents carry a balanced translocation, which puts them at high risk of recurrence. Karyotyping of parents should be considered after a Down syndrome pregnancy to exclude this risk. Nuchal translucency is a useful screening tool but is not specific for Down syndrome and can be a sign of Edwards' syndrome among others. It is therefore used as a screening test rather than a diagnostic test. In combination with serum screening as part of the 'integrated test', it is more sensitive and specific. Women with a risk of 1 in 200 or worse will usually be offered diagnostic tests such as CVS or amniocentesis. The risk of carrying a Down syndrome baby is 1 in 1400 at 25, 1 in 900 at 30, 1 in 400 at 35, 1 in 100 at 40 and 1 in 30 at 45. More babies are born with Down syndrome to women under 30 than to women over 40 due to the higher number of births in this age group.

6.6   D: The condition is inherited as an autosomal dominant trait and the risk of his sons developing the condition is 1 in 2

Huntington's disease usually manifests between 30 and 50 years of age and usually starts with chorea, with typical hemiballismus. Dementia develops later on, although there is often good insight, which leads to significant depression and suicide. The inheritance is autosomal dominant, giving offspring a 50% chance of developing the disease and their children a 25% chance of inheriting the disease, rising to 50% if their father develops the condition. The gene has been identified, so diagnosis is possible and although there is no cure this can be helpful in family planning.

6.7   D: The incidence is 1:2500 live births

Turner syndrome (45X) is seen in 1:2500 live births. Affected patients are often short, with wide-spaced nipples and a webbed neck. Coarctation of the aorta can occur and internal genitalia are abnormal, although the external genitalia and vagina are usually normal. This can present late as primary amenorrhoea. Oestrogen supplementation from puberty will encourage the development of normal secondary sexual characteristics. Learning disability is more commonly seen with Klinefelter syndrome in men. Many women with Turner syndrome live a normal life, albeit an infertile one.

6.8   A: Family trees are not helpful in counselling families affected by Down syndrome

Three generations of a family tree are needed, together with racial background, to identify genetic predisposition. Down syndrome arises in the parent as a balanced translocation (rare, <1% of cases) or spontaneously during meiosis, so family history is irrelevant. A basic working knowledge of genetics should be sufficient for GPs to advise on inheritance risks of different disorders, particularly with regard to pre-conception counselling. Conditions with variable penetrance or complex inheritance should be dealt with by the genetic counselling service because prediction of risk is complicated. Most people understand risk better as a proportion (eg 1 in 20 children would be affected and 19 in 20 would not be affected), rather than as a percentage (eg 5% are affected).

6.9   **C:**   **Phenylketonuria is an autosomal recessive trait, so both parents must be carriers**

Phenylketonuria is an autosomal recessive disorder which affects 1 in 10 000 live births. The risk of recurrence of the condition is 1 in 4 and risk of future children being carriers is 1 in 2, whereas the risk of having a child free from the gene is 1 in 4. Screening at birth is important because early phenylalanine exclusion will lead to normal mental development. Where unusual patterns of inheritance are seen, the possibility of biological versus stated parenthood should be considered but there are many other causes, such as incomplete penetrance and new mutation, so this area is best broached by an expert rather than risk causing offence.

6.10   **B:**   **The risk of affected offspring is 50%**

This picture shows café-au-lait patches and neurofibromas, so the patient has neurofibromatosis, which is inherited as an autosomal dominant trait. Offspring therefore have a 50% risk of being affected, but if they are not affected they will not be carriers. The condition is associated with brain tumours, including acoustic neuromas.

6.11   **A:**   **The condition is inherited as an autosomal dominant trait**

The condition is expressed in three consecutive generations and is therefore most likely to be a dominant trait. It affects men and women and therefore is unlikely to be an X-linked trait, which tends to affect only males, whereas women are usually carriers or free of the trait. Affected males with X-linked traits cannot pass the condition to sons, whereas all daughters of affected males will be carriers. There are very few conditions associated with the Y chromosome and these would obviously affect only males.

6.12   **D:**   **3, 1, 4, 2**

Ranking – 3: Klinefelter syndrome; 1: Down syndrome; 4: Turner syndrome; 2: fragile X syndrome

The incidence of Klinefelter syndrome is 1:500, Down syndrome 1:1000, Turner syndrome 1:2500, fragile X syndrome 1:4000.

EXTENDED MATCHING ANSWERS

Prevalence of genetic disease

An excellent resource for information on the frequency of genetic disease for patients and healthcare workers is available at www.geneticalliance.org.uk

6.13   **E:**   **5 per 1000 births**

6.14   **A:**   **0.05 per 1000 births**

6.15   **C:**   **0.4 per 1000 births**

6.16	B:	0.1 per 1000 births
6.17	B:	0.1 per 1000 births
6.18	C:	0.4 per 1000 births

Modes of inheritance

6.19   B: Autosomal recessive

Cystic fibrosis is inherited as an autosomal recessive with a 1 in 4 risk of two carriers having an affected child, a 2 in 4 risk of having a carrier child and a 1 in 4 risk of an unaffected child.

6.20   F: X-linked recessive

Duchenne muscular dystrophy is inherited as an X-linked recessive disorder. Women are very rarely affected (1 in 50 000 000) when both parents are carriers. Up to 30% of patients have the condition as a result of a new mutation.

6.21   D: Non-dysjunction

Non-dysjunction in meiosis causes the genotype 47XXY, the additional X chromosome coming from either parent. There is an association with increased maternal age.

6.22   A: Autosomal dominant

Huntington's disease is inherited as an autosomal dominant trait but does not usually present until middle age, by which time most patients have already had children. There is a 50% risk of children being affected.

Diagnostic tests in genetics

6.23   G: Heel-prick test

Shortly after birth a heel-prick blood sample is taken to test for TSH levels and a Guthrie test for phenylketonuria. In some areas, blood is also tested for immunoreactive trypsin, a marker for cystic fibrosis.

6.24   B: Carrier testing

Individuals of Ashkenazi Jewish extraction are tested for serum enzyme levels to detect carriers.

6.25   F: Guthrie test

Early diagnosis of phenylketonuria allows treatment of affected homozygotes, allowing normal neurological development.

6.26   J: Ultrasound

An anomaly scan at 18–20 weeks allows the prenatal diagnosis of congenital heart disease, allowing treatment in the immediate postnatal period or, in some cases, the prenatal period.

6.27   D: Fetoscopy

Fetoscopy allows cordocentesis for haemoglobinopathies at 16–20 weeks, as well as biopsies of skin and liver biopsy where relevant.

Cancer genetics

6.28   A: Acoustic neuroma

Neurofibromatosis is associated with acoustic neuromas, which usually present with sensorineural hearing loss or unilateral tinnitus.

6.29   E: Glioma

Tuberous sclerosis is an autosomal dominant inherited condition characterised by ash-leaf macules appearing on the skin in early childhood, followed by the development of red angiofibromatous papules on the face. The condition is also associated with seizures, interstitial lung disease and gliomas.

6.30   B: Acute lymphoblastic leukaemia

People with Down syndrome have an increased risk of acute lymphocytic leukaemia, whereas lymphoma is common in people with X-linked agammaglobulinaemia and ataxia telangiectasia.

6.31   C: Colonic cancer

Colonic cancer is seen at an early age (20s) in patients with the autosomal dominant condition, familial adenomatous polyposis, and these patients should all have regular colonoscopic screening from a young age.

6.32   L: Thyroid cancer

Multiple endocrine neoplasia is associated with pancreatic and pituitary tumours, peptic ulcer disease, phaeochromocytoma and medullary carcinoma of the thyroid. It has autosomal dominant inheritance and is inherited as a mutation in a tumour-suppressor gene, so patients are born as heterozygotes for that gene. Subsequent mutation of the other allele during the patient's lifetime then results in the development of cancer in that organ.

Antenatal testing

6.33	L:	Screening
6.34	G:	10–13 weeks
6.35	D:	0.5–1%
6.36	C:	0.25–0.5%
6.37	L:	Screening

Investigation	Screening or diagnostic test?	Gestation (weeks)	Risk of adverse effects (%)
Nuchal translucency	Screening	10–12	0
Chorionic villous sampling	Diagnostic	10–13	0.5–1
Amniocentesis	Diagnostic	15–18	0.25–0.5
Triple test	Screening	15–20	0
Anomaly scan	Screening	18–20	0

Chapter 7
Haematology

SINGLE BEST ANSWER QUESTIONS

7.1 Sickle cell anaemia
You are called to the minor injury unit see a 24-year-old woman suffering an acute painful sickle cell episode. She has already tried paracetamol, codeine and ibuprofen for the pain but still rates the pain as 9/10. Which one of the following would be the most appropriate course of action in this situation?

○ A   Administer oxygen at 2 l/min

○ B   Give morphine as an intramuscular bolus

○ C   Give pethidine as an intramuscular bolus

○ D   Give rectal diclofenac 100 mg

○ E   Phone her surgery to check that she does have sickle cell anaemia and is not a drug seeker

7.2 Leg pain
A 76-year-old woman with a history of treated hypertension had a deep vein thrombosis 12 months ago after a flight from Miami. She complains that over the last few months she has a painful itchy leg. Examination reveals unilateral varicose veins with some hyperpigmentation and oedema. What is the single most likely underlying diagnosis?

○ A   Cellulitis

○ B   Peripheral arterial disease

○ C   Post-thrombotic syndrome

○ D   Recurrent deep vein thrombosis

○ E   Varicose eczema

7.3 Well's score

A 53-year-old woman with no previous history of note presents with a swollen left leg. She has no erythema but is slightly tender posteriorly on the upper calf, and has no risk factors for deep vein thrombosis. You calculate her Well's score as 3. Which of the following would be the most appropriate action in this situation?

- ○ A Check her CRP levels
- ○ B Check her D-dimer levels and refer for imaging only if elevated
- ○ C Reassure her that a deep vein thrombosis is unlikely on the basis of her Well's score
- ○ D Refer for imaging
- ○ E Start anticoagulation as the diagnosis of deep vein thrombosis is confirmed by the Well's score

7.4 Thrombophillia

A 32-year-old woman suffered a deep vein thrombosis after breaking her leg skiing. She has been on warfarin for 6 months, but is concerned about the possibility of recurrence and asks you if you will test her for thrombophilia. She has no relevant family history, takes no regular medications and has no previous medical history of note. According to NICE guidance, which one of the following is an appropriate course of action in this situation?

- ○ A Do full thrombophilia screen before stopping warfarin
- ○ B Refer for pelvic ultrasound
- ○ C Refer her to haematology outpatients
- ○ D Stop warfarin and after 4 weeks carry out a full thrombophilia screen
- ○ E Stop warfarin and reassure her that no further testing is indicated at this time

7.5 Spherocytosis

A child has just registered with your practice because his family has moved to the area. He has recently been diagnosed with hereditary spherocytosis. Which one of the following statements about this condition is true?

- ○ A It is an X-linked recessive condition
- ○ B It is associated with aplastic crises
- ○ C It is usually diagnosed incidentally in adulthood on routine blood testing
- ○ D Patients should be treated with vitamin B_{12} supplementation
- ○ E There are usually no clinical signs

7.6 Sickle cell anaemia

You start a new job in a practice with a large African–Caribbean population, many of whom are affected by sickle cell anaemia. Which one of the following statements about this condition is true?

○ A   Infarction of the bone marrow causes severe pain

○ B   Osteomyelitis is rarely seen in patients with sickle cell disease

○ C   Sickle cell crises should usually be treated with paracetamol or non-steroidal drugs rather than with opiates because of the risk of addiction

○ D   The condition is exclusively seen in African–Caribbean populations

○ E   The condition is inherited as an autosomal dominant trait

7.7 Leukaemia

A 19-year-old man comes to see you after being diagnosed by the haematology department with leukaemia. Which one of the following statements about acute leukaemia is true?

○ A   Of adults aged <50 with acute myeloid leukaemia (AML) 70% are treated successfully

○ B   Acute lymphoblastic leukaemia (ALL) is invariably associated with a white cell count (WCC) $>20 \times 10^9$/l

○ C   ALL is usually diagnosed as an incidental finding on a routine full blood count (FBC)

○ D   AML is usually seen in children

○ E   Platelets are unaffected in acute leukaemia

7.8 Back pain

A 62-year-old man presents with a 6-month history of back pain and weight loss. He is a lifelong non-smoker and has no gastrointestinal symptoms. Examination is unremarkable, with no hepatosplenomegaly and no lymphadenopathy, but blood tests show an erythrocyte sedimentation rate (ESR) of 92 mm/h, raised calcium and creatinine levels, and a haemoglobin of 9.8 g/dl with normal white cells and platelets. The film has been reported as showing rouleaux. Which one of the following is the most likely diagnosis?

○ A   Acute myeloid leukaemia (AML)

○ B   Chronic lymphocytic leukaemia (CLL)

○ C   Chronic myeloid leukaemia (CML)

○ D   Multiple myeloma

○ E   Myelodysplasia

7.9 Fatigue

A 78-year-old woman complains of several months of increasing fatigue and, more recently, bleeding gums. She has had no weight loss and no other symptoms. She takes no regular medication. Examination shows her to be pale, with no hepatosplenomegaly or lymphadenopathy. Blood tests show normal renal function and liver function and normal calcium and ESR, but an FBC shows: neutrophil count 0.4×10^9/l, platelets 18×10^9/l and reticulocyte count <1%. Which one of the following statements is true about this situation?

○   A   This woman has aplastic anaemia

○   B   This woman has chronic lymphocytic leukaemia

○   C   This woman has iron deficiency

○   D   This woman has myeloma

○   E   This presentation is typical of myelofibrosis

7.10 Mouth lesions

A 62-year-old man comes to see you 24 hours after being discharged from hospital where he had been admitted for a suspected myocardial infarction. He complains that shortly after discharge he started to get blood blisters in his mouth (shown below).

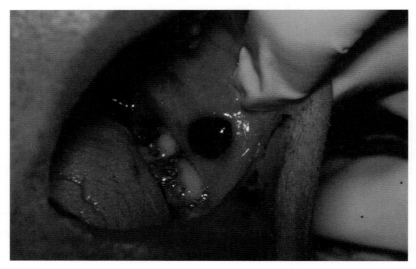

What is the likely diagnosis?

○   A   Aphthous ulceration

○   B   Behçet syndrome

○   C   Immune thrombocytopenia

○   D   Lichen planus

○   E   Trauma

7.11 Well man check

A 53-year-old man with a history of treated hypertension has routine blood tests carried out as part of a 'well man' check. He smokes 10 cigarettes a day and drinks 10–15 units of alcohol a week. His blood results are shown below:

	Result (normal range)
Haemoglobin	20.7 g/dl (12.0–18.0 g/dl)
Platelets	196×10^9/l (150–450×10^9/l)
WCC	2.43×10^9/l (0.9–4.5×10^9/l)
Neutrophils	5.58×10^9/l (1.9–9.0×10^9/l)
Haematocrit	0.58 (0.4–0.5)
Mean corpuscular volume (MCV)	90 fl (80–99 fl)
Mean corpuscular haemoglobin (MCH)	31.7 pg (27–32 pg)

Which one of the following is the most likely diagnosis?

- A Acute myeloid leukaemia
- B Vitamin B_{12} deficiency
- C Chronic lymphocytic leukaemia
- D Essential thrombocythaemia
- E Polycythaemia rubra vera

EXTENDED MATCHING QUESTIONS

Anaemia

Options

A Alcoholism
B Anaemia of chronic disease
C Vitamin B$_{12}$ deficiency
D Folate deficiency
E Glucose-6-phosphate dehydrogenase deficiency
F Hereditary spherocytosis
G Iron-deficiency anaemia
H Sickle cell anaemia
I Thalassaemia major
J Thalassaemia trait

For each of the clinical scenarios below, select the most appropriate diagnosis from the list above. Each option can be used once, more than once or not at all.

7.12 A 47-year-old, perimenopausal woman complains of fatigue and shortness of breath on exertion. On examination, she has glossitis and angular stomatitis, and she complains of brittle nails, which you find are spoon shaped.

7.13 A 36-year-old man with long-standing Crohn's disease complains of fatigue. A routine FBC shows a macrocytosis and a haemoglobin level of 10.5 g/dl. Intrinsic factor antibodies are negative.

7.14 A 25-year-old woman from Iran is given nitrofurantoin for a urinary tract infection. Three weeks later she presents with fatigue and shortness of breath. Urine testing reveals haemoglobinuria and an FBC shows a haemoglobin level of 7.6 g/dl with reticulocytosis.

7.15 A 67-year-old woman with long-standing hypothyroidism and vitiligo has a routine FBC, which shows a macrocytic anaemia. Further blood tests are positive for parietal cell autoantibodies and intrinsic factor antibodies.

7.16 A 32-year-old woman has an FBC done as part of pre-conceptual counselling. She is noted to have a mild microcytic/hypochromic anaemia with normal ferritin levels.

Clotting disorders

Options

A   Antiphospholipid syndrome
B   Autoimmune thrombocytopenia
C   Disseminated intravascular coagulopathy
D   Factor V Leiden
E   Haemophilia
F   Idiopathic thrombocytopenia
G   Thrombocythaemia
H   Vitamin K deficiency
I   Von Willebrand's disease

For each scenario described below, select the most appropriate diagnosis from the list above. Each option can be used once, more than once or not at all.

7.17   A 4-day-old breastfed baby whose mother has noticed bleeding from his umbilical stump.

7.18   A 36-year-old woman with recurrent miscarriages who has been treated by her GP for suspected rheumatoid arthritis for 10 years.

7.19   A 4-year-old girl is brought in by her parents with recurrent bruising. She has previously been fit and well and, apart from multiple bruises on her arms and legs, seems well.

7.20   A 14-year-old boy comes to see you after a traumatic dental extraction that resulted in a significant amount of bleeding. On reflection, his mother reports that he does seem to bruise more than his peers and also comments that his father and paternal uncle have had similar experiences at the dentist.

7.21   A 23-year-old girl experiences pain, swelling and erythema of her right calf after a flight to Hong Kong. Her only medication is the contraceptive pill and she does not smoke. On further questioning, she reports that her mother had a similar experience some years before.

Investigation of microcytic anaemia

7.22–7.26

Options

A	α-Thalassaemia trait
B	β-Thalassaemia trait
C	Ferritin
D	HbA$_2$
E	Low
F	No
G	Normal
H	Oral iron
I	Raised
J	Sickle cell trait
K	Transfusion
L	Yes

The following flow chart has been designed to simplify the investigation of microcytic anaemia (Hb = haemoglobin). From the list of options above, select the most appropriate choice for each numbered step in the flow chart. Each option can be used once, more than once or not at all.

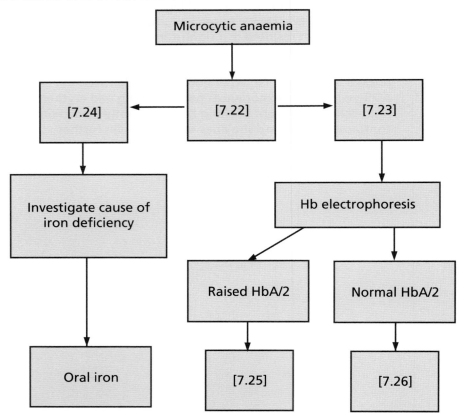

SINGLE BEST ANSWER

7.1   B: Give morphine as an intramuscular bolus

Patients with acute sickling crisis suffer extreme pain and should be treated accordingly. Although some drug addicts have used this condition as a way of obtaining drugs, patients should be given prompt adequate analgesia when presenting. Most patients manage their crises at home but where they present with severe pain not responding to oral medication parenteral opioids should be used. Supplementary oxygen helps, but the primary concern should be controlling pain. Pethidine should not be used due to a tendency to develop addiction.

7.2   C: Post-thrombotic syndrome

Post-thrombotic syndrome affects 25 % of patients suffering a deep vein thrombosis within 12 months and is due to venous obstruction with secondary venous hypertension. Patients are at increased risk of venous ulcers. Compression hosiery has been shown to reduce the risk of this condition by 50% and should be started as soon as possible after diagnosis of a DVT.

7.3   D: Refer for imaging

A Well's score estimates the probability of a deep vein thrombosis using clinical markers, including swelling, tenderness and oedema, as well as risk factors in the history such as previous DVT or cancer. It is not a diagnostic test. A Well's score ≥2 should prompt imaging. Point of care testing of D-dimer together with use of Well's score have been estimated to reduce demand for imaging by up to 90% (*Br J Gen Pract* 2010:**60**;742).

7.4   E: Stop warfarin and reassure her that no further testing is indicated at this time

NICE guidance (*Venous thromboembolic diseases: the management of venous thromboembolic diseases and the role of thrombophilia testing*, 2012) suggests the following:

- Do not offer testing to patients who are continuing anticoagulation treatment
- Consider testing patients who have had unprovoked DVT or PE (pulmonary embolus) if it is planned to stop anticoagulation treatment
- Consider testing patients who have had unprovoked DVT or PE with a first-degree relative who has had DVT or PE if it is planned to stop anticoagulation treatment
- Do not offer testing to patients who have had provoked DVT or PE
- Do not routinely offer thrombophilia testing to first-degree relatives of people with a history of DVT or PE and thrombophilia.

In this patient her DVT was provoked, so no further investigation is necessary unless she has a further DVT or PE. If there is a suspicion of malignancy (eg smoker) consider screening for occult malignancy.

7.5 B: It is associated with aplastic crises

Hereditary spherocytosis is an autosomal recessive condition that affects 1 in 5000 live births. It usually presents in childhood as jaundice or with aplastic crises, often triggered by parvovirus infections. Most children receive folic acid supplementation. Splenomegaly is common. It is rarely diagnosed in adulthood.

7.6 A: Infarction of the bone marrow causes severe pain

Sickle cell anaemia affects 1 in 4 West African and 1 in 10 African–Caribbean individuals. It is inherited as an autosomal recessive trait and is also carried in Mediterranean and Middle Eastern populations. Homozygotes suffer from infarction of bone marrow and haemolysis during times of low oxygen levels (eg with infections), causing a haemolytic anaemia and extreme bone pain, often requiring opiates. Infection of infarcted bone marrow is common.

7.7 A: Of adults aged <50 with acute myeloid leukaemia (AML) 70% are treated successfully

In ALL, 50% of patients have a normal WCC but typically have blasts present on the film and a normocytic anaemia. AML is rarely seen in children, whereas ALL is usually seen in children and young adults. The prognosis in AML is better for the under-50s, those with a WCC $<50 \times 10^9$/l and those without extramedullary disease at presentation. ALL usually presents with signs of marrow failure or bone pain. Platelets are usually reduced and a diagnosis of leukaemia should always be considered in children with apparent thrombocytopenia.

7.8 D: Multiple myeloma

Myeloma often presents with bone pain and examination findings are usually rare. At presentation, many patients will have biochemical evidence of nephropathy and bone destruction, and hyperviscosity is often seen, with a raised ESR and rouleaux formation. Bence Jones protein is characteristically raised. AML and ALL tend to present with signs of bone marrow failure and extramedullary infiltration (eg meningeal signs in AML). CLL presents as a routine finding on an FBC in most cases, whereas CML is usually associated with signs of bleeding and hepatosplenomegaly. Myelodysplasia generally presents with fatigue.

7.9 A: This woman has aplastic anaemia

Myelofibrosis typically presents over a longer period of time and is associated with hepatosplenomegaly due to extramedullary haematopoiesis. Aplastic anaemia is idiopathic in at least 70% of cases and has a poor prognosis, with <50% of patients surviving 6 months.

7.10 C: Immune thrombocytopenia

Immune thrombocytopenia is typically caused by heparin, sulphonamides, chloramphenicol, sulfasalazine, quinine and quinidine. It typically comes on 2–3 days after taking a drug that has been taken in the past, or 7 days after taking a new drug. It is reported to occur in up to 25% of patients on heparin. The platelet count typically rises 7–10 days after stopping the medication.

7.11   E: Polycythaemia rubra vera

The raised haematocrit and haemoglobin, with normal MCH and MCV suggest that the diagnosis is polycythaemia. These results, with a normal plasma volume and raised red cell mass, suggest true polycythaemia, rather than dehydration. Secondary causes include hypoxia, smoking and chronic lung disease. Patients should have a bone marrow biopsy to exclude myeloproliferative disease. Treatment is usually regular venesection to keep the haematocrit <0.45.

EXTENDED MATCHING ANSWERS

Anaemia

7.12   G: Iron-deficiency anaemia

Iron deficiency can be caused by blood loss through heavy menstrual bleeding or parasitic infection, or by poor iron intake. An FBC will usually show a microcytosis.

7.13   D: Folate deficiency

Folate deficiency can be due to poor intake or to malabsorption (eg coeliac disease, Crohn's disease). Bloods show a macrocytic anaemia and low folate levels. Treatment is with folate supplementation.

7.14   E: Glucose-6-phosphate dehydrogenase (G6PDH) deficiency

G6PDH deficiency affects up to 25% of people from southern Africa and the Middle East. Haemolysis can follow infection, fava bean ingestion and drugs (eg dapsone, quinine, antibiotics). Hospital admission is required to avoid renal damage and correct the haemolysis.

7.15   C: Vitamin B_{12}

Vitamin B_{12} is found in animal foods, including milk and eggs, but not in vegetables, so vegans are at risk of deficiency. Other causes of vitamin B_{12} deficiency include malabsorption (eg after gastrectomy) and autoantibodies. There is a strong association with vitiligo and Hashimoto's thyroiditis. Treatment is with 3-monthly vitamin B_{12} injections.

7.16   J: Thalassaemia trait

Thalassaemia trait is usually symptomless and is really of significance only if both partners in a relationship are affected.

Clotting disorders

7.17   H: Vitamin K deficiency

Vitamin K deficiency in babies is seen in exclusively breastfed babies who have not received vitamin K and manifests as bleeding, usually between days 2 and 4 of life. The cause is a combination of low natural levels at birth coupled with lack of bacterial vitamin K synthesis in the gut and immature liver function. Breast milk is low in vitamin K, whereas formula milk has vitamin K added.

7.18   A: Antiphospholipid syndrome

Antiphospholipid syndrome can be primary or secondary to connective tissue disease, most commonly SLE. It causes recurrent fetal loss, thrombocytopenia and recurrent ischaemic events. It is characterised by the presence of high titres of IgG antiphospholipid antibodies and is thought to be due to a coagulopathy rather than to a vasculitis.

7.19   F: Idiopathic thrombocytopenia

Idiopathic thrombocytopenia is the most likely diagnosis in children, although child abuse and leukaemia should be excluded. In adults taking medication, autoimmune thrombocytopenia is more likely.

7.20   I: Von Willebrand's disease

Von Willebrand's disease is inherited as an autosomal dominant trait and is characterised by excessive bleeding after dental extractions and prolonged bleeding time. The bleeding is usually much less severe than in haemophilia and can usually be controlled with tranexamic acid.

7.21   D: Factor V Leiden

Factor V Leiden is a variant of factor V that predisposes to venous thromboembolism. Patients with a suspicious family history should be tested before prescribing the combined oral contraceptive pill.

Investigation of microcytic anaemia

7.22   C: Ferritin
7.23   G: Normal
7.24   E: Low
7.25   B: β-Thalassaemia trait
7.26   A: α-Thalassaemia trait

HbA_2 is raised in β-Thalassaemia trait, but is normal in α-Thalassaemia trait.

Chapter 8
Immunology

SINGLE BEST ANSWER QUESTIONS

8.1 Vaccination in pregnancy
A woman in week 23 of her second pregnancy asks you if you would recommend her to have a flu vaccine this winter. Which of the following statements is true with regard to this situation?

○ A   All influenza vaccines available in the UK are live vaccines

○ B   All vaccines are contraindicated in pregnancy

○ C   Immunity lasts up to 5 years so patients vaccinated before becoming pregnant do not need a booster during pregnancy

○ D   Pregnant women are considered an 'at risk' category for influenza vaccination in the UK

○ E   Vaccination of pregnant women with H1N1 vaccine is associated with a higher risk of miscarriage than H1N1 infection

8.2 Rabies vaccination
A 19-year-old man is due to leave for a gap year travelling around Asia and asks your advice about rabies vaccination. Which one of the following statements is correct with regard to this vaccine?

○ A   Three doses of rabies vaccine provide lifelong protection against rabies

○ B   Patients attacked by animals in rabies endemic countries need treatment only if skin is broken

○ C   Patients receiving animal bites in the UK may be reassured that they do not need rabies vaccination

○ D   Patients receiving animal bites in endemic countries do not need further treatment if they have received a full vaccination course before exposure

○ E   Patients receiving animal bites in endemic countries should seek urgent medical attention for wound treatment, regardless of the extent of the injury

8.3 Immunotherapy
Which one of the following statements about the use of immunotherapy in allergic conditions is true?

○ A   Grazax is effective in patients with allergic rhinitis due to house-dust mite only where RAST tests are positive

○ B   Sublingual immunotherapy can be used on an as-needed basis

○ C   Sublingual immunotherapy is effective in patients with allergic rhinitis only

○ D   Sublingual immunotherapy results in angioedema in 15% of patients

○ E   Use of sublingual grass allergen tablets results in a significant reduction in medication use

8.4 Pneumococcal vaccination
You are updating the protocols for pneumococcal vaccination in the practice. Which one of the following patient groups needs a booster vaccination after routine primary immunisation?

○ A   Patients with asthma

○ B   Patients with chronic kidney disease

○ C   Patients with chronic obstructive pulmonary disease

○ D   Patients with diabetes

○ E   Patients with stable ischaemic heart disease

8.5 Allergic rhinitis
With regard to the drug management of allergic rhinitis, which one of the following statements is true?

○ A   Anticholinergics are effective for rhinorrhoea

○ B   Antileukotrienes are effective for ocular but not nasal symptoms

○ C   Nasal steroids are effective for nasal symptoms, but not for ocular symptoms

○ D   Oral antihistamines are the most effective treatment for nasal symptoms

○ E   Treatment of asthma has no effect on allergic rhinitis

8.6 Interpretation of skin changes
Consider the picture below:

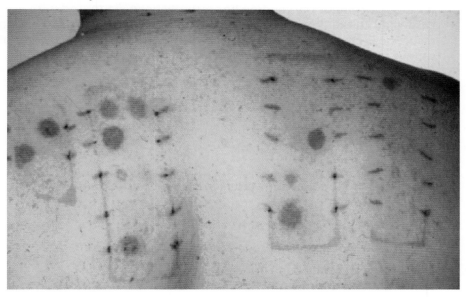

Which one of the following statements about this situation is true?

○ A   This patient has experienced a fixed drug reaction

○ B   This patient has had patch testing performed

○ C   This patient has had skin-prick testing

○ D   This patient is suffering from bullous pemphigoid

○ E   This patient is suffering from erythema multiforme

8.7 Chickenpox

A 24-year-old woman is 12 weeks pregnant. She works as a preschool teacher and one of the children has recently been diagnosed with suspected chickenpox. She feels as if she has a temperature but has no rash. She is not sure if she has had chickenpox in the past, and her mother cannot recall this either. Blood tests are carried out which show the following results:

Varicella IgG	Elevated
Varicella IgM	Normal
Measles IgG	Normal
Measles IgM	Normal

Which one of the following statements about this patient's varicella status is correct?

○ A   She has been infected with varicella in the past and is now immune

○ B   She has not been exposed in the past to chickenpox

○ C   She has recently been infected with chickenpox

○ D   She is measles immune

○ E   The results are most likely to be due to childhood vaccination

EXTENDED MATCHING QUESTIONS

Allergy testing

Options

A   Exclusion diet
B   IgE levels
C   None of these options
D   Patch testing
E   RAST
F   Skin-prick testing
G   Symptom diary

For each of the situations described below, select the most appropriate investigation from the list above. Each option may be used once, more than once or not at all.

8.8   A 35-year-old marketing executive complains of abdominal bloating and cramps after eating certain foodstuffs.

8.9   A 48-year-old woman who complains of 5 years of fatigue and myalgia, which she feels are due to mercury in her dental fillings.

8.10   A 13-year-old boy complains of rhinitis and wheeze for most days of the year, which are worse when he visits his father's house and better when he goes on holiday.

8.11   A 36-year-old paramedic complains of recurrent dermatitis affecting his hands when he is at work, which rapidly improves on holiday.

8.12   A 28-year-old man requests testing for wasp sting allergy.

Vaccines

Options

A   Inactivated
B   Immunoglobulins
C   Live attenuated
D   Recombinant antigen
E   Toxoid

For each of the vaccine types given below, select the most appropriate option to describe its mode of action from the list above. Each option may be used once, more than once or not at all.

8.13   **Pertussis**
8.14   **Measles, mumps and rubella (MMR)**
8.15   **Tetanus**
8.16   **Hepatitis B**
8.17   **Salk polio vaccine**

Allergy management in primary care

8.18–8.22

Options

A Admit
B β_2 Agonist
C β Blockade
D Depo-Medrone
E Intramuscular adrenaline
F Intravenous adrenaline
G Oral antihistamine
H Oral prednisolone

For each of the numbered gaps in the following allergy management flow chart, select the most appropriate option from the list above. Each option can be used once, more than once or not at all.

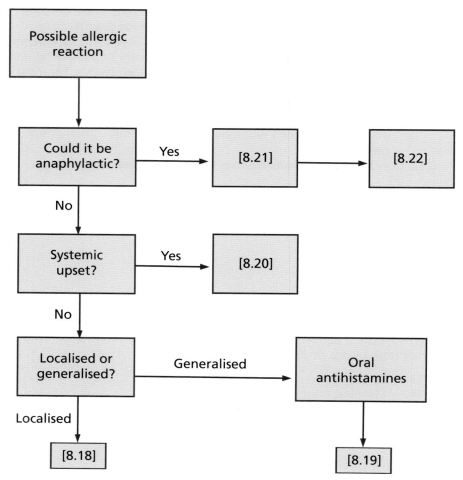

SINGLE BEST ANSWER

8.1   D: Pregnant women are considered an 'at risk' category for influenza vaccination in the UK

Patients developing influenza while pregnant are at increased risk of morbidity and mortality and therefore, since 2010, have been included in the clinical risk categories. Vaccination is safer than infection, and all but one of the vaccines available in the UK are inactivated. There is a theoretical risk from using live vaccines in pregnancy so they are usually avoided, unless risk outweighs benefits.

8.2   E: Patients receiving animal bites in endemic countries should seek urgent medical attention for wound treatment, regardless of the extent of the injury

Management of animal bites in rabies endemic countries involves urgent wound debridement and management to avoid increasing the risk of infection, together with assessment of risk. All cases should be discussed with a rabies specialist. Where mucous membranes have potentially been contaminated with saliva, even where there is no obvious wound, urgent irrigation is required to prevent infection through this route.

8.3   E: Use of sublingual grass allergen tablets results in a significant reduction in medication use

Grazax, a purified grass allergen extract in tablet form, is taken up to 16 weeks before the start of the allergy season in patients with proven IgE-mediated grass pollen sensitivity (through either RAST or skin-prick testing). It is well tolerated and results in a 30% reduction in symptoms and a 38% reduction in medication use. Serious side effects have not been reported in trials (*J Allergy Clin Immunol* 2006;**118**:434–40). Meta-analysis has shown that immunotherapy also reduces symptoms and medication use in children with asthma (*Chest* 2007;**133**:599–609).

8.4   B: Patients with chronic kidney disease

Patients with chronic kidney disease, hyposplenism or asplenia should have booster doses of pneumococcal vaccine and haemophilus vaccine every 5 years. Children vaccinated routinely should also have a booster dose at 13 months.

8.5   A: Anticholinergics are effective for rhinorrhoea

The ARIA (Allergic Rhinitis and its Impact on Asthma) guidelines for the treatment of allergic rhinitis suggest that oral antihistamines are effective for sneezing, rhinorrhoea and eye symptoms, but not for nasal obstruction. Intraocular antihistamines are effective only for eye symptoms. Corticosteroids are the most effective treatment for all symptoms, although they are not as effective for eye symptoms as intraocular antihistamines. Decongestants are effective only for nasal obstruction, whereas anticholinergics are effective only for rhinorrhoea. Antileukotriene antagonists are moderately effective for all symptoms except nasal itch. Treatment of asthma will often improve symptoms of allergic rhinitis and vice versa.

8.6   B: This patient has had patch testing performed

This patient has had patch testing, which is suitable for occupational allergies (eg contact dermatitis). Aeroallergens are better tested with skin-prick testing.

8.7   A: She has been infected with varicella in the past and is now immune

IgM is the first antibody to be produced in infection; IgG is produced later. Recent infection therefore results in raised virus-specific IgM, whereas historical infection results in raised IgG with normal IgM.

EXTENDED MATCHING ANSWERS

Allergy testing

8.8   A: Exclusion diet

Food intolerance is distinct from food allergy and can have a metabolic basis (eg lactase deficiency). Symptoms are distinct from food allergy, an IgE-mediated reaction characterised by nausea, vomiting, diarrhoea, urticaria and angioedema. Food intolerance can be diagnosed by exclusion diet but ideally this should be under the supervision of a dietician if there are multiple potential causes, to avoid malnutrition.

8.9   C: None of these options

These symptoms are not suggestive of allergy or intolerance. She should be questioned about other somatic symptoms and a diagnosis of depression considered. She would be best advised to seek dental advice regarding her fillings.

8.10   E: RAST

RAST will help to identify allergic reactions, which would allow some lifestyle modification, eg if cats or dogs are involved. If allergy to house-dust mite is detected this is often difficult to manage because of the prevalence of this allergen and the limited evidence for efficacy of house-dust mite elimination.

8.11   D: Patch testing

Patch testing will identify most T-cell-mediated delayed hypersensitivity contact allergens. Around 20–30 suspect allergens are tested as a batch and the responses used to identify which the culprits are. Appropriate precautions, eg hypoallergenic gloves or soaps, can then be taken.

8.12   F: Skin-prick testing

Skin-prick testing is suitable for insect stings. Where this is not available RAST may be used but may give a false negative if there has not been recent exposure.

Vaccines

8.13   A: Inactivated

The pertussis vaccine, either on its own or as part of a combination vaccine, contains inactivated *Bordetella pertussis*.

8.14   C: Live attenuated

MMR is a live attenuated vaccine.

8.15   E: Toxoid

Tetanus vaccine is a toxoid and is either given alone or in combination.

8.16   D: Recombinant antigen

Hepatitis B vaccine is a recombinant vaccine containing hepatitis B surface antigen (HBsAg) cultured from yeast cells.

8.17   A: Inactivated

Inactivated polio vaccines are now the norm, and oral live vaccine is no longer used routinely in the UK. The current vaccine in use contains three strains of poliovirus.

Allergy management in primary care

8.18   G: Oral antihistamine

8.19   H: Oral prednisolone

8.20   H: Oral prednisolone

8.21   E: Intramuscular adrenaline

8.22   A: Admit

Chapter 9
Infection

SINGLE BEST ANSWER QUESTIONS

9.1 Sore throat
A 13-year-old asylum seeker recently arrived from Georgia is brought to see you by her mother. She has had a sore throat for the last 48 hours but is now drowsy and restless, and cannot walk unaided. She has no previous history of note. On examination she is febrile and tachycardic, and has a thick white exudate over her tonsils. Which of the following is the single most likely diagnosis?

- A   Diphtheria
- B   Glandular fever
- C   Poliomyelitis
- D   Scarlet fever
- E   Vincent's angina

9.2 HIV
Which one of the following statements is correct with regard to HIV in the UK?

- A   Of people living in the UK with HIV 25% are undiagnosed
- B   Of cases of HIV diagnosed in the UK 75% were acquired abroad
- C   Foreign visitors to the UK are not entitled to NHS treatment for HIV-AIDS
- D   The incidence of new diagnoses in the UK is at a record high
- E   The risk of transmission from mother to child during pregnancy and childbirth is 10%

9.3 Jaundice

A 47-year-old man who works in a water treatment plant complains of flu-like symptoms of headache, myalgia and fever. He has been taking over-the-counter medication for this but after 6 days he becomes concerned because his skin looks yellow. On examination he has widespread lymphadenopathy and an enlarged liver, and is jaundiced. Reviewing his medical notes you see that he has been vaccinated against hepatitis A and hepatitis B and has no other risk factors. What is the single most likely diagnosis?

- ○　A　*Campylobacter* sp.
- ○　C　*Escherichia coli* O157
- ○　B　Epstein–Barr virus
- ○　D　Leptospirosis
- ○　E　Shigellosis

9.4 HPV vaccination

Your next patient is a 12-year-old girl who has come with her mother. The girl is due to have her human papillomavirus (HPV) vaccination at school soon. Her mother is very uneasy about this and asks your advice on whether it is worth having. Which one of the following statements is true with regard to this issue?

- ○　A　A single dose is given at age 13
- ○　B　The HPV vaccine will prevent her getting genital warts and cervical cancer
- ○　C　The vaccine is associated with potentially serious adverse reactions
- ○　D　Vaccination does not need to start until a girl becomes sexually active
- ○　E　Where three doses of vaccine are given it is >97% effective

9.5 Antimalarials in pregnancy
According to current guidelines, what are the recommendations for antimalarial chemoprophylaxis for pregnant women travelling to malarial areas? Select one option only.

○ A Doxycycline is safe in all trimesters of pregnancy

○ B Mefloquine is thought to be safe in treatment doses in the second and third trimesters

○ C Pregnant women are less at risk of developing malaria, so chemoprophylaxis should be avoided

○ D Pregnant women taking chloroquine should receive supplementation with 5 mg folic acid daily

○ E Women who have taken mefloquine before or during the first trimester should consider a termination

9.6 Dysuria
A 19-year-old woman presents with a burning sensation when passing urine and a yellow, blood-stained vaginal discharge. She admits to having had unprotected sexual intercourse 4 days ago. What is the single most likely diagnosis?

○ A Bacterial vaginosis

○ B Chlamydia infection

○ C Gonorrhoea

○ D Syphilis

○ E Trichomoniasis

9.7 Unwell child
A 4-year-old girl is brought in by her mother with a 3-day history of cough, runny nose and watery eyes. Today, mum has noticed red spots with white centres inside the girl's cheeks. Which one of the following is the single most likely diagnosis?

○ A Measles

○ B Rhinovirus

○ C Rubella

○ D Scarlet fever

○ E Varicella

9.8 Insects

A concerned mother comes to see you having found an insect in her daughter's sleeping bag after a school trip to the New Forest. She is concerned that her daughter may be at risk of disease and would like to know what action should be taken. Her daughter is asymptomatic and there are no abnormal findings on examination. The insect is shown below.

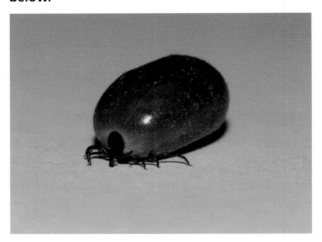

Which one of the following would be appropriate management in this situation?

- A   Prescribe amoxicillin
- B   Prescribe flucloxacillin
- C   Prescribe topical mupirocin to use on any insect bites
- D   Reassure the mother that in the absence of a rash or systemic symptoms no treatment is necessary
- E   Take blood for Lyme serology from the patient

9.9 Skin lesion

This 38-year-old soldier returned from a period in Iraq 2 weeks ago. He has developed a lesion on his skin that started as an erythematous papule:

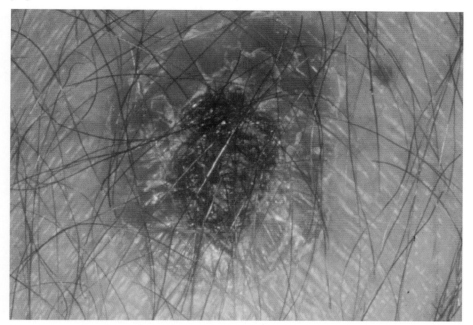

What is the single most likely diagnosis from the list below?

○ A Cutaneous leishmaniasis

○ B Cutaneous tuberculosis

○ C Leprosy

○ D Syphilis

○ E Systemic lupus erythematosus

9.10 Insect bite

A 39-year-old man complains of a sore insect bite. He thinks he was bitten 2–3 days ago while camping, and the bite is now very itchy. The bite is shown below.

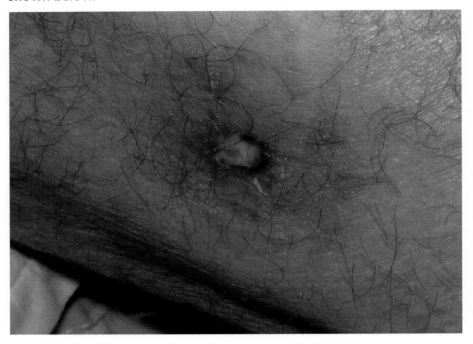

What is the most appropriate treatment?

- ○ A   Oral ampicillin
- ○ B   Oral doxycycline
- ○ C   Oral flucloxacillin
- ○ D   Oral loratadine
- ○ E   Topical Betnovate

9.11 Unwell child

A 9-month-old girl presents with a fever and vomiting. A urine sample was sent to the laboratory and you receive the following result:

White cells	>100 cells/µl
Red blood cells	>100 cells/µl
Organisms	3+
Epithelial cells	1+
Culture	*Escherichia coli* >10^8

Which of the following would be the single most appropriate initial management for this child?

○ A   Refer immediately for an urgent ultrasound scan of the kidneys

○ B   Repeat the urine sample to ensure that it is not a contaminated specimen

○ C   Start antibiotics, continue with a prophylactic dose and review in 2 months

○ D   Start antibiotics immediately and refer for urgent paediatric assessment

○ E   Start antibiotics immediately and repeat the urine sample in 7–10 days to confirm that the infection has cleared

EXTENDED MATCHING QUESTIONS

Antibiotics

Options

A   Admit for intravenous antibiotics
B   Amoxicillin
C   Co-amoxiclav
D   Flucloxacillin
E   Fusidic acid cream
F   Metronidazole
G   No treatment necessary
H   Trimethoprim for 3 days
I   Trimethoprim for 7 days
J   None of the above

For each of the following scenarios select the most appropriate antibiotic from the list of options. Each option can be used once, more than once or not at all.

9.12   **A 4-year-old boy has had a yellow, crusted lesion on his chin for a few days and has now developed a similar one on his right arm.**

9.13   **A woman with dysuria and frequency is currently 32 weeks pregnant.**

9.14   **A 64-year-old man comes to consult after a cat scratch to his face. On examination, he is afebrile with cellulitis around the scratch.**

9.15   **High vaginal swab results for a 38-year-old woman show bacterial vaginosis.**

Management of respiratory tract infections

9.16–9.19

Options

A 5 years
B 65 years
C 80 years
D Facial pain
E Postnasal drip
F Symptoms persisting for more than 5 days
G Significant co-morbidity
H Systemically unwell

Complete the algorithm below identifying patients in need of antibiotics in respiratory tract infection using the options above. Each option may be used once, more than once or not at all.

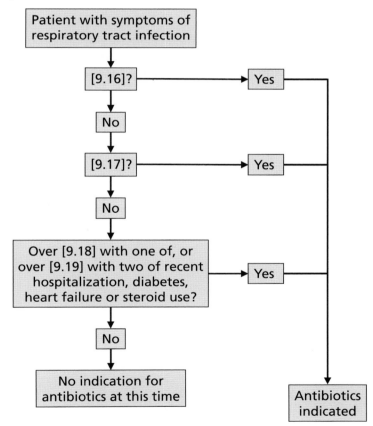

FREE TEXT QUESTIONS

9.20 Insect bites

You see a 25-year-old with no previous medical history of note who has been backpacking around southern Europe for the last 3 months, during which time he suffered extensively with tick bites while hiking in the forest. He complains of general malaise and reports that he has a rash on his back. On examination you note a circular rash with central clearing. He has no other symptoms or signs. What would be the most appropriate management in this case? Write your answer in the box below.

9.21 Dog bite

A 56-year-old woman with no previous medical history of note is bitten by her dog while breaking up a fight with another dog. She has a small puncture wound on her hand that is bleeding. She takes no regular medications and has no allergies. What would be the single most appropriate antibiotic, if any, to use in this situation? Write your answer in the box below.

SINGLE BEST ANSWER

9.1 A: Diphtheria

Diphtheria is uncommon in the UK but is prevalent in the former Soviet republics and South Africa. It is caused by a diphtheria toxin produced by the bacteria infecting the throat. It may be carried asymptomatically, cause a mild pharyngitis without the pharyngeal pseudomembrane, or cause systemic illness with myocarditis and cardiac failure. Treatment is with anti-toxin and macrolide or β-lactam antibiotics to clear the organism and prevent infection of others. Vaccination is effective to prevent the disease, but many of the UK population are not fully immunised.

9.2 A: Of people living in the UK with HIV 25% are undiagnosed

Health Protection Agency data show that, in 2011, 6280 new diagnoses were made of HIV in the UK. They estimated at that time that 25% of the 96 000 people living in the UK at the end of 2011 are undiagnosed. The number of cases diagnosed per annum is down 21% from its peak in 2005, largely due to reduced migration of people with HIV into the UK. New diagnoses in gay men are increasing, whereas around 50% of new diagnoses were acquired in the UK. Perinatal transmission occurs in 2% of HIV-positive mothers.

9.3 D: Leptospirosis

Leptospirosis can be spread by a number of different rodents but is usually associated with rats. People who work in environments with large numbers of rats are most at risk (eg sewage workers). Infection causes an initial flu-like illness, after which a proportion of patients go on to develop jaundice, renal failure and meningism. Most patients make an uneventful recovery. Diagnosis is by complement fixation of urine culture for *Leptospira* sp. Penicillin or tetracycline is usually effective treatment.

9.4 E: Where three doses of vaccine are given it is >97% effective

The HPV vaccination programme aims to prevent infection with the strains of HPV (16 and 18), which are associated with genital warts and cervical cancer in the UK. These vaccines are given in three doses from age 13 and provide 97–99% coverage. There have been no reports of serious adverse reactions. The vaccine covers some wart viruses but not all, so patients can still develop genital warts. There are currently two vaccines available in the UK, Gardasil and Cervarix. Gardasil also provides coverage against HPV6 and HPV11, so it is likely to provide additional cover against warts. Vaccination should start before sexual activity begins to ensure adequate protection before first exposure.

9.5   B: Mefloquine is thought to be safe in treatment doses in the second and third trimesters

There is no strong association between mefloquine in treatment doses and stillbirths or miscarriages in the second and third trimesters, although lack of data on its use in the first trimester has encouraged caution. Pregnant women have an increased risk of developing severe malaria and have a higher risk of fatality. Doxycycline is contraindicated in pregnancy and those taking proguanil should also take folic acid. Women who have taken mefloquine before or during the first trimester should be advised that this is not an indication to terminate the pregnancy.

9.6   C: Gonorrhoea

The early signs of gonorrhoea can be mild and are often missed, but symptoms in women can include a painful and burning sensation when passing urine and a yellow, blood-stained, vaginal discharge. Symptoms usually appear 2–10 days after becoming infected. Chlamydia infection usually presents 1–3 weeks after becoming infected. Symptoms include bleeding between periods, an unusual vaginal discharge and lower abdominal pain. Around 70% of women have no symptoms at all. The symptoms of syphilis are generally non-specific and it usually presents with a painless but infectious sore anywhere on the body, which resolves spontaneously in 2–6 weeks. Bacterial vaginosis presents with a typical grey–yellow, fishy, offensive discharge and it is not a sexually transmitted infection. Trichomoniasis presents with a typical yellow–green, frothy discharge and is less common than other sexually transmitted infections.

9.7   A: Measles

Tiny, bluish-white spots with surrounding erythema seen on the buccal mucosa of the cheek, known as 'Koplik's spots', are pathognomonic of early stage measles. The first symptoms of measles include cough, coryza, conjunctivitis, fever and malaise. A florid erythematous maculopapular rash, which starts at the head, appears 3–4 days later. Koplik's spots can appear 1–2 days before the rash.

9.8   D: Reassure the mother that in the absence of a rash or systemic symptoms no treatment is necessary

Ticks are frequently found in areas of long grass and woodland and prophylactic treatment in the absence of symptoms is not usually justified. Patients should be reassured and advised to report a rash of systemic symptoms. If these occur antibiotics should be used. Doxycycline, amoxicillin or cefuroxime is commonly used but advice from local microbiology services should be obtained before treatment.

9.9   A: Cutaneous leishmaniasis

Leishmaniasis is a parasitic disease spread by infected female sandflies and is mainly seen in the tropics and subtropics. It can be visceral, cutaneous or mucocutaneous. Visceral leishmaniasis is serious and can be fatal. Cutaneous leishmaniasis presents with one or more skin lesions that start as red papules and develop into ulcers. These can change in shape and appearance over time. There can be associated lymphadenopathy. With no treatment these ulcers will heal themselves, usually within 10 months, but can leave depigmented scars or go on to cause mucocutaneous leishmaniasis, which is very disfiguring. It is therefore advisable to treat after seeking advice from the local centre for disease control.

9.10   C: Oral flucloxacillin

This lesion is a secondarily infected insect bite. When these bites are very itchy, patients often scratch and introduce staphylococcal infection. Patients who have been in areas where deer are found can contract Lyme disease from tick bites, but these usually present with annular erythema rather than pus at the bite site. Non-infected bites can be treated with antihistamines or in severe cases with topical steroids. Lyme disease is treated with doxycycline in adults or a macrolide antibiotic in children.

9.11   D: Start antibiotics immediately and refer for urgent paediatric assessment

This result indicates a genuine bacterial infection. The risk of ascending infection and renal damage are high from birth to 6 years of age. Infection at this age suggests a structural renal abnormality.

EXTENDED MATCHING ANSWERS

Antibiotics

9.12   D: Flucloxacillin

This is impetigo that has spread. As a result of increasing resistance, current advice is for topical treatment to be reserved for very localised lesions.

9.13   I: Trimethoprim for 7 days

Current guidelines for urinary tract infections in pregnancy suggest that trimethoprim is unlikely to cause problems in the fetus in the third trimester, so first-line antibiotics for urinary tract infections in pregnancy are trimethoprim and nitrofurantoin; second-line antibiotics are cefalexin and amoxicillin. All these antibiotics should be given for 7 days in pregnancy.

9.14   C: Co-amoxiclav

Co-amoxiclav is used for facial cellulitis, and is the drug of choice for animal scratches and bites. Flucloxacillin or erythromycin (if penicillin allergic) can be used for cellulitis elsewhere, unless the infection is due to an animal scratch or bite. A febrile or ill patient should be admitted for intravenous antibiotics.

9.15   F: Metronidazole

Bacterial vaginosis can be treated with oral or vaginal metronidazole or vaginal clindamycin cream.

Management of respiratory tract infections

9.16   H: Systemically unwell
9.17   G: Significant co-morbidity
9.18   C: 80 years
9.19   B: 65 years

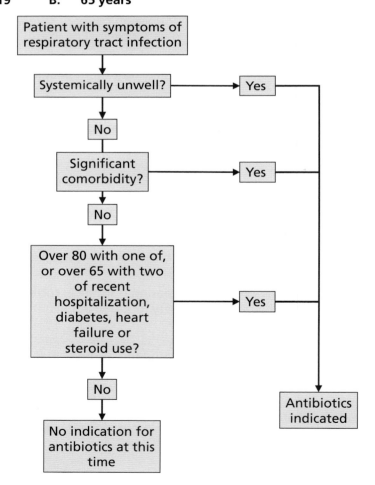

FREE TEXT ANSWERS

9.20   **Doxycyline 100 mg twice daily for 14 days**

This patient has signs and symptoms consistent with Lyme disease. In the absence of neurological or cardiological symptoms serological testing is not necessary, and most patients respond to doxycyline

9.21   **Co-amoxiclav**

All animal bites should be treated with prophylactic antibiotics. Where patients are penicillin allergic, metronidazole or doxycyline is a suitable alternative.

Chapter 10
Mental health and learning disability

SINGLE BEST ANSWER QUESTIONS

10.1 Suicide

One of your patients attempts suicide after suffering an acute postnatal psychotic illness. None of the professionals involved was aware of any problems and before discussion at your significant event meeting you wish to do some research into the subject. Which one of the following statements is correct with regard to this situation?

○   A   Education to A level or degree level is protective against severe postnatal depression

○   B   Most women suffering severe postnatal depression have a history of mental illness

○   C   Severe postnatal depression is more common in women under the age of 25 years

○   D   Severe postnatal depression is more common in woman without a current partner

○   E   Women suffering severe postnatal depression who attempt suicide tend to choose violent methods, eg hanging or jumping from a bridge

10.2 Psychosis

You see a 21-year-old patient who has recently been discharged from a mental health unit after a psychotic incident. His mother thinks that it has been caused by smoking cannabis. Which one of the following statements with regard to this association is correct?

- A Cannabis use moderates pre-existing psychotic symptoms
- B Patients with recent psychosis are twice as likely to have used cannabis as patients without psychosis
- C Skunk is associated with psychosis, but cannabis is not
- D There is no evidence of long-term harm from cannabis use
- E There is unequivocal proof that smoking cannabis causes psychosis

10.3 Schizophrenia

Which one of the following statements about the risk factors for schizophrenia is correct?

- A Development of schizophrenia is not associated with physical health
- B Genetic factors account for 90% of the risk of developing schizophrenia
- C Patients with premorbid schizoid personality traits are more likely to develop schizophrenia
- D Studies have failed to show any genetic factors in schizophrenia
- E There are no known biochemical triggers for the development of schizophrenia

10.4 Mental Capacity Act 2005

You work in an area with a number of care homes and are approached to give a talk on the Mental Capacity Act 2005, which has recently come into force. Which one of the following statements is true with regard to this legislation and its impact on everyday practice?

- A It allows for the establishment of a lasting power of attorney (LPA), which allows both financial and treatment decisions to be made on behalf of patients
- B It can be used to make treatment decisions on behalf of severely brain-damaged children
- C Next of kin are automatically nominated to make decisions in the event of incapacity
- D The Act specifies that advance directives are legally binding, whether verbal or written, as long as they are witnessed
- E Where a decision about place of residence needs to be made and there is no close relative to make it, the decision can be made by the treating doctor

10.5 Mental illness
Which one of the following statements about physical health in mental illness is correct?

○ A Physical health improves during manic periods in patients with bipolar disorder

○ B Physical health is at risk in patients with mental health problems

○ C Physical health is significantly better in obsessive–compulsive disorder (OCD) when compared with the general population

○ D Physical health is unaffected by depression

○ E Physical health is unaffected by schizophrenia

10.6 Alcohol dependency
Which one of the following is suggestive of alcohol dependency?

○ A Binge drinking

○ B Drinking alone

○ C Family history of alcohol dependency

○ D Salience of drinking habits

○ E The drinking of clear spirits only

10.7 Delirium
Which one of the following statements about delirium is correct?

○ A Delirium is best treated with antipsychotics

○ B Delirium is categorised as an organic disorder

○ C Delirium is typified by auditory hallucinations

○ D Delirium occurs only in elderly people

○ E Delirium occurs only in those with a pre-existing psychiatric diagnosis

10.8 Obsessive–compulsive disorder
Which one of the following statements about obsessive–compulsive disorder (OCD) is correct?

○ A OCD involves unpleasant thoughts that the individual does not recognise as being his or her own

○ B OCD is commonly associated with anxiety and depression

○ C OCD is commonly associated with mania

○ D OCD raises the risk of suicide in sufferers

○ E The onset of OCD tends to be earlier in men than in women

10.9 Childhood autism
Which one of the following statements about childhood autism is true?

○   A   It involves a preference for consistency and routine

○   B   It involves the normal early development of social interactions

○   C   It is a subtype of psychosis

○   D   It is associated with a reciprocal 'social smile'

○   E   It is not associated with self-harm

10.10 Suicide
Which one of the following statements about suicide is correct?

○   A   Rates are highest over the Christmas and New Year holiday period

○   B   Suicide by dangerous methods is more common in women

○   C   Suicide is more common in men

○   D   The incidence is 1/100 000 per year

○   E   The risk of suicide is reduced in schizophrenia when accompanied by akathisia

10.11 Management of depression
According to the NICE guidance, *Management of depression in primary and secondary care*, which one of the following statements is most accurate?

○   A   'Doing nothing' is an appropriate course of action in an initial presentation of mild depression

○   B   CBT is more effective than antidepressants in the treatment of an initial presentation of a severe depressive episode

○   C   SSRIs are the first choice in the management of mild depressive episodes

○   D   Tricyclic antidepressants are more effective than SSRIs

○   E   Venlafaxine can be introduced in primary care for patients who have failed to respond to other agents

10.12 Treatments for depression
This is a Kaplan–Meier survival plot for the number of patients maintaining remission after a severe depressive episode treated with antidepressants compared with placebo.

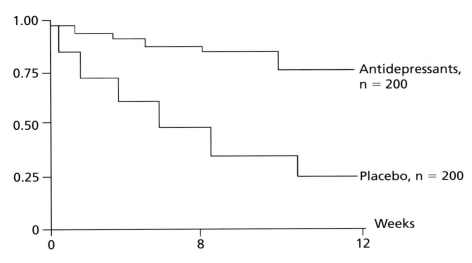

Which of the following best describes the data as they are represented?

A   All patients taking antidepressants maintain their initial improvement after 12 weeks of treatment

B   Approximately 150 patients taking antidepressants remain in remission at the end of the treatment represented by the graph

C   Approximately 75% of patients in the placebo arm remain in remission at the end of the treatment represented by the graph

D   Patients taking placebo and patients taking antidepressants show a similar rate of relapse after 12 weeks of treatment

E   Placebo and antidepressants are ineffective for maintaining long-term remission

EXTENDED MATCHING QUESTIONS

Side effects of antidepressants

Options

A   Amisulpiride
B   Citalopram
C   Fluoxetine
D   Lamotrigine
E   Mirtazepine
F   St John's wort
G   Tryptophan
H   Venlafaxine

For each of the descriptions of side effects below, select the most likely drug from the list above. Each option can be used once, more than once or not at all.

10.13   **Sedation and weight gain are common side effects.**
10.14   **This antidepressant can cause a rise in anxiety levels during initial titration.**
10.15   **Blood pressure should be monitored during initiation of this antidepressant.**
10.16   **Gastrointestinal side effects often occur with this antidepressant.**
10.17   **Caution should be exercised when choosing an antidepressant in a patient who is self-medicating with this.**

Learning disability

Options

A   Mild learning disability
B   Moderate learning disability
C   No learning disability
D   Profound learning disability
E   Severe learning disability
F   Suggestive of Down syndrome

For each of the intelligence quotient (IQ) scores below, select the most appropriate statement from the list above. Each option can be used once, more than once or not at all.

10.18   **IQ: 100**
10.19   **IQ: 38**
10.20   **IQ: 63**
10.21   **IQ: 28**

Mental Health Act assessment in the community

10.22–10.26

Options

A   1
B   2
C   3
D   4
E   135(2)
F   136
G   A clinical psychologist
H   A community psychiatric nurse
I   A consultant psychiatrist
J   A layperson
K   An approved social worker
L   Section 12

The following algorithm describes the process for detention under the Mental Health Act 1983. Using the list of options above, select the most appropriate option for each stage in the flow chart. Each option can be used once, more than once or not at all.

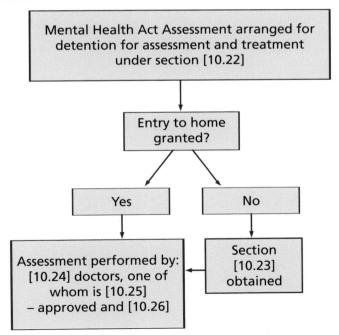

FREE TEXT QUESTION

10.27 Postnatal depression

You see a new mother who has been referred by the health visitors over concerns that she has postnatal depression. After assessing her you agree with her request for antidepressants. She is breastfeeding and keen to continue doing so and has previously had side effects with tricyclic antidepressants, so you decide to use a selective serotonin reuptake inhibitor. Which one of these drugs would be most appropriate in this situation? Write your answer in the box below.

SINGLE BEST ANSWER

10.1 E: Women suffering severe postnatal depression who attempt suicide tend to choose violent methods, eg hanging or jumping from a bridge

The Confidential Enquiry into Infant and Maternal Deaths has identified a significant number of deaths due to suicide in women with severe postnatal depression. The demographics of high-risk groups are different from other depressive or psychotic illness, however, and this group are more likely to choose violent suicide methods. They are typically aged >30, have supportive backgrounds, no history of mental illness and often well educated. A high index of suspicion and proactive screening for depression is recommended

10.2 B: Patients with recent psychosis are twice as likely to have used cannabis as patients without psychosis

There is clear evidence of a link between cannabis use and psychosis, although it is not clear whether this is causal or represents self-medication of pre-existing low-grade symptoms. A prospective study of cannabis use in Swedish conscripts showed that regular cannabis use before the age of 18 was associated with a sevenfold increase in risk of developing psychosis in the next 15 years. Cannabis use has increased from 10% of people ever having used it in the late 1960s to 50% in the twenty-first century but the incidence of psychosis has not increased this much, suggesting that any influence is likely to be multifactorial. Stronger strains of cannabis such as skunk seem to be more likely to produce mental health problems, but these are seen with all types of cannabis.

10.3 C: Patients with premorbid schizoid personality traits are more likely to develop schizophrenia

There are numerous associations with the development of schizophrenia. Premorbid schizoid personality traits (fanaticism, hypochondriasis, excessive shyness, eccentricity) and a positive family history are both associated with increased risk of developing schizophrenia, as is drug use (both cannabis and LSD/amphetamines). Twin studies show a 10–15% concordance for dizygotic twins and 30–60% concordance for monozygotic twins. Life events such as bereavement or losing a job, or brain injury (eg after a head injury) can be associated with the onset of schizophrenia.

10.4 A: It allows for the establishment of a lasting power of attorney (LPA), which allows both financial and treatment decisions to be made on behalf of patients

The Act includes provision for an LPA, which, unlike an enduring power of attorney (EPA), allows for both welfare decisions (eg where to live, payment of bills) and health decisions (eg treatment) to be made by the nominated person. These must be prearranged when the patient has capacity and registered with the Office of the Public Guardian. The Act applies only to those aged >16, and advance directives are covered only if they are written, if they do not have an appointed attorney at the time that they come into force and if the patient does not have capacity at the time that this comes to be enforced.

10.5   B: Physical health is at risk in patients with mental health problems

Physical health is often a significant concern in mental disorder, eg schizophrenia is associated with a lower life expectancy, and this is unrelated to the effects of antipsychotic medication. This is generally well known, but depression is also associated with significant co-morbidity and health risks, including a greater risk of myocardial infarction (MI). OCD does not protect physical health, but is the only mental disorder that is thought to protect against suicide.

10.6   D: Salience of drinking habits

Binge drinking is an increasing problem in the UK, especially in younger age groups and including under-age drinkers. Although it is not without health consequences, it is not specifically associated with the factors that Edwards and Gross (1976) classically described as being associated with alcohol dependence syndrome. These include reinstatement after abstinence, salience of drinking habits, relief drinking to avoid withdrawal, increasing tolerance to the effects of alcohol, a compulsion to drink and the experience of withdrawal symptoms.

10.7   B: Delirium is categorised as an organic disorder

Delirium is listed under 'Organic mental disorders' in ICD-10. It is also commonly referred to as an 'acute confusional state'. It is a non-specific syndrome characterised by concurrent disturbances of consciousness, perception, cognition, behaviour, emotion and the sleep–wake cycle. Although its frequency rises with age, it is not unique to elderly people. The highest frequency is seen in terminally ill patients (American Psychiatric Association, 1999). Disorientation in time and place is almost universal. Patients have a marked difficulty in sustaining concentration. These two points often make the assessment challenging. It is best treated by the management of the underlying cause, which can be as simple as a urinary tract infection or a recent change in medication. Low-dose antipsychotics and benzodiazepines can be used to treat the disorder symptomatically. Visual hallucinations are typical and the presence of these should always alert one to the possibility of an organic cause.

10.8   E: The onset of OCD tends to be earlier in men than in women

OCD comprises the experience of intrusive obsessional thoughts and the compulsion to do something in response. It is commonly associated with depression (30%), anxiety and depersonalisation. The obsessional thoughts experienced are recognised as being the individual's own, are unpleasant, and at least one must still be resisted in order for the diagnosis to be made. The mean age of onset is 20 years but it often occurs earlier in men, who can experience it in their early teens. The best treatment is through gradual exposure to environmental cues combined with response prevention, although in practice (serotoninergic) antidepressant therapy is also required.

10.9   A: Involves a preference for consistency and routine

Autism is typified by abnormalities of language and social interaction, which are marked and early. There is a strong preference for routine and alterations to routines already established will often be met with an abnormal behavioural response, which can include forms of self-injurious behaviour. Children with autism develop unusual preoccupations with objects and this will extend to toys, which will typically be played with in a way that suggests interest in function rather than fantasy. Compulsions are common and there can be poor speech comprehension. There is a lack of normal attachment behaviour, including reciprocal smiling (a 'social smile'), which is often deeply distressing for parents.

10.10   C: Suicide is more common in men

Suicide has an incidence in the UK of approximately 1/10 000 per year. The risk is raised in all mental disorders with the exception of OCD, and in schizophrenia the risk is higher in those who experience akathisia as a side effect of antipsychotic medication. The rates are highest during the summer and the spring in both hemispheres. It is more common in men, who are also more likely to choose dangerous or violent methods such as shooting. Jumping from structures is more commonly a method used in young than in elderly people. Remember that an individual does not need to have a mental disorder to commit suicide and that sociopolitical solutions are often more important than psychiatric ones.

10.11   A: 'Doing nothing' is an appropriate course of action in an initial presentation of mild depression

'Watchful waiting' is often the most appropriate course of action in such a presentation. The natural history of low mood dictates that over the following 2 weeks it might resolve (in which case the diagnosis of an adjustment disorder might be considered), stay the same or worsen. SSRIs are as effective as tricyclic antidepressants with a more favourable side-effect profile, and should be considered as first-line therapy for moderate and severe episodes treated in primary care. Venlafaxine should be initiated only by specialist mental health medical practitioners, including GPs with a special interest in mental health. For those presenting with severe depression, a combination of cognitive–behavioural therapy (CBT) and an SSRI should be considered as this is considered more cost-effective. There is no evidence to suggest that CBT alone is a superior management strategy.

10.12   B: Approximately 150 patients taking antidepressants remain in remission at the end of the treatment represented by the graph

This graph shows the number of patients maintaining improvement on antidepressants compared with placebo after 12 weeks of initial treatment. It shows that after this 12-week treatment period only 25% maintain their improvement on placebo, whereas approximately 75% (ie 150 patients) of those on antidepressants maintain their treatment response.

EXTENDED MATCHING ANSWERS

Side effects of antidepressants

10.13	E:	Mirtazepine
10.14	B:	Citalopram
10.15	H:	Venlafaxine
10.16	C:	Fluoxetine
10.17	F:	St John's wort

Mirtazepine's action at the histamine receptor is greater than at the noradrenergic receptor at the starting dose (15 mg). This is outweighed at higher doses so that the initial sedation experienced by most patients generally subsides. This can be usefully taken advantage of in patients with insomnia and a predominantly anxious presentation. Anxiety is a common side effect on starting citalopram, which might require symptomatic treatment, but patients should be advised that this is likely to pass after the first week or two. St John's wort is available over the counter. It is an enzyme inducer and possesses serotoninergic activity, which, when combined with selective serotonin reuptake inhibitors (SSRIs) or other serotoninergic drugs, can give rise to the serotonin syndrome. Fluoxetine frequently causes diarrhoea in the first 2–3 weeks but this usually settles in time.

Learning disability

10.18	C:	No learning disability
10.19	B:	Moderate learning disability
10.20	A:	Mild learning disability
10.21	E:	Severe learning disability

The IQ ranges for the determination of the severity of learning disability are: mild 50–69, moderate 35–49, severe 20–34, profound <20. Lower IQ has an association with lower social class of parents. With increasing severity there are an increasing number of organic causes associated with learning difficulty, the vast majority of which are detectable *in utero* or during the perinatal and postnatal period. The cause (eg Down syndrome) cannot be elucidated by IQ measurement, however.

Mental Health Act assessment in the community

10.22	C:	3
10.23	E:	135(2)
10.24	B:	2
10.25	L:	Section 12
10.26	K:	An approved social worker

The Mental Health Act is currently in the process of being revised to allow indefinite detention for people with personality disorders but for the time being the above rules apply.

FREE TEXT ANSWER

10.27 Sertraline

SSRIs are not licensed for use when lactating but data suggest that sertraline is probably the safest. Fluoxetine has a license for use during pregnancy but excessive sleepiness has been reported in children whose mothers breastfeed while taking this drug. Paroxetine has a discontinuation effect of jitteriness and citalopram has been reported to cause problems with weight gain and sleepiness. Studies of 30 babies have shown no harm from sertraline, although all of these drugs would be used off-licence.

Chapter 11
Musculoskeletal

SINGLE BEST ANSWER QUESTIONS

11.1   Rheumatoid arthritis
A 67-year-old woman with long-standing rheumatoid arthritis has recently started taking etanercept. She feels that this is working very well but has developed an acutely swollen, red knee. She comes to see you and asks if she can have this aspirated and steroid injected, which has always worked well in the past for exacerbations of her arthritis. Which one of the following would be an appropriate action in this situation?

○   A   Aspirate the joint and inject with steroid

○   B   Increase the dose of etanercept

○   C   Prescribe oral non-steroidal anti-inflammatories

○   D   Prescribe oral steroids

○   E   Stop the etanercept, check blood for inflammatory markers and send aspirate for microscopy

11.2   Back pain
A 34-year-old IT worker comes to you with a 6-month history of back pain, with no recent history of trauma and no red flag symptoms. He has presented in the past with intermittent episodes of back stiffness and occasional neck ache and was treated for plantar fasciitis last year. On examination he has no neurological signs but does have reduced range of movement in his cervical spine, particularly for extension. Which one of the following options is the most likely diagnosis?

○   A   Ankylosing spondylitis

○   B   Mechanical back pain

○   C   Osteoarthritis

○   D   Rheumatoid arthritis

○   E   Wedge fracture

11.3 Hip pain

A 72-year-old man presents with a 1-week history of a pain around his hip, which he tells you he feels most prominently in his right buttock, especially when he is gardening and when he turns on that side in bed. He is normally well and rarely comes to the surgery. He denies trauma, although he has spent the past few weeks digging his new allotment. On examination, leg lengths are equal and straight-leg raising is normal. He is markedly tender over the right hip but he has a normal range of movement in the hip. There is no rash. What is the single most likely diagnosis?

○ A Myeloma

○ B Osteoarthritis of hip

○ C Osteoarthritis of lumbar spine

○ D Sciatica

○ E Trochanteric bursitis

11.4 Pain in hands

A 53-year-old schoolteacher presents with a history of gradually increasing deformity of the small joints of both her hands, associated with stiffness and swelling. She has found it increasingly difficult to carry textbooks and is often clumsy with coffee cups and pens. She also tells you that she feels tired all the time. There is no relevant medical history and no family history of note. Her metacarpophalangeal joints are red and swollen. What is the single most likely diagnosis?

○ A Gout

○ B Osteoarthritis

○ C Pseudogout

○ D Rheumatoid arthritis

○ E Systemic lupus erythematosus

11.5 Ankle injury

Using the Ottawa rules in a patient with ankle pain after an injury, what findings would indicate the need for an X-ray? Select one option only.

○ A Bone tenderness 4 cm above the lateral malleolus

○ B Bone tenderness at the head of the fifth metatarsal

○ C Bone tenderness over the cuboid bone

○ D Patient unable to weight bear at the time of injury but now managing despite some pain

○ E Tenderness and swelling inferior to the lateral malleolus

11.6 Management of shoulder pain
Which of the following statements about new developments in the management of shoulder pain is true? Select one option only.

○ A   Adhesive capsulitis usually settles after 6 months

○ B   All patients with shoulder pain seen in primary care should have an X-ray performed

○ C   In the management of rotator cuff disorders, short-term outcomes are superior for physiotherapy compared with steroid injection

○ D   Red flag symptoms include unexplained wasting and sensory loss

○ E   Steroid injections should not be repeated due to the risk of cartilage damage

11.7 Hip pain
A 67-year-old man with a history of prostate cancer treated with Zoladex complains of persistent pain in his right hip for the last few weeks. He thinks that this might have started after he fell over while playing golf. On examination, he has a reduced range of movement in his hip and you arrange an X-ray at the local cottage hospital. The X-ray is shown below.

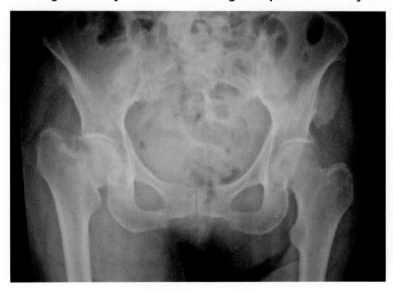

Which one of the following is the most likely diagnosis?

○ A   Constipation

○ B   Fractured neck of femur

○ C   Fractured pubic ramus

○ D   Osteoarthritis of the hip

○ E   Perthes' disease

11.8 Hand injuries

At which site would tenderness be felt in a scaphoid fracture? Select one option from A to E shown on the image below.

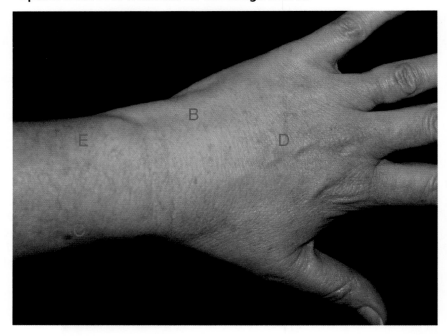

11.9 Foot pain

Indicate which one of the options A to E on the diagram below is the most likely site of tenderness in plantar fasciitis.

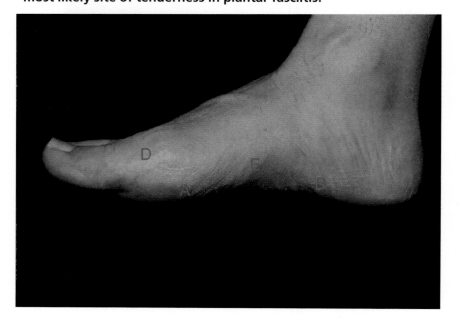

11.10 Interpretation of blood results
What is the most likely metabolic bone disease in a patient with the following results?

- Serum levels of calcium, phosphate, vitamin D and parathyroid hormone (PTH) all normal
- Markedly raised levels of alkaline phosphatase

○   A   Osteomalacia

○   B   Osteoporosis

○   C   Paget's disease

○   D   Primary hyperparathyroidism

○   E   Renal disease

EXTENDED MATCHING QUESTIONS

Management of fibromyalgia

Options

A   Amitriptyline
B   Codeine
C   Cognitive–behavioural therapy
D   Exercise
E   Fluoxetine
F   Ibuprofen
G   Pregabalin
H   Risperidone
I   Tramadol
J   Zopiclone
K   None of the above

For each of the statements below regarding management of symptoms in fibromyalgia, select the most appropriate option from the list above. Each option may be used once, more than once or not at all.

11.11   Useful where there is coexistent mood disorder.

11.12   First-line treatment where sleep disturbance occurs.

11.13   Useful for short-term use in acute exacerbations of pain.

11.14   Used under supervision over 12 weeks reduces pain, trigger points and depression.

Soft-tissue rheumatism

Options

A   De Quervain's tenosynovitis
B   Dorsal tenosynovitis
C   Fibromyalgia
D   Flexor tenosynovitis
E   Golfer's elbow
F   Osgood–Schlätter disease
G   Polymyalgia rheumatica
H   Tennis elbow
I   Trigger finger
J   Trochanteric bursitis

For each of the scenarios below, select the most appropriate diagnosis from the list above. Each option may be used once, more than once or not at all.

11.15   A 53-year-old woman complains of pain in her back, neck and abdomen over a period of several months. This seems to be worse in cold weather and she reports being very tender, particularly over her bony prominences. She gets headaches and sleeps badly. Examination is unremarkable apart from generalised tenderness. Blood tests are normal.

11.16 A 34-year-old baker complains of pain in the medial part of his elbow. On examination he is tender over the medial epicondyle, with pain on resisted pronation.

11.17 A 45-year-old housewife complains of pain and reduced movement of her thumb after spending the afternoon pruning roses. On examination there is pain on resisted abduction of the thumb and pain and tenderness on the radial side of the thumb proximal to the thumb base.

Rheumatological problems

11.18–11.21

Options

A Gout
B Polymyalgia rheumatica
C Primary nodal osteoarthritis
D Pseudogout
E Systemic lupus erythematosus
F Rheumatoid arthritis
G None of the above

For each of the signs shown below select the condition from the list above most often associated with this sign. Each option may be used once, more than once, or not at all.

[11.18]   [11.19]

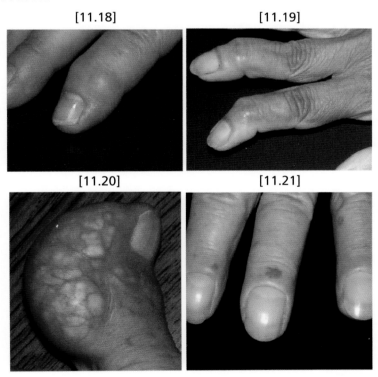

[11.20]   [11.21]

Management of osteoarthritis of the knee

11.22–11.27

Options

A   Chondroitin
B   Exercise
C   Glucosamine
D   Intra-articular hyaluronic acid injections
E   NSAID
F   Opioids
G   Paracetamol
H   Refer for surgery
I   Sibutramine
J   Weight loss

In conjunction with the local physiotherapy service, your practice has developed a flow chart to standardise the management of osteoarthritis of the knee. Complete the following flow chart with the most appropriate item from the list of options given above. Each option can be used once, more than once or not at all.

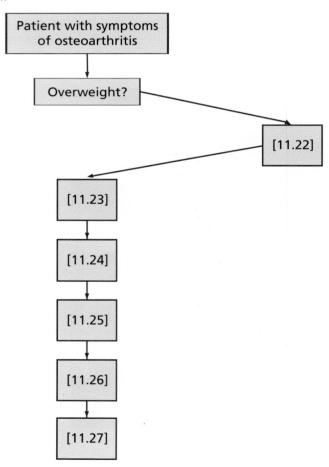

SINGLE BEST ANSWER

11.1 **E:** **Stop the etanercept, check blood for inflammatory markers and send aspirate for microscopy**

Anti-tumour necrosis factor (anti-TNF) treatments are associated with septic arthritis and can mask the severity of this complication. In any patient on anti-TNF treatment where infection is suspected, the treatment should be stopped and the infection investigated and treated. Before starting treatment with an anti-TNF you should ensure that vaccinations are up to date and patients should be warned of the possibility of infection and advised what to do if they develop symptoms and/or signs of infection. There should be a low threshold for admission in these patients.

11.2 **A:** **Ankylosing spondylitis**

Ankylosing spondylitis has a prevalence of approximately 1 in 2200 and affects men twice as frequently as women. It tends to present in young men with morning back pain and stiffness. As progressive spinal fusion occurs there can be reduced spinal movement, with kyphosis and sacroiliac joint pain. It is associated with plantar fasciitis, lung fibrosis, inflammatory bowel disease and amyloidosis. X-ray of the spine might show a 'bamboo spine', with vertebral fusion. The disease is associated with HLA-B27 positivity.

11.3 **E:** **Trochanteric bursitis**

Trochanteric bursitis is the most likely diagnosis, given the information provided in the history. One would expect to find tenderness on palpation of the affected side but a full range of movement. The pain is often felt deep in the buttock. Repeated trauma can result in inflammation of the bursa. Treatment options include NSAIDs and physiotherapy; corticosteroid injections can be useful for chronic episodes.

11.4 **D:** **Rheumatoid arthritis**

This is a classic presentation of rheumatoid arthritis in a middle-aged woman – symptoms affecting the small joints of her hands symmetrically, with pain, stiffness, swelling and loss of function. This can be associated with tiredness, malaise and other non-articular features, such as fever, weight loss, pleural effusion, mouth ulcers and dry eyes. Gout usually affects only one joint and pseudogout more typically affects the knee. This woman needs to be referred to a rheumatologist because early treatment with disease-modifying drugs can alter the progression of the disease and help to minimise the progression to involvement of larger joints.

11.5   A: Bone tenderness 4 cm above the lateral malleolus

X-ray if there is pain in the malleolar area or midfoot and bone tenderness in one or more of the following:

- Lower 6 cm of the distal fibula above the lateral malleolus
- Distal tibia above the medial malleolus
- The navicular bone
- The fifth metatarsal base.

Also X-ray if the patient is unable to weight bear at the time of the injury and subsequently.

11.6   D: Red flag symptoms include unexplained wasting and sensory loss

Adhesive capsulitis usually resolves after 18–24 months. Red flag symptoms include systemic signs of infection, bony abnormality (eg undisplaced fracture), history of cancer and neurological signs. Systematic reviews suggest equivalent short-term benefit for steroids and physiotherapy. Steroid injections can be repeated up to three times, but should not be used in the presence of a large tear.

11.7   B: Fractured neck of femur

This X-ray shows a right-sided fractured neck of femur. In the context of minor trauma there should be a high degree of suspicion that this is a pathological fracture. In this case it was due to bony metastases and he received radiotherapy to the hip after a surgical repair of the fracture.

11.8   A

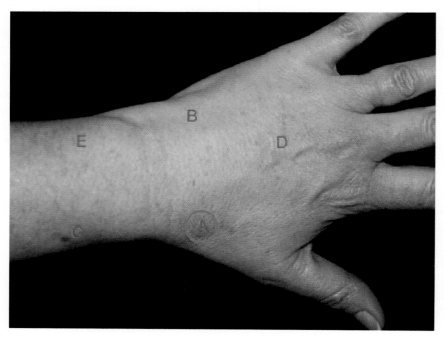

Tenderness in the anatomical snuffbox is suggestive of scaphoid fracture. Tenderness at D would suggest a metacarpal injury whereas tenderness at C or E would suggest the possibility of a radial or ulnar injury.

11.9   B

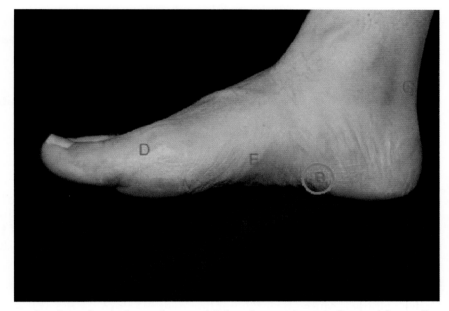

A represents the site of pain in patients with bunions, whereas D would usually be seen in a patient with gout. Tenderness at C is seen in Achilles tendinitis.

11.10   C: Paget's disease

Paget's disease is characterised by excessive and disorganised resorption and formation of bone. This is reflected by high levels of alkaline phosphatase. Osteomalacia often shows low calcium, phosphate and vitamin D levels. Alkaline phosphatase and PTH levels can be raised in osteomalacia but the best marker of disease is the serum vitamin D level. In osteoporosis there are usually normal levels of all these minerals and hormones.

EXTENDED MATCHING ANSWERS

Management of fibromyalgia

11.11   E: Fluoxetine

Patients with fibromyalgia often have symptoms of low mood, and in this situation SSRIs are helpful. Duloxetine is often used, but is not licensed for this indication in the UK.

11.12   A: Amitriptyline

Amitriptyline should be used where pain and sleep disturbance predominate, with pregabalin or gabapentin as second line if tricyclics are not tolerated. Hypnotics should be avoided due to the long-term nature of the condition.

11.12   I: Tramadol

Tramadol has been shown to be effective for short-term use in exacerbations of pain.

11.14   D: Exercise

Graded exercise therapy has been shown to significantly improve physical and psychological symptoms in fibromyalgia.

Soft-tissue rheumatism

11.15   C: Fibromyalgia

Fibromyalgia is usually diagnosed on the basis of the history and lack of any evidence of other causes of symptoms. The American College of Rheumatology diagnostic criteria state that pain should be present in all 4 quarters of the body and should be present in at least 11 of 18 trigger points. Graded exercise and low-dose amitriptyline are helpful.

11.16   E: Golfer's elbow

Golfer's elbow is caused by inflammation over the flexor origin at the medial epicondyle. Treatment involves rest and support. If this doesn't help (together with the avoidance of exacerbating factors), steroid injections might help.

11.17   A: De Quervain's tenosynovitis

De Quervain's tenosynovitis is caused by inflammation of the extensor pollicis brevis and abductor pollicis longus tendons resulting from repetitive activity. It usually settles with rest and sometimes steroid injection, but surgery might be needed if it becomes chronic.

Rheumatological problems

11.18   C: Primary nodal osteoarthritis

Primary nodal osteoarthritis affects the distal interphalangeal joint, causing Heberden's nodes to form. It affects women (10:1) predominantly and there is usually a positive family history.

11.19   F: Rheumatoid arthritis

Rheumatoid arthritis causes swan neck deformity, hyperextension of the PIP joint with flexion of the DIP joint.

11.20   A: Gout

Untreated hyperuricaemia will in time cause gouty tophi to develop.

11.21   E: Systemic lupus erythematosus

SLE is often associated with a vasculitic rash.

Management of osteoarthritis of the knee

11.22   J: Weight loss

11.23   B: Exercise

11.24   G: Paracetamol

11.25   E: NSAID

11.26   F: Opioids

11.27   H: Refer for surgery

Chapter 12
Neurology

SINGLE BEST ANSWER QUESTIONS

12.1   Swallowing problems
A 57-year-old woman complains that for the last few months she has
been getting increasingly frequent attacks of choking when eating and
drinking. Her family have also commented that she is losing weight and
her voice sounds more nasal than usual. She is otherwise fit and well
and takes no regular medications. On examination her tongue looks thin
and fasciculated, and she is unable to poke her tongue out for you to
examine her throat. Her speech sounds slurred and you notice twitching
in her eyelids. Which one of the following is the single most likely
diagnosis?

- A   Brain tumour
- B   Guillain–Barré syndrome
- C   Motor neurone disease
- D   Multiple sclerosis
- E   Myasthenia gravis

12.2   Headache
A 34-year-old man with no previous medical history of note complains
that over the last 3 weeks he has had repeated acute severe headaches,
always on the right-hand side of his head behind his eye. These make
him feel sick and he describes them as the worst pain he can remember.
At the time of the attacks he also reports that his right eye waters and
his nose runs. Examination is normal. Which one of the following would
be appropriate management in this situation?

- A   Low-dose amitriptyline
- B   Pizotifen
- C   Propranolol
- D   Refer urgently to neurology
- E   Topirimate

12.3 Epilepsy

You are asked to do a tutorial for your final year medical student on the impact on patients and their families of a diagnosis of epilepsy. Which one of the following statements is correct with regard to epilepsy?

A Epilepsy is a rare condition in the UK

B Epilepsy is usually an isolated diagnosis

C Most cases of epilepsy are inherited as autosomal recessive traits

D Up to 75% of patients become seizure free on treatment

E With good treatment compliance patients with epilepsy have normal morbidity and mortality when compared with patients without epilepsy

12.4 Blurred vision

A 35-year-old woman complains that for the last few weeks she has been aware of blurred vision and slurred speech when she is tired, and has noticed that her eyelids seem to be droopy. She is easily fatigued, but reports that she feels well when she wakes in the morning. She has no history of recent travel and no previous medical history of note. Examination shows normal reflexes and tone, and normal sensation, but bilateral ptosis and no cranial nerve signs. What is the single most likely diagnosis?

A Depression

B Lyme disease

C Motor neurone disease

D Multiple sclerosis

E Myasthenia gravis

12.5 Pins and needles

A 34-year-old man complains of 6 months of gradual onset of burning pain in both feet with numbness on both sides. He takes no regular medicine although he has been treated in the past for intravenous drug abuse. Examination shows reduced sensation on both feet but normal reflexes power and tone. Which one of the following statement with regard to his management is correct?

A He should be admitted as an emergency

B He should be reassured that his symptoms will settle in time

C He should be referred for an outpatient MRI

D He should be referred initially for nerve conduction studies

E He should be tested for HIV infection

12.6 **Amnesia**
A 65-year-old man who has struggled with alcohol addiction all his life has been found to be confused 2 weeks after attempting to detox himself by going cold turkey. When you see him he does not recognise you or his carers, and on detailed testing he has both retrograde and anterograde amnesia. He has no other neurological signs and no signs of infection. He is noted to be confabulating throughout the consultation. What is the single most likely diagnosis?

○ A Alzheimer's disease

○ B Cerebrovascular accident

○ C Delirium tremens

○ D Korsakoff's psychosis

○ E Wernicke's encephalopathy

12.7 **Management of Gilles de la Tourette syndrome**
Which of the following statements is correct with regard to the management of patients with Gilles de la Tourette syndrome?

○ A Aripiprazole is the drug of choice in children

○ B Cognitive–behavioural therapy is the only treatment modality proven to be effective

○ C Eye movement desensitisation and reprocessing are effective in patients with tics

○ D Haloperidol is effective but may cause unacceptable side effects

○ E There is no place for pharmacological therapy in management

12.8 **Twitching**
A 23-year-old girl presents with recurrent twitching of her face and abdomen, which started after one of her friends gave her a pill for travel sickness. On examination, she has repetitive twitching movements of her face and both arms and abdomen, every 20–30 seconds. Examination is otherwise normal. Which of the following is the most likely diagnosis? Select one option only.

○ A Jacksonian epilepsy

○ B Multiple sclerosis

○ C Non-organic symptoms

○ D Tardive dyskinesia

○ E Temporal lobe epilepsy

12.9 Treatment of Alzheimer's disease
Which one of the following statements about drug treatment of Alzheimer's disease is true?

    A   Cholinesterase inhibitors are available only in oral formulation

    B   Cholinesterase inhibitors have been shown to reverse cognitive impairment in patients with Alzheimer's disease

    C   Cholinesterase inhibitors can be initiated in primary care

    D   Long-acting benzodiazepines are useful in prevention of irritability and aggression

    E   Regular exercise has been shown to maintain performance in activities of daily living

12.10 Pins and needles
A 40-year-old man complains of numbness and paraesthesia of the left thumb, index and middle fingers, and half of the ring finger over a period of several weeks. Initially the symptoms were present only at night, but now he is starting to get symptoms in the daytime and is getting pain in his shoulder. On examination he has wasting and weakened abduction of the thumb, but no fasciculation. He has diet-controlled diabetes but no other history of note. What is the most likely diagnosis?

    A   Carpal tunnel syndrome

    B   Cervical radiculopathy

    C   Diabetic neuropathy

    D   Motor neurone disease

    E   Multiple sclerosis

12.11 Motor neurone disease
One of your patients has just been diagnosed with motor neurone disease and comes to see you to discuss the diagnosis. Which one of the following statements about the management of this condition is true?

    A   All patients should have a tracheostomy performed to prevent aspiration

    B   Baclofen does not help in the treatment of spasticity

    C   NICE guidance does not support the use of riluzole in motor neurone disease

    D   Riluzole has been shown to bring about remission in 25% of patients

    E   Riluzole increases the period of time to need for ventilation but does not improve prognosis

12.12 Suspected meningitis
Which of the following statements about the initial management of suspected meningitis is correct? Select one option only.

○   A   A stat dose of ciprofloxacin is effective prophylaxis in close contacts

○   B   Cefotaxime can be used safely in patients known to have anaphylaxis with penicillin

○   C   Dexamethasone should be given with the first dose of antibiotics

○   D   Intravenous amoxicillin is the first-line empirical treatment for suspected meningitis

○   E   Treatment should be guided by the results of blood culture

12.13 Trigeminal neuralgia
Which of the following statements about trigeminal neuralgia is true? Select one option only.

○   A   Amitriptyline is the most effective treatment

○   B   It always affects the mandibular branch of the trigeminal nerve

○   C   It can be associated with a facial nerve palsy

○   D   It is typically relapsing and remitting

○   E   Paroxysms of pain usually last at least 30 minutes

12.14 Facial weakness
A 76-year-old man who had a parotid tumour removed last year complains that he has developed a lopsided smile. He feels fine in himself. His picture is shown below.

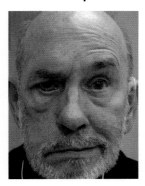

What is the most likely cause?

○   A   Cerebrovascular accident

○   B   Malignant infiltration

○   C   Meningioma

○   D   Motor neurone disease

○   E   Multiple sclerosis

12.15 Epilepsy

Consider the graph shown below, which illustrates the epidemiology of epilepsy.

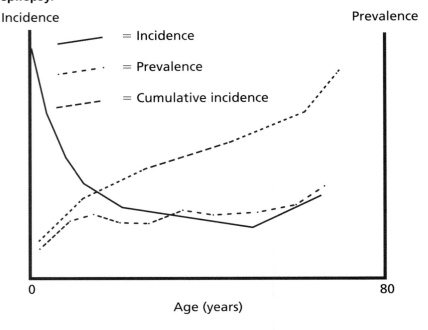

Which one of the following statements about these data is true?

○ A The fact that the cumulative incidence is higher than the prevalence in middle to older age suggests that most people enter remission at some stage

○ B The fall in incidence in early to middle age is due to the high mortality of childhood epilepsy

○ C The graph shows that most patients with epilepsy have the condition all their lives

○ D The increase in incidence in old age is due to an increase in idiopathic epilepsy

○ E The increase in prevalence in old age is due to physiological changes affecting seizure threshold

EXTENDED MATCHING QUESTIONS

Headache

Options

A   Analgesic overuse headache
B   Brain tumour
C   Chronic paroxysmal hemicrania
D   Chronic sinusitis
E   Cluster headache
F   Giant-cell arteritis
G   Migraine
H   Postcoital cephalgia
I   Subarachnoid haemorrhage
J   Temporal lobe epilepsy
K   Tension-type headache
L   Transient global amnesia
M   Transient ischaemic attack

For each of the descriptions below, select the most appropriate diagnosis from the list above. Each option can be used once, more than once or not at all.

12.16   A 67-year-old man with a history of several weeks of malaise, now complains of headache and scalp tenderness on the sides of his head, together with pain in his scalp on eating.

12.17   A 44-year-old man complains of daily headaches that are centred around his right eye over the past 2 months. These are severe and are not improving despite taking paracetamol and ibuprofen every day. They are associated with nasal congestion and epiphora.

12.18   A 73-year-old woman presents with 2 months of headaches, worse in the morning, but usually improve by mid-afternoon. They are getting gradually worse, and seem particularly bad when she bends over. She feels nauseous with them and experiences visual disturbances at times.

12.19   A 23-year-old woman who takes the combined oral contraceptive pill complains of severe headache with flashing lights and loss of vision in one eye. She reports that she felt 'out of sorts' immediately before with hypersensitivity to lights and sound started.

Peripheral nerve disorders

Options

A   Carpal tunnel syndrome
B   Charcot–Marie–Tooth disease
C   Diabetic neuropathy
D   Drug-induced peripheral neuropathy
E   Polio
F   Vitamin B deficiency

For each of the scenarios below, select the most likely cause from the list above. Each option may be used once, more than once or not at all.

12.20   A 29-year-old woman complains of progressive problems with walking. She had pes cavus diagnosed in childhood. On examination her legs have a champagne-bottle appearance. Reflexes are reduced on both sides. She reports other affected family members.

12.21   A 73-year-old man complains of pins and needles and numbness in both feet. He takes amiodarone and warfarin for atrial fibrillation but is otherwise well.

12.22   A 21-year-old woman with a long history of anorexia complains of paraesthesia and numbness of her feet. Blood tests are taken and these show a macrocytic anaemia.

New-onset seizure

12.23–12.27

Options

A   Epilepsy likely
B   Epilepsy unlikely
C   Incontinence
D   No
E   Petit mal
F   Syncope likely
G   Syncope unlikely
H   Tongue biting
I   Yes

The differentiation of epilepsy from syncope can be difficult. The following flow chart has been developed to simplify the diagnosis. From the list of options above, select the most appropriate choice for each question in the flow chart.

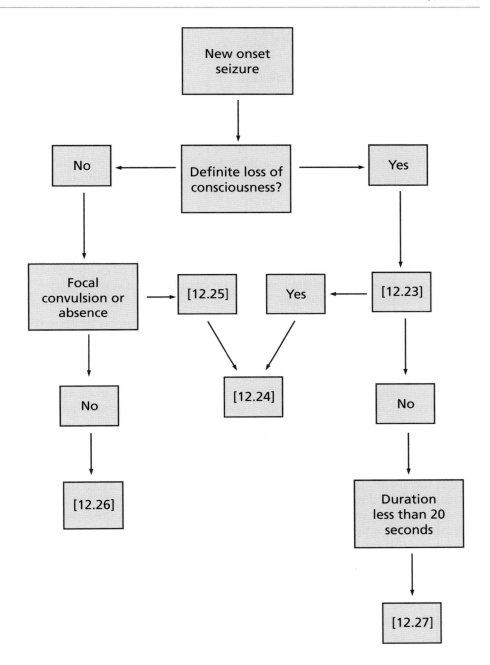

SINGLE BEST ANSWER

12.1   C: Motor neurone disease

This patient has symptoms of a bulbar palsy. The progressive nature suggests that this is most likely to be due to motor neurone disease. Guillain–Barré usually causes an ascending paralysis rather than starting with bulbar symptoms. Unlike multiple sclerosis there is no sensory or cognitive loss and the sphincters and ocular muscles are unaffected, distinguishing the condition from myasthenia gravis. A brain tumour would normally cause symptoms of raised intracranial pressure.

12.2   D: Refer urgently to neurology

Patients presenting for the first time with cluster headache should be referred for urgent assessment due to the risk of an underlying lesion, such as an arteriovenous malformation or tumour. Acute treatment of cluster headache consists of triptans or high-flow oxygen. Prophylaxis with verapamil or glucocorticoids is often effective.

12.3   D: Up to 75% of patients become seizure free on treatment

Epilepsy affects 400 000 people in the UK. It is often seen in association with other conditions such as cerebral palsy or tuberous sclerosis, or in later life as a result of cerebrovascular disease. About 40% of cases of epilepsy have a generic component. Epilepsy is associated with two to three times higher morbidity and mortality rates due to both epilepsy itself (sudden unexpected death and seizures) and to accidents, eg drowning.

12.4   E: Myasthenia gravis

Myasthenia gravis typically presents with weakness, usually of the ocular, bulbar, facial and girdle muscles. Patients are easily fatigued and usually first notice blurred vision or ptosis. The condition affects 1:20 000 people and can be associated with thymoma. Autoantibodies against acetylcholinesterase receptors are positive in 75% of cases, and diagnosis can be confirmed with a Tensilon test. Treatment is with oral pyridostigmine with treatment of any associated thymoma. Where thymoma is present, the 5-year survival rate is 30%; for non-thymoma cases 80% respond well to oral treatment.

12.5   E: He should be tested for HIV infection

Peripheral neuropathy is common, and investigation should be directed to the most common causes. Patients should have a history and examination to identify potential underlying disease and be tested accordingly. The most common causes are diabetes, alcohol use, vitamin B_{12} deficiency and HIV. All patients should have a biochemical screening and treatment initiated with either a tricyclic antidepressant or anticonvulsant. Nerve conduction studies may be helpful where there is diagnostic doubt. Cauda equina symptoms should prompt emergency admission.

12.6   D: Korsakoff's psychosis

Korsakoff's psychosis is characterised by both retrograde and anterograde amnesia, frequently with marked confabulation. It is seen in 80% of untreated patients with Wernicke's encephalopathy and can be precipitated by delirium tremens in patients who suddenly cease drinking. It can also be caused by subarachnoid haemorrhage and stroke, and these should be excluded. Diagnosis is clinical and one of exclusion, and treatment is with thiamine. Wernicke's encephalopathy is characterised by acute onset of confusion, nystagmus, partial ophthalmoplegia and ataxia due to thiamine deficiency.

12.7   D: Haloperidol is effective but may cause unacceptable side effects

There is good evidence for the use of neuroleptics alongside CBT in Gilles de la Tourette syndrome, with the strongest evidence for haloperidol and pimozide. Aripiprazole is effective with a favourable side-effect profile but is unsuitable for use in children. Eye movement desensitisation is used in post-traumatic stress disorder. Where haloperidol is not tolerated atypical neuroleptics such as risperidone may be useful.

12.8   D: Tardive dyskinesia

Tardive dyskinesia is characterised by repetitive facial grimaces and choreoathetoid movements of the upper limbs, and is usually seen after neuroleptic use, although it can occur after taking antiemetics or over-the-counter medications. It is more common in females and usually settles with drug withdrawal, although 40% still have symptoms after 3 years. Anticholinergics (eg Kemadrin) or benzodiazepines usually help with symptoms. Jacksonian epilepsy is a condition where seizures are initially localised but spread to become a generalised tonic–clonic seizure; temporal lobe epilepsy is characterised by unusual behaviour or hallucinations.

12.9   E: Regular exercise has been shown to maintain performance in activities of daily living

Alzheimer's disease should be treated using a multidisciplinary approach, including regular exercise and group activities, which have been shown to slow the decline in performance of activities of daily living. Cholinesterase inhibitors are useful in mild-to-moderate disease and NICE guidance suggests that they should be initiated only by specialists. Sedatives and alcohol should be avoided because of the risk of falls and increased confusion. Cholinesterase inhibitors are available as patches, which are useful where nausea or vomiting occurs with the oral form or in more advanced cases for control of agitation.

12.10   A: Carpal tunnel syndrome

Carpal tunnel syndrome is caused by compression of the median nerve at the wrist. Diagnosis can be confirmed by Phalen's or Tinel's tests, or by nerve conduction studies where there is doubt. Treatment is with steroid injection, although surgery is often required when there is muscle wasting.

12.11   E: Riluzole increases the period of time to need for ventilation but does not improve prognosis

Riluzole has been shown to increase the mean time to need for ventilation but does not affect the final outcome. The multidisciplinary approach involving occupational therapy and physiotherapy as well as speech and language therapy can lead to significant benefits, and symptomatic drug treatments such as benztropine for drooling and baclofen or diazepam for spasticity are very helpful. The decision to ventilate is one that must be made with the patient because this will often be seen as simply prolonging the patient's suffering.

12.12   A: A stat dose of ciprofloxacin is effective prophylaxis in close contacts

Rifampicin is traditionally used for prophylaxis but ciprofloxacin has fewer side effects and interactions, although is it is unlicensed for this use. Intravenous or intramuscular benzylpenicillin should be used for suspected meningitis, or cefotaxime if there is a history of drug reaction with penicillin. In cases of anaphylaxis, however, chloramphenicol should be used. Amoxicillin is the treatment of choice for listeria meningitis. Meningitis is a life-threatening condition and treatment should not be delayed for blood cultures. Polymerase chain reaction (PCR) testing will often confirm the diagnosis after initiation of therapy, regardless of antibiotic use.

12.13   D: It is typically relapsing and remitting

Trigeminal neuralgia is a relapsing and remitting neuralgic pain in any of the branches of the trigeminal nerve, nearly always unilateral and characterised by paroxysms lasting <2 minutes. Associated neurological signs suggest the presence of alternative causes such as tumour. Carbamazepine is effective in 70% of patients and gabapentin is often used as an alternative. Refractory cases can be treated with surgery.

12.14   B: Malignant infiltration

This man has a lower motor neurone lesion, as evidenced by the fact that he cannot furrow his brow (the brow is innervated bilaterally). Causes of this include Bell's palsy, Lyme disease, herpesvirus infection (zoster or acute infection) and cholesteatoma. Trauma, Guillain–Barré syndrome, diabetes and sarcoidosis are other common causes. Lower motor neurone facial nerve palsy can be seen in patients with a history of parotid gland tumours, due to either iatrogenic damage or tumour infiltration. Upper motor neurone causes include central nervous system tumours, multiple sclerosis, syphilis and cerebrovascular disease. Bell's palsy is a diagnosis of exclusion.

12.15 **A:** **The fact that the cumulative incidence is higher than the prevalence in middle to older age suggests that most people enter remission at some stage**

The risk of recurrence after a single seizure is approximately 50–70% but the long-term prognosis is good. Retrospective studies suggest that, after 20 years, 76% of patients had at least one 5-year period of complete freedom from seizures, and 70% remained seizure free. Approximately 50% were in remission of at least 5 years' duration and had been off all antiepileptic drugs for at least 5 years. The cumulative incidence of epilepsy is considerably higher than the prevalence, suggesting that most patients enter long-term remission at some stage.

EXTENDED MATCHING ANSWERS

Headache

12.16 **F:** **Giant-cell arteritis**

Giant-cell arteritis causes a prodromal illness of malaise, anorexia and weight loss, followed by temporal headache and scalp tenderness. Jaw claudication is pathognomonic of this condition. Late features include visual loss and severe temporal tenderness.

12.17 **E:** **Cluster headache**

Cluster headache typically affects men in their 40s and causes daily severe headaches, often with associated watering of the eye and nasal symptoms. The headaches are severe and last 1–2 hours. They are often triggered by alcohol.

12.18 **B:** **Brain tumour**

These symptoms are consistent with raised intracranial pressure (ICP). Common chronic causes include brain tumour but, when presenting acutely, a colloid cyst or intracranial bleed should be excluded.

12.19 **G:** **Migraine**

This is a typical history of focal migraine, with a prodrome, aura and headache, followed by resolution. Treatment is aimed at avoiding provoking factors (including the pill) where appropriate and treating symptoms, often with a triptan.

Peripheral nerve disorders

12.20   B: Charcot–Marie–Tooth disease

Charcot–Marie–Tooth disease is a hereditary peripheral neuropathy that usually presents with walking difficulties in the first or second decade. There are reduced reflexes and sensorimotor neuropathy, and peripheral nerves can be palpably thickened. It is inherited as an autosomal dominant condition and usually causes mild disability with a normal lifespan.

12.21   D: Drug-induced peripheral neuropathy

Many drugs can cause peripheral neuropathy, but the most common causes are amiodarone, phenytoin, isoniazid, vincristine, nitrofurantoin and gold. The neuropathy is often irreversible.

12.22   F: Vitamin B deficiency

Vitamin B_{12} deficiency causes peripheral neuropathy and can cause subacute combined degeneration of the cord if it is not treated. It also causes megaloblastic anaemia, glossitis, alopecia and malabsorption, and can cause optic neuritis. It is rare in developed countries in people who are otherwise healthy, but might be seen in people with malabsorption, eg patients with pernicious anaemia or patients who have had bowel resection (eg for Crohn's disease).

New-onset seizure

12.23   H: Tongue biting
12.24   A: Epilepsy likely
12.25   I: Yes
12.26   B: Epilepsy unlikely
12.27   F: Syncope likely

Syncope can cause stiffening of the body, twitching of the limbs and occasional incontinence. These symptoms are not therefore always useful in differentiating epilepsy from syncope. Attempt to identify a precipitating factor for syncope, such as standing for long periods (particularly if the ambient temperature is high), pain, strong emotion, micturition, diarrhoea or vomiting. It is uncommon for syncope to occur without some warning symptoms, usually including some combination of nausea, blurred vision, light-headedness and a sensation of muffled hearing. Syncope is often accompanied by pallor and sweating, whereas cyanosis is usual in the early stages of generalised tonic–clonic seizures. The actual duration of the loss of consciousness in syncope usually amounts to a few seconds only; it can, however, be longer if the patient is supported in the upright position after fainting. The postictal phase after syncope does not involve prolonged drowsiness and confusion, and recovery is generally rapid, although the patient might feel a sense of malaise for some time. Tongue biting suggests a seizure.

Chapter 13
Ophthalmology

SINGLE BEST ANSWER QUESTIONS

13.1   Altered vision
A 47-year-old, short-sighted woman complains of a 1-week history of flashes of light at the edge of her vision in her left eye. Today she has noticed a dark curtain over one side of her visual field, which does not go away with head movements. The single most likely diagnosis is:

○   A   Migraine

○   B   Retinal detachment

○   C   Uveitis

○   D   Vitreous haemorrhage

○   E   Vitrous detachment

13.2   Loss of vision
A 70-year-old woman complains of several weeks of generalised aches and pains and difficulty getting out of a chair. Over the last 24 hours she has become aware of loss of vision in her left eye, with pain in her jaw on chewing. On examination, she has a visual acuity of 6/60 and a left relative afferent pupillary defect. Her left disc appears pale and swollen. The single best option in the management of this patient is:

○   A   A 7-day course of 15 mg prednisolone and then review

○   B   Conservative management as the vision has already been lost

○   C   Refer to neurology with an MR scan

○   D   Start 80 mg prednisolone and refer to ophthalmology

○   E   Urgent temporal artery biopsy

13.3 Double vision

An 80-year-old man complains of sudden-onset double vision. He is otherwise well and not known to have high BP or high cholesterol, but he does smoke. On examination, he appears to have restricted lateral gaze in the left eye. His double vision is horizontal and worse on looking to the left and into the distance. His pupils react normally and there is no headache or ptosis. Which one of the following statements about his management is correct?

○ A   Advise him to attend his optometrist, who will prescribe glasses with prisms

○ B   Do nothing – it is likely that this will resolve in a few weeks

○ C   Start aspirin and investigate for cardiovascular risk

○ D   Start aspirin, investigate for cardiovascular risk and refer to ophthalmology

○ E   Urgent referral to neurosurgery

13.4 Painful red eye

A 68-year-old man complains of a painful red eye. He had cataract surgery 2 days ago and, aside from some mild grittiness, his eye was comfortable. Since then his eye has become very red and painful, and he is no longer able to see properly. The single most likely diagnosis is:

○ A   Acute angle-closure glaucoma due to the drops used to dilate the pupil before the surgery

○ B   Endophthalmitis

○ C   Postoperative iritis

○ D   Severe allergic reaction to the anaesthetic injection

○ E   Severe conjunctivitis

13.5 Visual deterioration

A 79-year-old woman complains of relatively sudden deterioration of vision in her left eye. She has very poor vision in her right eye because of macular degeneration. She states that over the past 2 weeks when she looks at straight edges they appear bent. Also, when looking at a fence or a brick wall, all the straight lines appear wavy. Which one of the following statements about this condition is correct?

○ A   She has developed wet macular degeneration in her left eye and needs laser treatment

○ B   She has dry macular degeneration in her left eye and needs to start taking oral anti-VEGF tablets

○ C   She has macular degeneration in her left eye. There is no treatment other than recommending vitamins and stopping smoking

○ D   She has wet macular degeneration and is eligible for intravitreal anti-VEGF therapy on the NHS

○ E   She has wet macular degeneration and needs surgery

13.6   Visual problems

A myopic man complains of seeing flashing lights and floaters.
The appearance of his fundus is shown below:

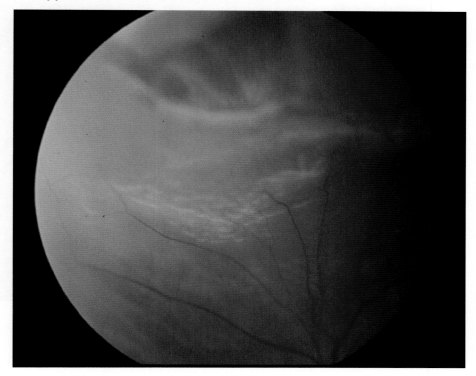

Which one of the following statements about this patient is correct?

○ A   Being short-sighted usually reduces the risk of this condition

○ B   He has a retinal tear that can be treated with laser in the outpatient department

○ C   He has already lost vision and therefore surgery is not urgent

○ D   He will need an urgent operation to prevent irreversible visual loss

○ E   He will need surgery within 1 week

13.7 Visual deterioration

A 70-year-old woman complains of a gradual deterioration in vision in both eyes. Her visual acuity is 6/9 and 6/12. She has been told by her optician that she has macular degeneration and has heard of new treatments available for this condition. She would like your advice about treatment. Examination findings are shown below:

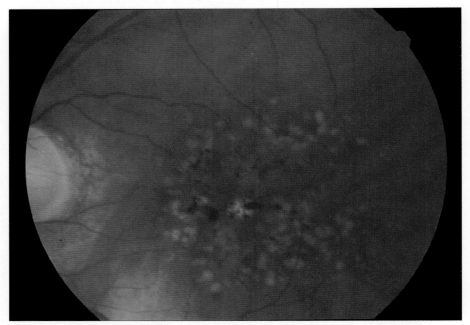

Which one of the following statements is correct with regard to this clinical situation?

○   A   She has evidence of diabetic maculopathy and needs to have her diabetes managed

○   B   She requires an urgent referral to ophthalmology for intravitreal Lucentis

○   C   She would be a suitable candidate for laser treatment

○   D   She would be a suitable candidate for photodynamic therapy

○   E   You should advise her to stop smoking and ensure a diet high in fresh fruit and vegetables

13.8 Diabetic eye problems

You see a young diabetic patient in your clinic. He is in his early 20s and has very poorly controlled type 1 diabetes. He doesn't like taking his insulin and he drinks and smokes to excess. His BP is slightly elevated. Fundoscopic findings are shown below:

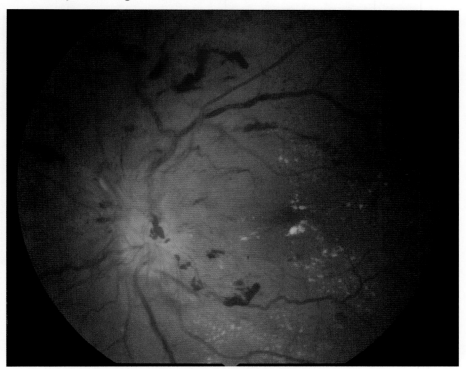

Which one of the following statements is true with regard to his visual prognosis?

- A   After laser treatment his vision should remain stable
- B   He is at risk of visual loss due to retinal detachment
- C   He needs surgery to maintain his vision
- D   Regardless of the amount of laser treatment given, he is likely to be registered blind in 5 years
- E   With adequate laser and optimisation of diabetic control and risk factors, his vision can be maintained

13.9 Eye conditions

Which area of the eye would you expect to see a pterygium develop? Select the most appropriate option from A to E on the photo below.

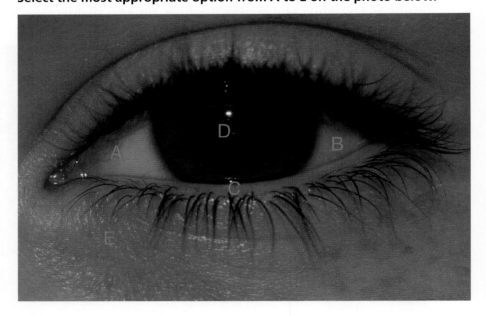

EXTENDED MATCHING QUESTIONS

Patients presenting with ptosis

Options

A   Bilateral ptosis in a patient with excessive skin around the eyes
B   Bilateral ptosis in a patient with frontal balding and a prolonged hand-shake
C   Bilateral ptosis, worse at the end of the day, with associated intermittent diplopia
D   Unilateral ptosis with the eye deviated down and out, with a large pupil
E   Unilateral ptosis with a history of orbital cellulitis
F   Unilateral ptosis with a small pupil, anhidrosis and enophthalmos

For each of the diagnoses below, select the most likely findings from the list of options above. Each option can be used once, more than once or not at all.

13.10   Third nerve palsy
13.11   Myotonic dystrophy
13.12   Myasthenia gravis
13.13   Horner syndrome

Eye problems

13.14–13.17

Options

A   Acute conjunctivitis
B   Blepharitis
C   Ectropion
D   Entropion
E   Pinguecula
F   Pterygium
G   Subconjunctival haemorrhage
H   None of the above

For each of the conditions below, select the most likely diagnosis from the list above. Each option may be used once, more than once or not at all.

[13.14]   [13.15]

[13.16]   [13.17]

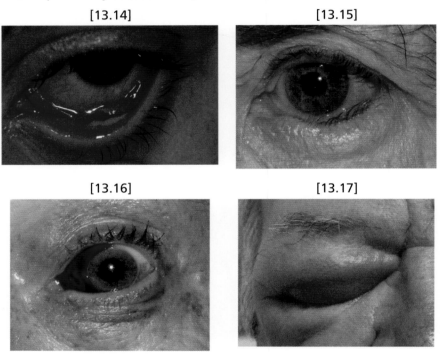

Visual fields

Options

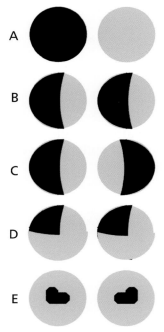

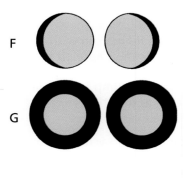

For each of the following patients, select the most likely visual field defect from the options above. Each option can be used once, more than once or not at all.

13.18   An elderly woman who has had a stroke
13.19   A homeless, alcoholic smoker
13.20   A man with acromegaly
13.21   A diabetic who has had panretinal photocoagulation
13.22   A patient with glaucoma

Management of eyelid problems

13.23–13.25

Options

A   Clean lid margin with cotton tip
B   Hot flannels applied for 10 minutes
C   Lubricants
D   Massage lump for 10 minutes
E   Oral antibiotics
F   Topical antibiotics

Complete the flowchart below describing the daily routine for self-management of chalazion and blepharitis from the list of options above. Each option may be used once, more than once or not at all.

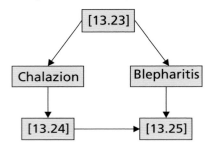

FREE TEXT QUESTION

13.26 Interpretation of ophthalmological investigations
You receive a letter from a local optometrist regarding one of your
patients. The results are summarised below:

Visual acuity right eye:	6/7
Visual acuity left eye:	6/6
Intraocular pressure right eye:	28
Intraocular pressure left eye:	27

In the box below write the most likely diagnosis based on these results.

SINGLE BEST ANSWER

13.1 B: Retinal detachment

Although all of the options can cause 'flashes and floaters', the complaint of a dark, constant, peripheral shadow demands an exclusion of retinal detachment. Myopic (short-sighted) people are more at risk because of their relatively large eyes. The treatment of retinal detachment is surgical. In the early stages vision can be maintained at normal levels but if the detachment is left and the macula detaches (a macula-off retinal detachment) the visual prognosis is poor.

13.2 D: Start 80 mg prednisolone and refer to ophthalmology

Giant-cell arteritis is an emergency. The patient has a high risk of blindness. In a patient such as the one in the question, the risk is to the other eye, which can rapidly become affected if the condition is not treated. Characteristically, patients have a prodrome of temporal artery tenderness, jaw claudication, malaise, weight loss and fatigue, and might have already been diagnosed with polymyalgia rheumatica. Classically, the ESR is very elevated, and is accompanied by a rise in the C-reactive protein (CRP). This is by no means always the case, however, and giant-cell arteritis can still occur in the absence of a very high ESR. Treatment comprises high-dose steroids, which are very slowly tapered down. To confirm the diagnosis, a temporal artery biopsy is performed by the ophthalmologist.

13.3 D: Start aspirin, investigate for cardiovascular risk and refer to ophthalmology

The patient has developed a left nerve VI palsy. The most common reason for this to occur in a patient of this age is microvascular disease and cardiovascular risk factors should be addressed. Referral to ophthalmology is necessary to:

- confirm the diagnosis and exclude involvement of other cranial nerves (including the optic disc)
- obtain an orthoptic assessment in order to quantify the diplopia and prescribe the correct prisms
- arrange relevant investigations and follow-up.

It is also possible to develop cranial nerve palsies in association with giant-cell arteritis and so, if there is any suspicion of polymyalgia rheumatica, this diagnosis should be considered.

13.4 B: Endophthalmitis

This is an emergency and the patient needs urgent referral to ophthalmology. This condition, where there is intraocular infection, can rapidly progress to irreversible blindness and retinal detachment. The classic presentation is one of a painful red eye developing a few days after surgery. There might be a hypopyon (pus in the anterior chamber) and slit-lamp examination will reveal significant intraocular inflammation. Deterioration to irreversible blindness or retinal detachment is rapid and prognosis is poor, even with prompt treatment.

Management includes intravitreal sampling and injection of antibiotics. Vitrectomy might be necessary to clear debris. If retinal detachment occurs due to necrosis of the retina, further vitreoretinal surgery is indicated.

13.5 D: She has wet macular degeneration and is eligible for intravitreal anti-VEGF therapy on the NHS

There are two main types of macular degeneration, wet and dry. Intravitreal injections of Lucentis (anti-VEGF) at 4- to 6-weekly intervals in patients with recently diagnosed wet macular degeneration can bring about dramatic improvement in vision. Referral to an ophthalmologist is indicated so that the patient can be fully assessed for eligibility for these drugs. There is no treatment for dry macular degeneration, although stopping smoking and ensuring a diet rich in fresh fruit and vegetables are recommended.

13.6 D: He will need an urgent operation to prevent irreversible visual loss

The photograph shows a large retinal tear and a peripheral retinal detachment. Small tears alone can be treated with laser in order to prevent retinal detachment but, once the retina has detached, surgery is necessary. The detachment is peripheral and the subretinal fluid has not reached the macula. This means that the patient's vision may be saved with urgent surgery to reattach the retina. Once the macula has detached, vision becomes poor – typically 6/60 or worse. Surgery can restore vision to some degree but not usually to previous levels. Myopic individuals are at higher risk of detachment because their eyes are relatively large.

13.7 E: You should advise her to stop smoking and ensure a diet high in fresh fruit and vegetables

The photo shows areas of drusen, pigment changes and atrophy consistent with dry macular degeneration. Dry macular degeneration is more common than wet macular degeneration and there is no treatment for this, with slowly progressive loss of central vision. Abstinence from smoking and a diet rich in fresh fruit and vegetables can help slow the progression of the disease. Wet macular degeneration is characterised by fluid leakage and subretinal oedema, resulting in visual distortion. Intravitreal Lucentis, an anti-VEGF drug, restores vision and prevents scarring. Photodynamic therapy destroys abnormal blood vessels near the macula. This treatment is aimed at preventing deterioration in vision, although the treatment itself causes significant scarring. It can be difficult to detect wet changes without a slit-lamp examination and therefore ophthalmology referral might be indicated. Most importantly, the patient should be aware that, if she starts to experience distortion of her vision, this could herald the development of wet changes and an urgent referral to ophthalmology would then be appropriate.

13.8   E: With adequate laser and optimisation of diabetic control and risk factors, his vision can be maintained

This photograph shows proliferative diabetic retinopathy with extensive neovascularisation at the optic disc. There are multiple dot-and-blot haemorrhages, microaneurysms and hard exudates. This patient is at high risk of visual loss due to vitreous haemorrhage and maculopathy. Urgent panretinal laser is indicated. It is likely that several sessions of laser will be needed to bring about regression and involution of the abnormal blood vessels. Management of the patient's risk factors is most important, including the psychological side of his condition. Surgery might be necessary if vitreous haemorrhage does not clear after several months, or if there is a progressive tractional retinal detachment. This type of detachment is different from that due to a retinal tear because it can remain stable for a long time, requiring monitoring only.

13.9   A

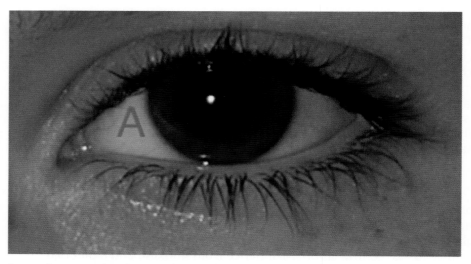

Pterygiums are benign overgrowths of the conjunctiva, usually seen at the medial canthus and growing laterally. They are thought to be due to exposure to heat, wind or dust. If they encroach on the cornea surgery may be indicated.

EXTENDED MATCHING ANSWERS

Patients presenting with ptosis

13.10	D:	Unilateral ptosis with the eye deviated down and out, with a large pupil
13.11	B:	Bilateral ptosis in patient with frontal balding and a prolonged handshake
13.12	C:	Bilateral ptosis, worse at the end of the day, with associated intermittent diplopia
13.13	F:	Unilateral ptosis with a small pupil, anhidrosis and enophthalmos

Eye problems

13.14	A:	Acute conjunctivitis
13.15	D:	Entropion
13.16	G:	Subconjunctival haemorrhage
13.17	H:	None of the above.

This is an allergic reaction to an insect bite.

Visual fields

13.18   B

Stroke usually causes a homonymous hemianopia.

13.19   E

Tobacco typically causes a caecocentral scotoma.

13.20   C

Optic chiasma compression (eg from a pituitary tumour) causes a bitemporal hemianopia.

13.21   G

Photocoagulation involves burning the peripheral visual field and results in constricted visual fields.

13.22   F

Glaucoma causes bilateral arcuate scotomas and delayed diagnosis can result in irreversible tunnel vision.

Management of eyelid problems

13.23 **B:** **Hot flannels applied for 10 minutes**

13.24 **D:** **Massage lump for 10 minutes**

13.25 **A:** **Clean lid margin with cotton tip**

This was described in the *British Medical Journal* (2010;**341**:c4044). Infected chalazia should be treated with oral antibiotics. Failure to resolve should prompt incision and drainage if affecting vision. Failure of blepharitis to improve should prompt oral doxycycline for 3 months.

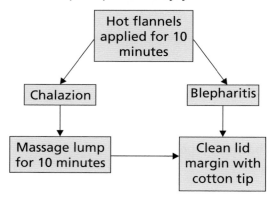

FREE TEXT ANSWER

Interpretation of ophthalmological investigations

13.26   Glaucoma

Raised intraocular pressure is the hallmark of glaucoma. Visual acuity is preserved until late in the disease due to relative preservation of the macula. Field testing is much more sensitive in picking up early glaucoma, whereas slit-lamp examination may show cupping of the optic disc.

Chapter 14
Paediatrics

SINGLE BEST ANSWER QUESTIONS

14.1 **Nosebleeds**
A 3-month-old baby boy is brought to see you by his mother. She came home from work after leaving him in the care of her older daughter and found that he had suffered a nosebleed. Her daughter does not recall this happening and says that he has been fine all morning. He was born at term after a normal delivery and is formula fed. On examination the child appears well but there is some dried blood in each nostril. There are no other signs of bleeding. Which one of the following would be the most appropriate action in this situation?

- A Admit under the on-call paediatrician
- B Give vitamin K
- C Prescribe topical antibiotics to use while the nose heals
- D Reassure his mother that the bleeding is likely to be due to a cold and should settle
- E Report the family to social services

14.2 **Six-week check**
While carrying out a routine baby check on a 6-week-old baby you note that there seems to be an absent red reflex in both eyes. The eyes look otherwise normal and the rest of the examination is unremarkable. The mother says that her pregnancy was unremarkable other than a flu-like illness in the second trimester. Which one of the following would be an appropriate action in this instance?

- A Admit under the on-call paediatrician
- B Inform the health visitor
- C Reassure mother that this is unlikely to be significant
- D Refer to ophthalmology outpatients
- E Refer to orthoptic clinic

14.3 Kawasaki's disease
You receive a telephone call from one of your patients whose son has been admitted to hospital with suspected Kawasaki's disease. She has been doing some research on the internet and has heard that it has fatal complications. She asks if this is true. Which one of the following statements is true in this situation?

- A   Of patients 70% develop cardiac complications
- B   Aspirin should not be used due to the risk of Reye syndrome
- C   Kawasaki's disease can cause myocardial infarction
- D   The mortality rate is approximately 20%
- E   Nephrotic syndrome is frequently seen in these patients

14.4 Self-harm
A 12-year-old girl is brought in to see you by her parents after an episode of deliberate self-harm the previous weekend. Her parents are obviously distraught and are terrified that she will do this again and be more successful next time. Which one of the following is a risk factor for successful suicide attempt after deliberate self-harm?

- A   Drug or alcohol abuse
- B   Early presentation after an episode of deliberate self-harm
- C   High performance at school
- D   Isolated episode of deliberate self-harm
- E   Spontaneous act of deliberate self-harm

14.5 Eating disorders
After a practice significant event, you decide to actively screen for patients with eating disorders. Which one of the following patients has a possible eating disorder?

- A   A 10-year-old girl who has started her periods a year earlier than her peers
- B   A 13-year-old girl with type 1 diabetes who is poorly compliant
- C   A 14-year-old boy who has lost 10 kg since becoming a vegan
- D   A 15-year-old girl with a BMI of 31 kg/m^2 who asks for help losing weight
- E   A 16-year-old girl with a BMI of 26 kg/m^2

14.6 Constipation

A 9-month-old boy has suffered from chronic constipation since birth. His mother had been told by his health visitor that this would improve with weaning but she finds that he is no better. He opens his bowels every few days and his mother tells you that it is usually liquid. When you examine him his abdomen is distended, although his mother says that he has always been like that. What is the most likely diagnosis in this case?

○   A   Anal fissure

○   B   Hirschsprung's disease

○   C   Hypothyroidism

○   D   Lactose intolerance

○   E   Simple constipation

14.7 Febrile seizure

An 18-month-old baby has been discharged after a febrile seizure. Which of the following statements about this condition is true? Select one option only.

○   A   Sixty per cent of children have recurrent febrile seizures during subsequent illnesses

○   B   A prolonged seizure is a risk factor for further prolonged attacks

○   C   In most cases the seizure lasts 10–15 minutes

○   D   Rigorous attempts should be made to reduce the temperature with ibuprofen and/or paracetamol

○   E   Seizures do not occur until the fever is apparent

14.8 Hip pain

A 4-year-old boy with no history of note comes to see you with a 24-hour history of pain in his right hip and refusal to weight bear. His temperature is 38°C. When you examine him he will not move his hip but there are no signs if bruising and no rash. The single most likely diagnosis is:

○   A   Henoch–Schönlein purpura

○   B   Juvenile rheumatoid arthritis

○   C   Perthes' disease

○   D   Septic arthritis

○   E   Slipped upper femoral epiphysis

14.9 Childhood development

A health visitor asks you to see a 9-month-old child with regard to his development. Which one of the following statements about him would be of concern?

○ A He does not say 'mama' or 'dada'

○ B He first smiled at 8 weeks of age

○ C He has never crawled

○ D He is unable to pull himself up to stand

○ E He shows a preference for using his right hand

14.10 Henoch–Schönlein purpura

A 9-year-old boy has been given a diagnosis of Henoch–Schönlein purpura and has now had the rash for 2 weeks. With regard to his outpatient follow-up, which one of the following statements is most appropriate?

○ A The boy needs no further paediatric follow-up

○ B The boy needs to be followed up by the paediatric team until his rash has resolved

○ C The boy needs to be seen by an ophthalmologist and a paediatrician within 2 weeks

○ D The boy should be followed up by the paediatric team for at least 6 months after the rash has resolved

○ E The boy needs no follow-up now that he has had the rash for 2 weeks

14.11 Croup

A 14-month-old child is brought to see you out of hours with croup. It is 2am. The child started with symptoms 2 hours ago. He has a barking cough and stridor at rest. He has no other signs of respiratory distress. The single most appropriate course of action would be:

○ A Explain the diagnosis to parents and send him home with advice to return if he gets worse

○ B Give oral dexamethasone and send him home with advice to return if he gets worse

○ C Give oral dexamethasone and send him home with a further dose to be given in a further 12 hours

○ D Give oxygen and send to hospital in an ambulance

○ E Refer for paediatric assessment

14.12 Rash

The child in the photograph below attends the surgery. He has had a febrile illness for several days and today this rash has appeared. The child is now afebrile and well in himself.

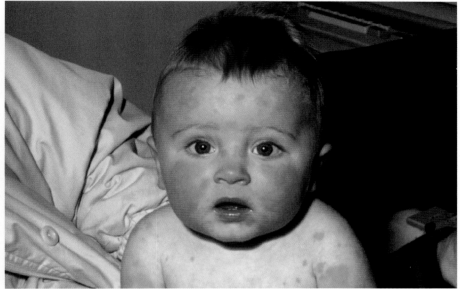

Credit: DR H.C. ROBINSON/ SCIENCE PHOTO LIBRARY

Which is the single most appropriate advice to give the family?

○   A   The child is at high risk of renal impairment over the next few days

○   B   The child is currently infectious and should not attend nursery

○   C   The child requires oral antibiotics

○   D   The disease is self-limiting and requires no treatment

○   E   The rash is very rare and might indicate an underlying problem with immunity

14.13 Unwell child

This 10-year-old boy attends the surgery. He has been unwell for 4 days, with a high fever, conjunctivitis, sore throat and harsh cough. He is lethargic. The rash started yesterday behind his ears and has now spread to his body. The child is normally well but it is noted that he has never received any immunisations.

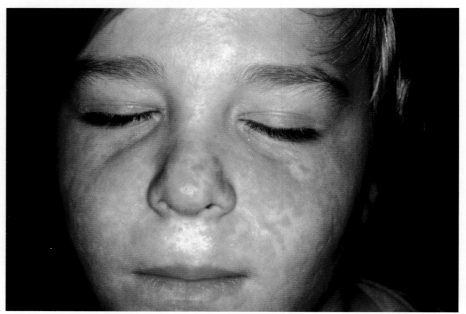

Credit: CNRI/SCIENCE PHOTO LIBRARY

What is the single most likely diagnosis?

○ A Measles

○ B Mumps

○ C Parvovirus

○ D Pertussis

○ E Rubella

14.14 Growth monitoring

A 9-week-old baby is brought to see you by his mother. She is concerned about the baby's feeding and feels that he has been unsettled and irritable for the last 5 days. He has started to vomit forcefully over the past 24 hours. You cannot find any abnormality on examination. The baby is thriving and height and weight are both on the 25th centile today. The boy's head circumference chart is shown below; the latest measurement is from today.

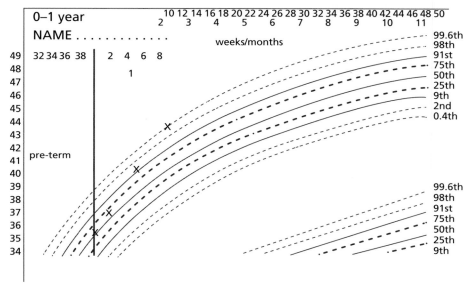

The single most appropriate action would be:

○   A   Ask the health visitor to review the child's head circumference in 1 week

○   B   Paediatric admission

○   C   Reassure mum that all is well

○   D   Review the child yourself in 1 week

○   E   Routine paediatric outpatient referral

EXTENDED MATCHING QUESTIONS

Vomiting

Options

A   Cows' milk protein intolerance
B   Gastroenteritis
C   Gastro-oesophageal reflux
D   Hiatus hernia
E   Hirschsprung's disease
F   Lactose intolerance
G   Overfeeding
H   Posseting
I   Pyloric stenosis
J   Reduced gastric motility

For each of the following clinical situations, choose the single most likely diagnosis from the list of options given above. Each option can be used once, more than once or not at all.

14.15   **A 1-week-old baby is brought by his mother. He was born at home. Mum is concerned that he is vomiting and not feeding well. On questioning, his mother tells you that she cannot remember her child opening his bowels. On examination, the child appears grey, and his abdomen is distended and firm. He vomits forcefully when you palpate his abdomen.**

14.16   **A 6-week-old baby is brought to see you with increasing vomiting. His mother reports that he feeds very well and is always hungry. Initially he vomited small amounts after some feeds. Over the last week, he has had large vomits after every feed. On examination, the baby is alert and hungry but appears to have lost weight.**

14.17   **A 6-week-old baby has a history of vomiting. His mother reports that from the age of 1 week her child has vomited after almost every feed. He is distressed when he vomits and if he is laid flat after a feed. He is thriving and examination is unremarkable.**

14.18   **A 6-week-old baby has a history of vomiting. His mother reports that he vomits after feeds, two or three times a day. He is described as a hungry baby. He takes 300 ml every 3 hours during the day, having seven feeds in 24 hours. His weight is above the 99th centile. Examination is otherwise unremarkable.**

Wheeze

Options

A   Anaphylaxis
B   Asthma
C   Bronchiolitis
D   Chronic lung disease
E   Croup
F   Cystic fibrosis
G   Foreign body inhalation
H   Primary ciliary dyskinesia
I   Recurrent aspiration
J   Virus-induced wheeze

For each of the following clinical situations, choose the single most likely diagnosis from the options given above. Each option can be used once, more than once or not at all.

14.19   A 2-year-old child is brought to see you with sudden onset of wheeze and shortness of breath. The symptoms started when the child was at nursery this morning. She has been otherwise well. There is no significant past medical or family history. On examination, she is distressed, with mild subcostal recession; there is an audible wheeze. On auscultation, you can hear wheeze on the right side of the chest, with good air entry throughout.

14.20   A 20-month-old boy is brought to see you with respiratory distress. He has been unwell for 2 days with a runny nose, cough and reduced feeding. He is normally fit and well. On examination, the child is coryzal and has a temperature of 38.1°C. His respiratory rate is 32/min, with mild subcostal recession. Wheeze can be heard throughout the chest with good air entry. He has a blanching maculopapular rash on his trunk.

14.21   A 22-month-old boy is brought to see you by his mother. They have recently moved to the area. His mother tells you that he often needs antibiotics for his chest and that this is why she has brought him in now. On examination, the child is small and thin (weight and height are on the 0.4th centile) with visible Harrison's sulci. He has mild subcostal recession. Wheeze can be heard throughout the chest.

14.22   A 6-week-old baby is brought to see you with breathing difficulties. She was born at 33 weeks' gestation and was discharged home 2 weeks ago. She has a 24-hour history of fast, noisy breathing and reduced feeding and the mother thinks that she might have stopped breathing just now in the waiting room. On examination, there is subcostal recession and wheeze is heard bilaterally.

Telephone triage

14.23–14.29

Your practice is planning to use a telephone triage process for assessment of unwell children. You decide to base this on the NICE guidance CG47 *Feverish Illness in Children*, based on red, amber and green features of the child's illness.

Complete the flowchart below from the list of options. Each option may be used once, more than once or not at all.

Options

A   999 ambulance
B   All features green
C   Amber features present
D   Any red features
E   Face-to-face assessment
F   Manage at home
G   No
H   Urgent face-to-face assessment
I   Yes

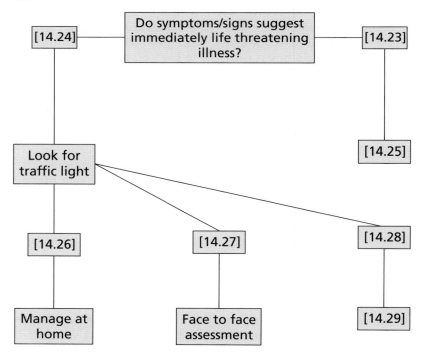

Vital signs

14.30–14.34

Options

A	10–15
B	20–25
C	25–35
D	60–90
E	60–100
F	90–120
G	95–140
H	110–160
I	110–180

Complete the table below of normal vital signs for children, from the list above. Each option may be used once, more than once or not at all.

Age (years)	Heart rate	Respiratory rate
<1	**14.30**	30–40
1–2	100–150	**14.31**
2–5	**14.32**	25–30
5–12	80–120	**14.33**
>12	**14.34**	15–20

Vesicular rash in children

14.35–14.42

Options

A   Central dimple
B   Contact with disease
C   Crops of lesions
D   Face and hands
E   Limbs
F   May be seriously ill
G   No
H   Trunk
I   Yellow crusting
J   Yes

Complete the table below from the list of options listed above.

	Fever	Malaise	Distribution	Pruritus?	Features
Chickenpox	Mild to moderate	Mild	Mainly truncal	Yes	**14.35** **14.36**
Dermatitis herpetiformis	No	No	**14.37**	**14.38**	Sporadic cases
Eczema herpeticum	Moderate to high	Moderate	In areas of eczema	**14.39**	**14.40**
Hand, foot and mouth disease	Mild	Mild	Palms, soles and inside mouth	No	Minor epidemics
Impetigo	No	No	Face and hands	Yes	Vesicles replaced by **14.41**
Molluscum contagiosum	Nil	Nil	Variable	No	Pearly vesicles with **14.42**

FREE TEXT QUESTION

14.43 **Paracetamol dose in babies**

You see a child for his 8-week check. He is due to have his first course of vaccinations the next day and his mother asks you if he can take paracetamol if he gets a fever. In the box below, write the appropriate dose in milligrams, if any, that you would advise.

SINGLE BEST ANSWER

14.1   A: Admit under the on-call paediatrician

Spontaneous nosebleeds in infants are very rare and this presentation raises concerns over clotting disorders or non-accidental injury. Assessment by a paediatrician will rule out organic causes and allow assessment of possible abuse. Vitamin K-deficient bleeding would be unusual in a bottle-fed baby.

14.2   D: Refer to ophthalmology outpatients

Loss of red reflex can be a sign of congenital cataract or retinoblastoma. Congenital cataract is more likely than retinoblastoma in bilateral cases, although this can be bilateral. Causes of congenital cataract include maternal infection (eg rubella, varicella), hypercalcaemia, Down syndrome, myotonic dystrophy and Alport syndrome. Correction at an early age is necessary to avoid amblyopia.

14.3   C: Kawasaki's disease can cause myocardial infarction

Kawasaki's disease is a vasculitis of unknown origin. It causes a febrile illness in children aged under 5 years that is characterised by fever, polymorphous rash, cervical lymphadenopathy, conjunctival injection, and erythematous desquamation of the hands and feet. Up to a third of untreated patients will develop coronary artery stenosis and aneurysms, and these can lead to myocardial infarction. Treatment is with intravenous immunoglobulin and aspirin and, if aneurysms are found, this treatment should be lifelong. The mortality rate in the UK is <5%.

14.4   A: Drug or alcohol abuse

Risk factors for successful suicide after an episode of deliberate self-harm can be classified as relating to either the current episode or the background of the patient. Factors relating to the current episode that indicate high risk include efforts to avoid being found, planning, use of a dangerous method and refusal of help. Patients who have drug and/or alcohol problems, underlying mental illness or personality disorders, patients who are socially isolated or who have had previous episodes of deliberate self-harm, and older males are higher risk. Between 1% and 2% of patients who deliberately self-harm will be dead within 12 months, and 50% of those who die from suicide have taken a non-fatal overdose previously.

14.5   C: A 14-year-old boy who has lost 10 kg since becoming a vegan

Risk factors for eating disorders include late-onset or irregular periods, seeking advice on weight loss when the BMI is normal, signs of vomiting or laxative abuse, and poor compliance with insulin treatment in people with diabetes and vague gastrointestinal symptoms and poor growth. At least 10% of patients with eating disorders are male, although these are often under-diagnosed. The SCOFF questionnaire might be useful:

- Do you make yourself sick when you feel uncomfortably full?
- Do you fear that you have lost control over how much you eat?
- Have you lost more than 1 stone over a 3-month period?
- Do you believe yourself to be fat when others say you are thin?
- Would you say that food dominates your life?

A score >2 indicates a likely case of bulimia or anorexia.

14.6   B: Hirschsprung's disease

Hirschsprung's disease is caused by lack of parasympathetic innervations to a segment of bowel. It often presents as failure to pass meconium but in 6% of cases the infant will pass meconium, and go on to develop chronic constipation. Stools are often liquid and there is frequently failure to thrive. Treatment usually involves resection of the affected portion of bowel. Hypothyroidism is a cause of chronic constipation, as is cystic fibrosis, but these would normally be picked up by the neonatal screening programme. Anal fissure is associated with passage of hard stools accompanied by fresh blood and pain.

14.7   B: A prolonged seizure is a risk factor for further prolonged attacks

A clinical review of febrile seizures in children was published in the *British Medical Journal* in 2007. Seizures can occur before the fever is apparent and can occur early or late in the course of the febrile illness. The fever is usually at least 38°C. In 87% of cases the seizure lasts less than 10 minutes and only 30% of children have recurrent febrile seizures during subsequent illnesses. Rigorous attempts to reduce the temperature with paracetamol or ibuprofen are not recommended because there is no evidence that this decreases recurrence of seizures. Parents should be reassured. Febrile status epilepticus occurs in 5% of affected children and a prolonged seizure is a risk factor for further prolonged attacks.

14.8   D: Septic arthritis

The features of refusal to weight bear and fever warrant immediate referral to rule out septic arthritis. Transient synovitis ('irritable hip') can also present in this way but is a diagnosis of exclusion. Slipped upper femoral epiphysis and Perthes' disease both affect older children. Acute myeloid leukaemia and Henoch–Schönlein purpura can both present with bone and joint pain, but it would be unusual for there to be no other features.

14.9   E: He shows a preference for using his right hand

It is abnormal to show a hand preference before 18 months of age and this can indicate an underlying neurological problem such as cerebral palsy. Other warning signs at the 8-month developmental assessment include persistence of primitive reflexes (such as moro, stepping, grasp), fisting, squint, or parental concern about vision or hearing.

14.10   D: The boy should be followed up by the paediatric team for at least 6 months after the rash has resolved

Henoch–Schönlein purpura is a vasculitic disorder of unknown aetiology. The diagnosis is made clinically on the basis of a characteristic purpuric rash on the lower limbs and buttocks. The disease can affect many systems, most typically causing abdominal pain (which can be due to intussusception) and joint pain and swelling. Rare complications include seizures and strokes. The most common serious complication is renal disease. This occurs in 60% of cases and can progress to end-stage renal failure (1–2% of cases). Renal involvement can occur up to 6 months after the rash has disappeared. All children with Henoch–Schönlein purpura therefore require paediatric follow-up involving urine dipstick and BP monitoring for at least 6 months.

14.11   E: Refer for paediatric assessment

This child has acute laryngotracheobronchitis (croup). The presence of stridor at rest indicates that this child requires acute paediatric assessment and at least a period of observation in hospital. Treatment is with oral dexamethasone or nebulised budesonide. Clinical features that suggest at least moderate croup (requiring assessment and treatment in hospital) include: stridor at rest, subcostal recession, tachypnoea or altered conscious level/irritability. Cyanosis is a very late sign and is usually preceded by a period of significant respiratory distress.

14.12   D: The disease is self-limiting and requires no treatment

This child has fifth disease, also known as 'slapped cheek disease'. It is caused by parvovirus B19 and commonly affects children between the ages of 4 and 12 years.

The infectious period is 4–20 days before the appearance of the rash. The illness usually consists of a mild febrile illness with the development of a characteristic 'slapped cheek' rash. The child is usually very well, although the rash can be dramatic. Infection with parvovirus B19 is associated with miscarriage in woman who are <20 weeks pregnant, so he should be kept away from pregnant women.

14.13   A: Measles

This child has measles, which is a notifiable disease. It is highly infectious from 14 days before the rash appears to 5 days after the onset of the rash. Children are usually unwell, with a high fever. The rash usually starts on the face on day 3 or 4 of the illness, and spreads downwards. Koplik's spots are present before the onset of the rash and are consequently seen only rarely. There is no specific treatment for measles, although complications might require treatment. The illness usually lasts for 7–10 days and most children recover well. Serious complications include pneumonia, seizures, encephalitis, deafness, long-term neurological impairment and, in some cases, death.

14.14   B: Paediatric admission

This child has a rapidly increasing head circumference and symptoms of raised intracranial pressure. He needs to be seen urgently by a paediatrician. Physical signs associated with raised intracranial pressure in a baby can include dilated scalp veins, 'sun-setting' eyes and a bulging fontanelle, although these are usually late signs. A child should have a paediatric assessment if the head circumference crosses two centile lines, or is greater than the 98th centile and not in proportion with height and weight measurements. Children should be seen urgently if there is a rapid change in head circumference or associated physical symptoms or signs.

EXTENDED MATCHING ANSWERS

Vomiting

14.15   E: Hirschsprung's disease

Classically this presents in the neonatal period with failure to pass meconium within 24 hours and features of obstruction. It is caused by aganglionosis of the distal bowel. If only a small segment of large bowel is affected children can present several years later with chronic constipation. Diagnosis is made by rectal biopsy.

14.16   I: Pyloric stenosis

Caused by hypertrophy of the pyloric sphincter. Classically presents at 6 weeks with a preceding history of worsening vomiting as the pylorus becomes increasingly hypertrophied with use. Babies usually feed very well and are very hungry. Weight loss can be dramatic. Management includes stopping feeds, correction of electrolyte imbalance and surgical correction. The prognosis is very good.

14.17   C: Gastro-oesophageal reflux

Common in infancy, due to relatively poor muscle tone. Symptoms improve with age. This is due to stronger muscle tone, introduction of dietary solids and a more upright posture for the baby. In severe cases there can be failure to thrive and feeding aversion because of the distress associated with feeds. There are several management options:

- Keeping the child upright (no proven benefit)
- Propping up the head of the bed (no proven benefit)
- Thickening agents (proven benefit)
- Antacids, eg Gaviscon (no proven benefit)
- Ranitidine (proven benefit)
- Omeprazole and domperidone, often used but not licensed.

14.18   G: Overfeeding

Full-term babies normally require 150 ml/kg per day of milk. Particularly hungry babies might need more than this to settle them but volumes >200 ml/kg per day are not recommended. Overfeeding is common and often results in vomiting.

Wheeze

14.19   G: Foreign body inhalation

A sudden onset of respiratory distress in a child of 18 months to 3 years should raise the suspicion of an inhaled foreign body. If there is a suggestive history and/or unilateral clinical signs it is an important diagnosis to rule out. Urgent paediatric assessment is required.

14.20   J: Virus-induced wheeze

Many children aged <3 years wheeze with viral infections. No treatment is usually necessary. A trial of salbutamol via inhaler and spacer can be given to children aged >1 year if respiratory distress is severe or if there is a strong family history of atopy.

14.21   F: Cystic fibrosis

Recurrent lower respiratory tract infections and poor weight gain warrant further investigation. The most likely diagnosis in the white population is cystic fibrosis. Other pathologies such as immunodeficiencies, congenital lung abnormalities and rarer causes of bronchiectasis such as primary ciliary dyskinesia should be considered if cystic fibrosis testing is negative.

14.22   C: Bronchiolitis

Bronchiolitis is a viral illness affecting infants aged <1 year. It is predominantly caused by respiratory syncytial virus (RSV). Clinical features include respiratory distress, wheeze, coryzal symptoms, low-grade temperature and reduced feeding. Treatment is supportive. Those under the age of 2 months, ex-premature babies and those with existing pathology (eg cardiac disease) are at particular risk and can develop apnoeas. Paluvizumab, a monoclonal antibody against RSV, is now available, although it is very expensive. It is currently offered to premature babies with significant lung disease and to some children with cardiac problems.

Telephone triage

14.23	I:	Yes
14.24	G:	No
14.25	A:	999 ambulance
14.26	B:	All features green
14.27	C:	Amber features present
14.28	D:	Any red features
14.29	H.:	Urgent face-to-face assessment

Vital signs

14.30	H:	110–160
14.31	C:	25–35
14.32	G:	95–140
14.33	B:	20–25
14.34	E:	60–100

Age (years)	Heart rate	Respiratory rate
<1	110–160	30–40
1–2	100–150	25–35
2–5	95–140	25–30
5–12	80–120	20–25
>12	60–100	15–20

Vesicular rash in children

14.35	B:	Contact with disease
14.36	C:	Crops of lesions
14.37	D:	Face and hands
14.38	J:	Yes
14.39	J:	Yes
14.40	F:	May be seriously ill
14.41	I:	Yellow crusting
14.42	A:	Central dimple

	Fever	Malaise	Distribution	Pruritis?	Features
Chickenpox	Mild to moderate	Mild	Mainly truncal	Yes	Contact with disease Crops of lesions
Dermatitis herpetiformis	No	No	Face and hands	Yes	Sporadic cases
Eczema herpeticum	Moderate to high	Moderate	In areas of eczema	Yes	May be seriously ill
Hand, foot and mouth disease	Mild	Mild	Palms, soles and inside mouth	No	Minor epidemics
Impetigo	No	No	Face and hands	Yes	Vesicles replaced by yellow crusting
Molluscum contagiosum	Nil	Nil	Variable	No	Pearly vesicles with central dimple

FREE TEXT ANSWER

14.43   60 mg

Paracetamol is not licensed for regular use until after 3 months but a dose of 60 mg may be used for post-immunisation from 2 months.

Chapter 15
Renal

SINGLE BEST ANSWER QUESTIONS

15.1 Renal colic
A 37-year-old man with a history of renal calculi asks for a home visit for a severe attack of colic. He has tried some paracetamol and codeine but vomited. On examination he is flushed and tachycardic, and has tenderness in his right loin area. Urinalysis is strongly positive for blood. His blood pressure is 100/70 mmHg and his temperature is 37.6°C. Which one of the following would be the single most appropriate option in his management at this point?

- A Hospital admission
- B Intramuscular diclofenac 75 mg stat and review in 2 hours
- C Intramuscular morphine 2.5 mg stat and review in 2 hours
- D Oral morphine sulphate 10–20 mg 3 hourly and review if no better
- E Rectal diclofenac 100 mg stat and review if no better

15.2 Proteinuria
A 41-year-old woman sees the practice nurse complaining of urinary frequency and mild discomfort. Her mid-stream urine is dipped and recorded as positive for blood and nitrites, with protein strongly positive. Her blood pressure is normal. How would you manage her? Select one option only.

- A Carry out a 24-hour urine collection
- B Refer to a renal clinic
- C Send urine for albumin:creatinine ratio
- D Treat underlying urinary tract infection and repeat urinalysis in 2 weeks
- E Treat underlying urinary tract infection with instructions to return if symptoms recur

15.3 Renal side effects
Which one of the following statements is correct regarding the effect of analgesics on renal function?

○ A NSAIDs are safe if used on an as required basis only

○ B Co-prescription of ACE inhibitors or ARBs is associated with reduced risk of NSAID-associated acute kidney injury

○ C Dual therapy with ACE Inhibitors or ARBs and diuretics significantly increases susceptibility to NSAID-associated renal damage

○ D Risk of NSAID-associated renal damage increases with duration of use beyond 30 days

○ E Sustained-release NSAID preparations are associated with lower risk of renal damage than standard preparations.

15.4 Polycystic kidneys
One of your patients is in her second pregnancy and has just had a growth scan at 30 weeks which has shown that her baby has polycystic kidneys. She has researched this on the internet and is worried that her 6-year-old son will have inherited the condition. She comes to see you to discuss this situation. Which one of the following statements is true with regard to this situation?

○ A Childhood polycystic kidney disease is inherited as an autosomal recessive trait

○ B Many patients with polycystic kidneys are asymptomatic

○ C She can be reassured that infantile polycystic kidney disease is always present on prenatal ultrasound and so her other child will not be affected

○ D She should be advised that her other child has a 50% chance of being affected

○ E With medical treatment from an early age most children have a normal life expectancy

15.5 Chronic renal impairment
You see a 69-year-old man with diabetes for his annual review. He was noted to have stage 3 chronic renal impairment 2 years ago and, although his estimated glomerular filtration rate (eGFR) has been stable, his haemoglobin has dropped over that period to 10.1 g/dl. He has had a colonoscopy and gastroscopy, and been told that his anaemia is due to his chronic renal impairment. According to NICE guidelines, which one of the following statements about his management is correct?

○ A Anaemia in chronic renal disease is usually macrocytic, so folic acid should be prescribed

○ B He should be referred for erythropoietin injections

○   C   He should have regular blood transfusions

○   D   No treatment is necessary as long as his haemoglobin is >10 g/dl

○   E   Oral iron supplements should be prescribed

15.6 Urinary tract infection

A 67-year-old man comes to see you with his third proteus urinary tract infection in 3 months. These infections seem to settle down with antibiotics but he does report that he gets a persistent ache in his back between attacks, and often notices blood in his urine. Clinical examination is unremarkable apart from microscopic haematuria. Urine cytology is positive for blood but shows no atypical cells. You arrange an ultrasound scan, which shows unilateral hydronephrosis. What is the single most likely diagnosis?

○   A   Chronic renal failure

○   B   Prostatic enlargement

○   C   Schistosomiasis

○   D   Ureteric calculus

○   E   Urethral valves

15.7 Dysuria

A 19-year-old man has had perineal pain for the past 3 days and has developed a fever. He also describes dysuria. On rectal examination he is found to have a tender, boggy prostate gland. Which one of the following actions is the most appropriate next step?

○   A   An HIV test should be organised as soon as possible

○   B   A urine sample should be obtained for culture

○   C   Antibiotics should be started only after any culture results have been received

○   D   Rectal tissue should be swabbed and sent to the laboratory

○   E   The prostate should be massaged to obtain prostatic fluid for culture

15.8 Urinary tract infection

Which one of the following symptoms suggests upper urinary tract infection in women?

○   A   Fever

○   B   Haematuria

○   C   Pain on passing urine

○   D   Urinary frequency

○   E   Urinary urgency

15.9 Renal calculi

Which one of the following microorganisms is most likely to be associated with struvite (mixed infective) renal calculi?

○   A   *Candida albicans*

○   B   Enterococci

○   C   *Escherichia coli*

○   D   *Proteus* sp.

○   E   Streptococci

15.10 Monitoring renal function

A 78-year-old man comes to see you for his annual check-up. He has been treated for hypertension for some years and it has always been well controlled. On checking his BP you find the systolic persistently raised >170 mmHg. You arrange for some blood tests, which show a reduced eGFR. An ECG is normal and urine dipstick testing is negative for protein. Reviewing his records there seems to have been something of a decrease in his eGFR over the last 2 years. He is otherwise well, apart from some nocturia, dribbling and poor flow, which he feels is normal at his age. A graph showing his recent eGFR results is shown on the following page.

Which one of the following is the most appropriate action at this point?

○   A   Introduce a calcium antagonist to improve BP control

○   B   Refer for renal ultrasound

○   C   Refer to cardiology for advice on further antihypertensive treatment

○   D   Start finasteride

○   E   Start ramipril and repeat renal function test in 1 week

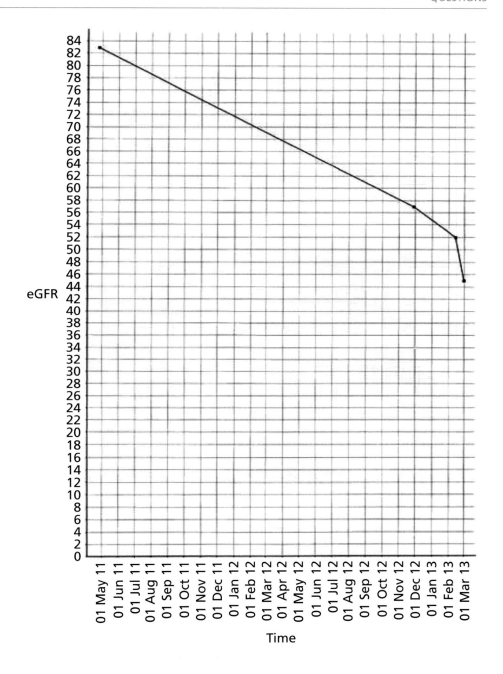

15.11 Discoloured urine

A 74-year-old man with no previous history of note complains of discoloured urine for the last 2 days. He has no other urinary symptoms and does not take any regular medications. His urine specimen is shown below.

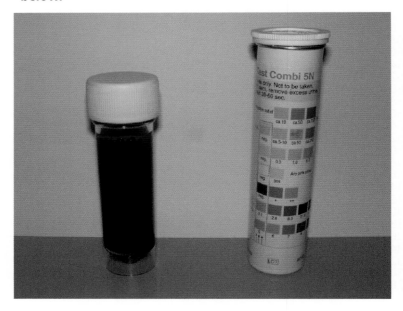

Which one of the following is the most appropriate initial stage in his management?

    A   Check platelet levels and prothrombin time

    B   Refer for plain KUB (kidneys, ureters and bladder) X-ray

    C   Refer under 2-week rule

    D   Start trimethoprim pending results of culture

    E   Treat with fluids and NSAIDs and refer for outpatient intravenous urogram

EXTENDED MATCHING QUESTIONS

Loin pain

Options

A   Adrenal cortical necrosis
B   Aortic aneurysm
C   Polycystic kidneys
D   Pelviureteric junction obstruction
E   Pyelonephritis
F   Renal adenocarcinoma
G   Renal haemangioma
H   Renal vein thrombosis
I   Retroperitoneal haemorrhage
J   Ureteric calculus

For each of the scenarios below, select the most appropriate diagnosis from the list above. Each option can be used once, more than once or not at all.

15.12   A 56-year-old man on long-term warfarin therapy after prosthetic heart valve replacement complains of right-sided back pain, hip weakness and malaise for the past week. He has a pulse of 110 beats/min, and a BP of 110/80 mmHg.

15.13   A 48-year-old man presents with a 3-month history of intermittent haematuria and discomfort in the left loin. A mass is palpable in the left upper quadrant.

15.14   A 30-year-old woman presents with acute right-sided loin pain, which comes in waves and radiates to her groin, with vomiting. Abdominal examination is negative and urinalysis shows microscopic haematuria.

15.15   A 67-year-old man presents with sudden-onset, severe left loin pain that is radiating to the left groin, with nausea and dizziness. He has a pulse of 136 beats/min and a BP of 90/60 mmHg.

The management of chronic renal impairment in primary care

15.16–15.20

Options

A Aim for BP <125/75 mmHg
B Aim for BP <130/80 mmHg
C Aim for BP <140/80 mmHg
D Aim for BP <150/90 mmHg
E Check phosphate levels
F Check urine for protein
G eGFR < 15 ml/min
H eGFR < 30 ml/min
I eGFR 30–60 ml/min
J eGFR > 60 ml/min
K eGFR > 90 ml/min
L Refer to renal physician

Complete the following algorithm, which describes the management of chronic renal impairment in primary care, from the list of options above (CKD is chronic kidney disease). Each option can be used once, more than once or not at all.

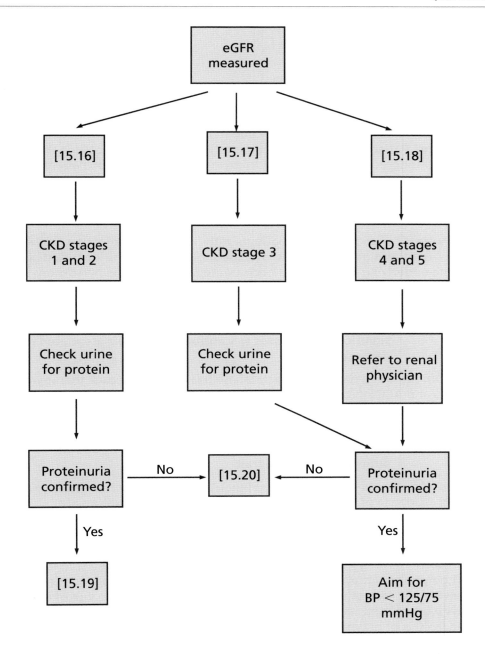

SINGLE BEST ANSWER

15.1   A: Hospital admission

Although most patients with renal colic can be managed at home with oral or rectal analgesics and NSAIDs, patients with symptoms or signs or urinary sepsis should be admitted as an emergency due to a high risk of overwhelming sepsis developing. Patients in whom the diagnosis of renal colic is uncertain should also be considered for admission, eg to exclude aortic aneurysm. Patients managed at home should have urgent outpatient imaging.

15.2   D: Treat underlying urinary tract infection and repeat urinalysis in 2 weeks

Proteinuria is commonly seen in patients with urinary tract infection. In the absence of other signs of renal disease, she should have her urine tested again once the underlying infection has been treated. If proteinuria persists on dipstick she should have a sample sent for albumin:creatinine ratio and be tested for diabetes. If this is raised she should be referred to a renal clinic.

15.3   C: Dual therapy with ACE inhibitors or ARBs and diuretics significantly increases susceptibility to NSAID-associated renal damage.

Data from the UK general practice database has shown that dual therapy with diuretics and ACE inhibitors/ARBs increases the risk of acute kidney injury by 31%, and the effect is most marked (twofold) in the first 30 days. Monotherapy with ACE inhibitors/ARBs does not increase risk compared with NSAIDs alone.

15.4   A: Childhood polycystic kidney disease is inherited as an autosomal recessive trait

Childhood polycystic kidney disease is inherited as an autosomal recessive trait, with an incidence of 1 in 40 000. Most children with the condition are diagnosed antenatally with ultrasound but, less commonly, they can present later in childhood with an abdominal mass. Prognosis is poor, with renal transplantation the only realistic option for most patients. There are often associated hepatic cysts and subsequent portal hypertension and splenomegaly. Adult polycystic kidney disease is inherited as an autosomal dominant trait. It is less severe but 45% of patients will develop renal failure by the age of 60. It is always bilateral and can be associated with liver cysts; berry aneurysms are found in 40% of patients with the adult form of the condition.

15.5   B: He should be referred for erythropoietin injections

NICE guidelines say that a target haemoglobin of between 10.5 g/dl and 12.5 g/dl is ideal, and patients should be referred to the renal anaemia team if their haemoglobin is <11 g/dl. If patients have low iron stores, supplementary iron might be needed and this is usually in the form of parenteral supplements. Folate supplements are not necessary unless there is coexistent folate deficiency (eg due to poor diet or alcoholism).

15.6   D: Ureteric calculus

Renal tract calculi cause different symptoms depending on their anatomical location. Lower ureteric stones can impact at the vesicoureteric junction and cause hydronephrosis. Other significant causes to consider in this case are tumour of the bladder or ureter. Prostatic hypertrophy (either benign or malignant) and urethral strictures can cause bilateral hydronephrosis. Proteus infections are associated with renal tract calculi. Schistosomiasis is a common cause of haematuria in north Africa but is not common in the UK.

15.7   B: A urine sample should be obtained for culture

This patient has symptoms consistent with acute prostatitis. Fever, arthralgia, low abdominal or perineal pain, and a urethral discharge are all common symptoms. Diagnosis is made by urine culture. Prostatic massage should be avoided because it can allow the infection to disseminate, and will be painful for the patient. Treatment with quinolone antibiotics is usually effective.

15.8   A: Fever

Lower urinary tract infections (cystitis) in women are common. Symptoms include pain on passing urine, urinary frequency and urgency, haematuria and suprapubic pain. Three days of antibiotic treatment is usually indicated in these patients. Upper urinary tract infections (pyelonephritis) cause fever, flank pain, nausea or vomiting. Urine should be sent for culture and antibiotic treatment is usually indicated for at least 7 days. Women who are systemically unwell might need admission to hospital.

15.9   D: *Proteus* sp.

Renal calculi are common, affecting approximately 2% of the UK population, although most are asymptomatic. Symptomatic patients often present with severe, colicky abdominal pain that causes difficulty lying still. The pain often radiates to the testes or labia; haematuria is also a common feature. Most calculi are composed of calcium oxalate or calcium phosphate. Around 15–20% of renal calculi are known as 'mixed infective' or 'struvite' calculi. They are associated with chronic urinary tract infection. These calculi are composed of magnesium ammonium phosphate. Urease-producing bacteria break down urea to form this compound. *Proteus* and *Klebsiella* spp. produce urease enzyme and are common causes of struvite calculi.

15.10   B: Refer for renal ultrasound

Unexplained deterioration in eGFR or an unexpected change in the BP should prompt a search for causes of secondary hypertension. This patient had an enlarged prostate causing bladder outflow obstruction and progressive hydronephrosis. Management of the hydronephrosis followed by treatment of the prostatism restored renal function to normal.

15.11   C: Refer under 2-week rule

This history is suspicious of a renal tract tumour. The lack of dysuria and frequency makes urinary tract infection unlikely and renal stones would normally cause colic. Clot retention from a bleeding lesion can cause colicky pain in patients with malignancies but the absence of colic makes a stone unlikely. Haematuria is very common in patients on warfarin and a drug history should be taken. The most likely site of a lesion in this instance is the bladder, and small lesions are not visible on plain X-ray or ultrasound.

EXTENDED MATCHING ANSWERS

Loin pain

15.12   I: Retroperitoneal haemorrhage

Poorly controlled anticoagulant therapy results in bleeding into the renal and gastrointestinal tracts. Retroperitoneal bleeding is uncommon and can present as hip weakness due to femoral nerve paresis. A retroperitoneal haematoma might be palpable over the psoas.

15.13   F: Renal adenocarcinoma

Renal cell carcinoma is usually of insidious onset. Loin pain occurs when the renal capsule is stretched or invaded, and haematuria occurs when the tumour erodes into the pelvicalyceal system.

15.14   J: Ureteric calculus

Ureteric colic from calculus obstruction can present as an acute abdomen with normal serum inflammatory markers and amylase. There is usually microscopic haematuria.

15.15   B: Aortic aneurysm

A leaking abdominal aortic aneurysm can present as left loin pain radiating to the groin and can be mistaken for ureteric calculus obstruction. There might be guarding/rigidity and a pulsatile mass is sometimes present. An absent or diminished femoral pulse on that side with early signs of hypovolaemia should point to an impending catastrophe.

The management of chronic renal impairment in primary care

15.16   J: eGFR >60 ml/min

15.17   I: eGFR 30–60 ml/min

15.18   H   eGFR <30 ml/min

15.19   A: Aim for BP <125/75 mmHg

15.20   B: Aim for BP <130/80 mmHg

Chapter 16 Reproductive: male and female

SINGLE BEST ANSWER QUESTIONS

16.1 **Management of menorrhagia**
What is the most effective non-surgical management strategy for menorrhagia?

○ A Combined oral contraceptive pill

○ B Mirena (levonorgestrel intrauterine system)

○ C Depo-Provera

○ D Progesterone-only pill

○ E Tranexamic acid

16.2 **Contraception**
A 26-year-old woman who recently had an ectopic pregnancy treated with laparoscopic salpingectomy visits her GP to discuss contraception. She is keen to try for a baby again but feels that she should leave this for 6 months to get over the operation. Which one of the following is the most appropriate contraceptive method for her?

○ A Barrier method

○ B Combined oral contraceptive (COC) pills

○ C Copper intrauterine contraceptive device (IUCD)

○ D Depo-Provera

○ E Mirena coil

16.3 Subfertility
Which one of the following statements about the cause of subfertility is true?

○   A   A cause is found after standard investigations in only 30% of cases

○   B   Endometriosis is found in about 25% of cases

○   C   Ovulatory failure accounts for about 20% of cases

○   D   Sperm defects are found in about 5% of couples

○   E   Tubal damage is the most common cause in women

16.4 Cervical screening
A 25-year-old woman recently diagnosed with HIV after donating blood attends for her first smear. She is a non-smoker and is otherwise fit. With regard to cervical screening, which of the following is correct in this case? Select one option only.

○   A   Cervical smear 3-yearly

○   B   Cervical smear yearly

○   C   Colposcopy and smear every 3 years

○   D   HPV vaccination and 3-yearly cervical smears

○   E   Initial colposcopy and yearly cervical smears

16.5 Contraception
A 15-year-old girl is attending with her 16-year-old boyfriend for contraceptive advice. She has been poorly compliant with the combined oral contraceptive in the past due to difficulty in taking it without her parents discovering. She is Gillick competent, medically fit and has no significant family history. Which one of the following contraceptives is the least appropriate for this patient?

○   A   Combined pills

○   B   Contraceptive patches

○   C   Depo-Provera

○   D   Implant

○   E   IUCD

16.6 Pyuria

A 40-year-old woman has recently emigrated to the UK from Asia. At her new patient check she reports that she has recently lost weight and feels tired. She is found to have leukocytes in her urine which persist despite antibiotic treatment. There is no significant bacterial growth on two consecutive urine cultures. What diagnosis do you suspect? Select one option only.

○ A Bladder carcinoma

○ B Bladder stones

○ C Contamination from vaginal discharge

○ D Interstitial cystitis

○ E Tuberculosis

16.7 Urethritis

Non-gonococcal urethritis may result from infection with which one of the following organisms?

○ A Bifidobacteria

○ B *Chlamydia psittaci*

○ C *Mycobacterium bovis*

○ D *Mycoplasma hominis*

○ E *Ureaplasma urealyticum*

16.8 Dysuria

A 45-year-old businessman complains of dysuria and discharge after returning from a business trip to Berlin. A swab confirms chlamydial infection but tests for other sexually transmitted infections are negative. What is the single most appropriate treatment for this condition?

○ A Azithromycin

○ B Benzylpenicillin

○ C Ciprofloxacin

○ D Fluconazole

○ E Trimethoprim

16.9 Amenorrhoea

A 30-year-old woman complains of several weeks of headaches. On further questioning she admits to secondary amenorrhoea of 12 months' duration. She has had an X-ray performed (shown below) which was reported as showing enlargement of the pituitary fossa.

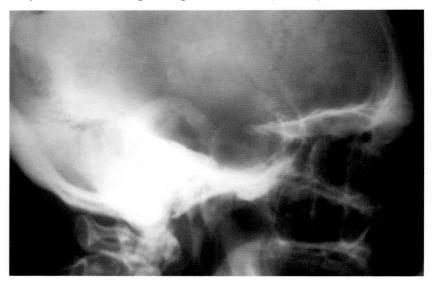

Which one of the following is the single most likely diagnosis?

- ○ A Cysticercosis
- ○ B Glioma
- ○ C Prolactinoma
- ○ D Sarcoidosis
- ○ E Tuberculosis

16.10 Interpretation of antenatal blood results

A 28-year-old primip who is 32 weeks pregnant complains of epigastric pain, nausea and pedal oedema. Her BP is 140/90 mmHg and her urine is showing 2+ of proteins. She feels unwell. Blood tests are taken, the results of which are shown below:

Haemoglobin	10.0 g/dl
Haematocrit	0.35
WCC	$12 \times 10^9/l$
Platelets	$95 \times 10^9/l$
Bilirubin	20 µmol/l
ALP	250 U/l
ALT	76 U/l
Protein	6.6 g/l
LDH	550 U/l
Amylase	35 U/l
Creatinine	60 µmol/l
Urea	4.0 mmol/l
Uric acid	442 µmol/l
Na^+	141 mmol/l
K^+	3.5 mmol/l
Glucose	5 mmol/l

Which one of the following is the single most likely diagnosis?

A   Acute liver failure

B   Cholecystitis

C   Fatty liver

D   HELLP syndrome

E   Renal failure

EXTENDED MATCHING QUESTIONS

Menstrual symptoms

Options

A *Agnus castus*
B Evening primrose oil
C Hysterectomy
D Hysterectomy with bilateral salpingo-oophorectomy
E Progesterone on days 14–25
F Referral to a gynaecologist for a trial of gonadotrophin-releasing hormone analogue
G SSRI on days 14–25 of the menstrual cycle
H Symptom diary
I Vitamin B$_6$

Select the most appropriate plan of management for the women with following presenting symptoms. Each option can be used once, more than once or not at all.

16.11 **A 35-year-old woman presents for the first time with bloating, breast pain and premenstrual headache.**

16.12 **A 40-year-old woman who is currently on Cerazette for symptoms of premenstrual syndrome, and who feels out of control, with mood swings, tension and irritability affecting her life.**

16.13 **The above-mentioned woman, after trying two different treatments, demands to have a hysterectomy.**

16.14 **A 45-year-old woman with a symptom diary suggestive of premenstrual syndrome but who wants to try natural treatment.**

16.15 **A 40-year-old woman with premenstrual breast tenderness requests non-hormonal treatment.**

Emergency contraception

Options

A Barrier contraception
B Barrier contraception for 7 days + emergency contraception
C Continue combined oral contraceptive and barrier contraception for 7 days
D Depo-Provera
E Offer IUCD
F Pregnancy test followed by emergency contraception (levonorgestrel) and screen for sexually transmitted infections (STIs)
G Reassurance
H Screen for STIs, emergency contraception (levonorgestrel) and barrier contraception for next 7 days
I Sterilisation

Please choose the best management option for the each of the women described in the scenarios below with regard to emergency contraception. Each option can be used once, more than once or not at all.

16.16 A 20-year-old student requests emergency contraception. She had unprotected sexual intercourse after a night out with friends 2 days ago. She does not remember when her last period was but thinks that it was about 3 months ago. She assures you that she has had no other unprotected sexual intercourse since her last period.

16.17 A weight-conscious, married mother of three, whose last child was born only 3 months ago, does not wish to have any further children. She reports a burst condom 24 hours ago, and requests emergency contraception and long-term family planning advice.

16.18 A 17-year-old girl had unplanned sex last night with a stranger. Her last period was 7 days ago. She is on the progesterone-only pill and she took her last pill 36 hours ago.

16.19 A 27-year-old married woman whose last period was 15 days ago is on a combined contraceptive pill. She forgot to take her last pill (which was due 12 hours ago) and had sex 3 hours ago.

16.20 A 30-year-old married woman on the COC pill has had an episode of diarrhoea and vomiting for the last 3 days. Her last period was 9 days ago. She has not had sex since being ill but wonders if it is safe to do so.

Gynaecological emergencies

Options

A Appendicitis
B Complete miscarriage
C Constipation
D Ectopic pregnancy
E Endometriosis
F Ovarian hyperstimulation
G Ovarian torsion
H Pelvic inflammatory disease
I Retroverted uterus
J Syncopal attack
K Threatened miscarriage
L Urinary tract infection

For each of the following scenarios, select the most appropriate diagnosis from the list of options above. Each option can be used once, more than once or not at all.

16.21 A woman who is 8 weeks into her first pregnancy and who had a small fresh vaginal bleed 2 days ago now presents with brownish loss. Her ultrasound scan performed in the early pregnancy assessment clinic 2 days ago showed an intrauterine gestational sac with a normal fetal heart.

16.22 A 20-year-old woman attends the out-of-hours treatment centre with abdominal pain and having fainted. Her last period was 5 weeks ago. Her urine pregnancy test is positive, her blood pressure is 70/40 mmHg and her pulse is 120 beats/min.

16.23 An 18-year-old presents with right iliac fossa pain, diarrhoea and a temperature of 38°C. Vaginal examination reveals slight tenderness on the right side with no palpable masses. She is tender in the right iliac fossa with guarding.

16.24 A 35-year-old being treated for infertility had embryo transfer 5 days ago. She now complains of feeling unwell and breathless. Abdominal examination shows distension and dullness to percussion in the flanks.

16.25 A 20-year-old primip presents with urinary retention. She also complains of tenderness in her loins. Urine dipstick testing is positive for protein. A booking scan 2 weeks ago showed a normal 12-week fetus.

Menopausal symptoms

16.26–16.31

Options

A   12 months postmenopause
B   Continue
C   Continuous combined estrogen/progestogen
D   Lifestyle advice
E   Estrogen only
F   Previous hysterectomy
G   Sequential estrogen/progestogen

Complete the flowchart below for the management of menopausal symptoms, using the list if options above. Each option may be used once, more than once or not at all.

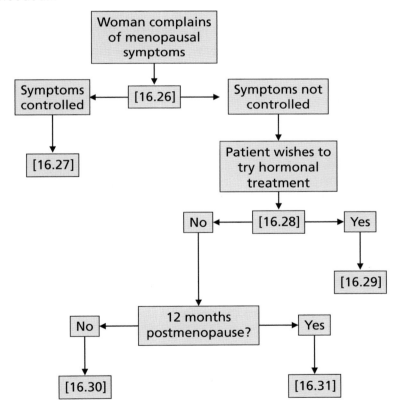

SINGLE BEST ANSWER

16.1   B: Mirena (levonorgestrel intrauterine system)

This has been shown in a 2-year RCT to be superior to pharmacological treatment with a drop-out rate half of that seen in conventional drug treatment, in patients with menorrhagia (ECLIPSE Study, *New England Journal of Medicine* 2013).

16.2   B: Combined oral contraceptive (COC) pills

IUCDs are not advisable for short-term contraception, and there is a theoretical increased risk of ectopic pregnancy. Depo-Provera is associated with secondary amenorrhoea and can cause delayed return to fertility. Barrier methods are less effective than the combined pill but can be useful if the contraceptive pill is contraindicated.

16.3   C: Ovulatory failure accounts for about 20% of cases

The main causes of infertility are shown below (remember that some couples can have more than one cause):

- Unexplained – 30%
- Sperm defects – 25%
- Ovulatory failure – 20%
- Tubal damage – 15%
- Other – 10%
- Endometriosis – 5%
- Mucus defects – 5%
- Other male problems – 2%
- Coital failure – 2%

16.4   E: Initial colposcopy and yearly cervical smears

HIV-positive patients are at increased risk of developing cervical intraepithelial neoplasia (CIN) and they can progress rapidly from CIN to cervical cancer. It is important to counsel these women adequately regarding the need for initial colposcopy and yearly cervical smears thereafter.

16.5   E: IUCD

Depot injection is useful for short-term use in teenagers, particularly those who have been poorly compliant in the past with oral medication. It is not suitable for long-term use due to effects on bone density. An IUCD would be difficult to fit in nulliparous woman, although is sometimes inserted at the time of termination of pregnancy.

16.6   E: Tuberculosis

Persistent pyuria with negative cultures in a woman from a high-prevalence area should raise the suspicion of tuberculosis. Carcinoma and stones would present with haematuria and can increase the risk of a UTI but cultures would be positive.

16.7   E: *Ureaplasma urealyticum*

Chlamydia trachomatis accounts for up to half of cases of non-specific urethritis. In the remainder, *Ureaplasma urealyticum* and *Mycoplasma genitalium* are pathogens, whereas *Mycoplasma hominis* is not. Bifidobacteria are commensal faecal organisms. *Mycobacterium bovis* causes infection in cattle and *Chlamydia psittaci* causes psittacosis.

16.8   A: Azithromycin

Often patients are infected with more than one pathogen at a time and consideration should be given to treating accordingly. *Chlamydia* sp. is sensitive to doxycycline and azithromycin. Any partners should be treated at the same time, as untreated chlamydia infection can cause infertility in females by damaging the fallopian tubes. Aciclovir is a treatment for herpes; benzylpenicillin can be used to treat syphilis or gonorrhoea. A high index of suspicion for other sexually transmitted infections should prompt screening for co-infection, including HIV. Ciprofloxacin is useful for the management of gonorrhoea but resistance is becoming a problem in some areas of the UK.

16.9   C: Prolactinoma

Enlargement of the pituitary fossa suggests the diagnosis of prolactinoma. Other symptoms could include subfertility and galactorrhoea. A glioma would not normally cause amenorrhoea and would not show on a plain X-ray. Cysticercosis can cause central nervous system lesions but these are visible on computed tomography, not on a plain X-ray.

16.10   D: HELLP syndrome

HELLP syndrome (**h**aemolysis, **e**levated **l**iver enzymes, **l**ow **p**latelets) is the diagnosis in this patient. The raised LDH and ALT, low platelets and raised bilirubin indicate the need for urgent action. Patients with pre-eclampsia can have this syndrome with even mild elevation of blood pressure. This patient should be delivered after being started on magnesium sulphate because, if it is left untreated, it is associated with high mortality rates.

EXTENDED MATCHING ANSWERS

Premenstrual syndrome (PMS)

16.11	H:	Symptom diary
16.12	G:	SSRI on days 14–25 of the menstrual cycle
16.13	F:	Referral to a gynaecologist for a trial of gonadotrophin-releasing hormone analogue
16.14	A:	*Agnus castus*
16.15	B:	Evening primrose oil

For confirmation of a diagnosis of premenstrual syndrome it is essential to keep a symptom diary for 3 months before starting any medical or surgical treatment. SSRIs are effective for psychological symptoms related to PMS. A trial of a gonadotrophin-releasing hormone analogue should be considered before hysterectomy. *Agnus castus* has been found to be effective for PMS symptoms in randomised controlled trials.

Emergency contraception

16.16	F:	Pregnancy test followed by emergency contraception (levonorgestrel) and screen for STIs
16.17	E:	Offer IUCD

This is the most suitable long-term option in this case.

16.18	H:	Screen for STIs, emergency contraception (levonorgestrel) and barrier contraception for next 7 days

Patients missing one or more progesterone pills will need emergency contraception and 7 days of additional cover with barrier contraception, and should also be advised on future barrier contraception use along with pills.

16.19	G:	Reassurance

Patients on the combined pill who forget their pill can take it up to 12 hours late without problems. If pills are more than 24 hours late or where antibiotics are being taken, the 7-day rule needs to be applied, with barrier precautions for 7 days.

16.20	C:	Continue COC and use barrier contraception for 7 days

Gynaecological emergencies

16.21	K:	Threatened miscarriage
16.22	D:	Ectopic pregnancy

Any female with vaginal bleeding or symptoms of internal bleeding and a positive pregnancy test should be considered to have an ectopic pregnancy until proven otherwise.

16.23   **A:**   **Appendicitis**

16.24   **F:**   **Ovarian hyperstimulation**

Ovarian hyperstimulation can present with pleural effusions and ascites.

16.25   **I:**   **Retroverted uterus**

Menopausal symptoms

16.26   **D:**   **Lifestyle advice**

16.27   **B:**   **Continue**

16.28   **F:**   **Previous hysterectomy**

16.29   **E:**   **Estrogen only**

16.30   **G:**   **Sequential estrogen/progestogen**

16.31   **C:**   **Continuous combined estrogen/progestogen**

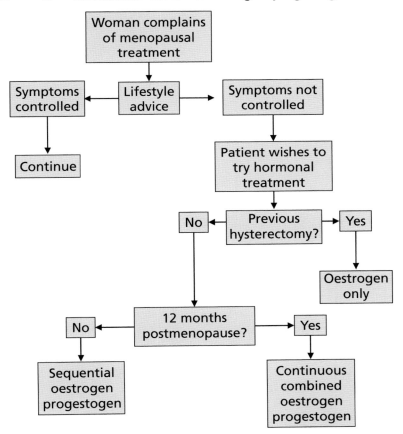

Chapter 17
Respiratory

SINGLE BEST ANSWER QUESTIONS

17.1   H1N1 prophylaxis
Your practice is updating its management plan for potential epidemics of swine flu in line with recent World Health Organization guidance. Which one of the following groups are considered at high risk and should be offered antiviral treatment in the event of developing a flu-like illness in an outbreak?

○   A   Adults aged >50 years

○   B   Adults aged >60 years

○   C   Children aged <12 years old

○   D   Healthcare workers

○   E   Pregnant women

17.2   Fibrosing alveolitis
A 57-year-old man is newly diagnosed with cryptogenic fibrosing alveolitis. He comes to see you to discuss his condition and asks about his prognosis. Which one of the following statements is correct with regard to this issue?

○   A   He has a significantly increased risk of developing lung cancer

○   B   Most patients do not experience any functional limitation

○   C   The majority of patients respond to treatment

○   D   The mean life expectancy from diagnosis is 6 months

○   E   Treatment should be aimed at the underlying cause

17.3 Chest tightness
A 24-year-old woman complains of intermittent chest tightness and wheeze over the past 3 months. Her symptoms have been getting worse and are troublesome at night. She smokes cigarettes socially. She has a past history of hay fever. Her respiratory examination is normal. What is the next best action? Select one option only.

- A Ask her to keep a diary of her symptoms and review her in 2 weeks

- B Issue her a prescription for a salbutamol metered-dose inhaler and arrange a review in 2 weeks

- C Refer her to the hospital as an outpatient for a chest X-ray

- D Show her how to use a peak flowmeter and request that she keeps a record of morning and evening readings for 1 week, then come for review

- E Show her how to use a peak flowmeter and request that she keeps a record of morning and evening readings for 2 weeks, then come for review

17.4 Sleep apnoea
A 40-year-old man has recently been diagnosed with mild obstructive sleep apnoea. He works as a handyman for a local school and part-time as a taxi driver. He attends for review. Which one of the following is the single most appropriate course of action?

- A Advise that he need not inform his car insurance company of his diagnosis as his obstructive sleep apnoea is mild

- B Ensure that he has been told verbally and in writing that he must inform the Driver and Vehicle Licensing Agency (DVLA) of the diagnosis

- C Inform him that for now he should not work as a taxi driver. He might be able do so in the future provided that he has no daytime sleepiness over the following month

- D Inform him that he has a legal obligation to inform the school that he has obstructive sleep apnoea and will not be able to operate machinery until further notice

- E Inform him that he is likely to require nasal CPAP treatment overnight

17.5 Hoarseness
A 42-year-old man who is an ex-smoker complains of right shoulder pain and hoarseness for 4 weeks. Examination of his shoulder reveals a normal range of movement. His chest is clear, he is not breathless and he has no lymphadenopathy. His voice is hoarse. He does not have finger clubbing. The single most appropriate course of action is:

○ A   Organise a chest physician to review him urgently as an outpatient

○ B   Organise an urgent cervical spine X-ray

○ C   Organise an urgent chest X-ray

○ D   Organise a routine chest X-ray

○ E   Organise a routine X-ray of his shoulder and review with results

17.6   Acute breathlessness
The practice nurse asks you to urgently assess a teenager who is in the waiting room. He has a history of asthma. On examination, his respiratory rate is 30/min with prolonged expiration; he cannot complete sentences on talking to you, is tachycardic and has wheeze heard throughout his chest. What is the single most appropriate course of action, given the following options?

○ A   Give 5 mg salbutamol via oxygen-driven nebuliser and send home if he feels completely back to normal

○ B   Give oxygen via facemask at 10 l/min and call an ambulance

○ C   Give six puffs of salbutamol via a spacer and if the patient starts to improve send him home with a 5-day course of prednisolone

○ D   Give salbutamol nebuliser and prednisolone 40 mg orally; arrange hospital assessment

○ E   Give 10 puffs of salbutamol and 10 puffs of ipratropium; arrange a review the next day with the asthma nurse

17.7   Respiratory emergencies
A 14-year-old boy is rushed into the surgery by his mother with sudden-onset abdominal pain and vomiting, and an urticarial skin rash. On examination, you note that he is very breathless with both stridor and wheeze. His lips and tongue are swollen. From the following options, what is the most appropriate initial drug management? Select one option only

○ A   Administer nebulised 1 in 1000 adrenaline, 2 ml via oxygen-driven nebuliser

○ B   Administer oxygen and give 1 in 1000 adrenaline, 0.1 ml intravenously

○ C   Administer oxygen and give 1 in 1000 adrenaline, 0.5 ml intramuscularly

○ D   Administer oxygen and give 10 puffs of salbutamol via a spacer

○ E   Give nebulised salbutamol 5 mg via oxygen-driven nebuliser

17.8 Drug treatment of COPD

Your practice holds a clinic for the treatment of patients with known COPD. Some patients who are reviewed find that they are still symptomatic despite taking single short-acting bronchodilators. According to NICE guidelines, what would the most appropriate next treatment option be? Select one option only.

○ A A 4-week trial of combination long-acting β agonist and inhaled corticosteroid

○ B Combined therapy of current short-acting β agonist and theophylline

○ C Long-acting bronchodilator (β agonist or anticholinergic)

○ D Mucolytic therapy to reduce the incidence of dry cough

○ E Oxygen therapy via nasal cannulae at 2 l/min for 15 hours each day

17.9 Chest X-ray

This 64-year-old man has had a productive cough, shortness of breath and intermittent fever for the past week. He is a non-smoker. He has had a chest X-ray and this is the AP film:

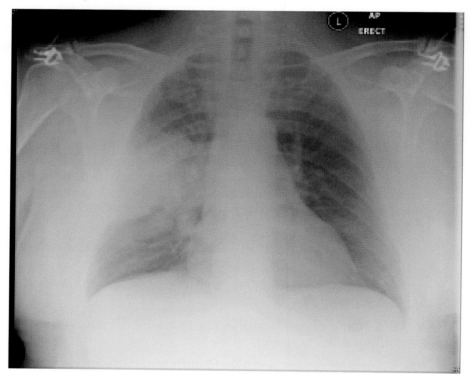

What is the most likely diagnosis? Select one option only.

○ A Foreign body aspiration

○ B Pneumonia

○ C Pneumothorax

○ D Pulmonary oedema

○ E Upper respiratory tract infection

17.10 Treatment of COPD
This 72-year-old woman has COPD. She has severe hypoxaemia (PaO_2 <7.3 kPa) and receives treatment at home using the machine shown below.

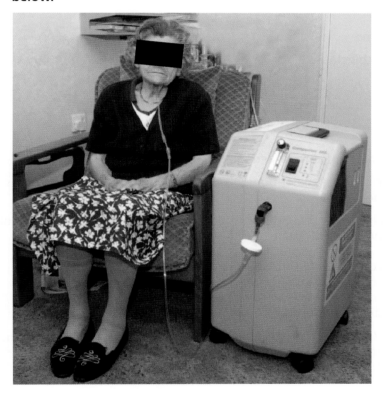

To benefit from this treatment, she should use it for a prolonged period each day. What minimum treatment duration is required each day to significantly reduce mortality rates in COPD? Select one option only.

○ A 8 hours

○ B 12 hours

○ C 15 hours

○ D 18 hours

○ E 22 hours

17.11 Spirometry

A 45-year-old woman presents with increasing exertional breathlessness over the past 6 months. She has scleroderma. Spirometry shows:

	Measured	Predicted
FVC (litres)	1.98	3.51
FEV$_1$ (litres)	1.64	2.82
FEV$_1$/FVC	83%	80%

FEV$_1$ = forced expiratory volume in 1 second; FVC = forced vital capacity.

Which of the following is the most likely diagnosis? Select one option only.

A Asthma

B Bronchiectasis

C Extrinsic allergic alveolitis

D Pulmonary fibrosis

E Tracheal stenosis

17.12 Management of chronic asthma

Select the rank order of the options (1–4) that best fulfils the requirements given in the question.

The following is a list of management steps in chronic asthma (1–4) for adults and children over 5 years of age:

1 Addition of inhaled corticosteroid
2 Addition of long-acting β agonist
3 Addition of regular oral steroids
4 Bronchodilator as needed

The responses (A–E) rank the management steps in chronic asthma in various orders. Select the response that places the options (1–4) in the order of **early** management first to **advanced** management last.

Select one rank order only.

A: 1, 2, 3, 4

B: 2, 1, 3, 4

C: 4, 3, 1, 2

D: 4, 1, 2, 3

E: 3, 1, 2, 4

EXTENDED MATCHING QUESTIONS

Shortness of breath

Options

A   Bronchial carcinoma
B   Bronchiolitis
C   COPD
D   Croup
E   Metastatic lung disease
F   Pneumonia
G   Pneumothorax
H   Pleural effusion
I   Pleurisy
J   Upper respiratory tract infection

Choose the most likely diagnosis for each patient described below from the list of options above. Each option can be used once, more than once, or not at all.

17.13   A 78-year-old man presents with cough, dyspnoea and weight loss over the past month. He has recent-onset haemoptysis and his nail beds appear spongy. He smokes regularly. On examination, his respiratory rate is 18/min at rest and he has crackles affecting his right lung.

17.14   A 55-year-old man has had a productive cough for the past 3 days. He has right-sided chest pain and feels short of breath. He is a non-smoker. On examination, his respiratory rate is 20/min at rest. Right low chest percussion is dull and he has inspiratory right lower zone crackles. His temperature is 38.5°C.

17.15   A 60-year-old woman complains of a dry cough and sore throat for the past 3 days. She says that she feels breathless for a short while after coughing. She smokes 10 cigarettes a day. On examination, her oropharynx looks injected, her respiratory rate is 14/min, her BP 150/90 mmHg and her pulse 70 beats/min. Her chest is clear to auscultation and she is apyrexial. She has had no previous chest problems.

17.16   A man asks to see one of the nurses at your practice to get a 'cough bottle'. On further questioning, he tells the nurse that he has had a productive cough intermittently for the past 4 years. He is in his late 40s. At present, he smokes cigars regularly and experiences shortness of breath when dressing or walking more than 100 yards on the flat. His weight is steady. He sometimes wheezes on exertion.

17.17   A 6-month-old baby is seen at a general practice with a 3-day history of shortness of breath, reduced feeding and cough. On examination, the child has a respiratory rate of 30/min and his chest examination reveals bilateral coarse inspiratory crepitations. He is afebrile.

Assessment of airflow obstruction in COPD

17.18–17.22

Options

A   Cough and sputum production common
B   Evening cough and sputum production problematic
C   50–80% predicted
D   50–70% predicted
E   33–49% predicted
F   30–49% predicted
G   <33% predicted
H   <30% predicted
I   Severe dyspnoea on minimal exertion
J   Severe dyspnoea prevents even minimal exertion

The following flow chart has been adapted from NICE guidance on classifying COPD.

For each stage of the flow chart, select the most appropriate option from the list above for measured FEV_1 and likely symptomatology. Each option can be used once, more than once or not at all.

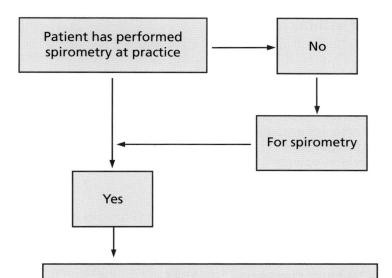

Mild airflow obstruction FEV$_1$ [17.18] predicted.
Moderate airflow obstruction FEV$_1$ [17.19] predicted.
Severe airflow obstruction FEV$_1$ [17.20] predicted.

Mild
- Little or no clinical signs usual at rest
- Morning cough

Moderate
- Dyspnoea on moderate exertion
- [17.21]

Severe
- [17.22]
- Productive cough and wheezing
- Life-threatening exacerbations

Management of asthma

17.23–17.29

Options

A   Inhaled steroid 200–800 µg/day
B   Inhaled steroid up to 2000 µg/day
C   Leukotriene receptor antagonist
D   Long-acting β_2 agonist
E   Refer for specialist opinion
F   Short-acting β_2 agonist as needed
G   Sustained-release theophylline

Complete the table below describing the stepwise approach to managing chronic asthma in primary care, using the list of options above. Each option may be used once, more than once or not at all.

Step 1	Intermittent mild symptoms	**17.23**
Step 2	Regular preventive treatment	Add in **17.24**
Step 3	Add-on treatment	Consider adding **17.25** if no improvement after 12-week trial of **17.26**
Step 4	Failure to control at step 3	Trial of **17.27** if no improvement after 12-week increase **17.28**
Step 5	Regular use of rescue oral steroids despite step 4	**17.29**

SINGLE BEST ANSWER

17.1   E: Pregnant women

The WHO advice prompt treatment of over-65s, under-5s, nursing home residents, pregnant women, patients with co-morbidity, and those with severe and progressive illness.

17.2   A: He has a significantly increased risk of developing lung cancer

Patients with cryptogenic fibrosing alveolitis have a 10-fold increased risk of developing lung cancer. Overall, the prognosis is poor, with only a small proportion responding to treatment and a 5-year survival rate of 40–50%. In most cases a cause cannot be identified and, where steroids and immunosuppression do not work, lung transplantation might be an option. For most patients, however, treatment is symptomatic, with oxygen when necessary.

17.3   E: Show her how to use a peak flowmeter and request that she keeps a record of morning and evening readings for 2 weeks, then come for review

The history is suggestive of asthma and her past history of hay fever suggests atopy, supporting the diagnosis. A 20% or greater diurnal variation in peak flow on 3 days a week for 2 weeks is highly suggestive of asthma. She is unlikely to be able to use an inhaler effectively without training by a healthcare professional. The British Thoracic Society (BTS) guidelines recommend objective tests to confirm the diagnosis of asthma before starting long-term therapy.

17.4   B: Ensure that he has been told verbally and in writing that he must inform the DVLA of the diagnosis

The Scottish Intercollegiate Guidelines Network (SIGN) have produced guidelines for the investigation and management of obstructive sleep apnoea (OSA). OSA can lead to an increased risk of the sufferer having an accident due to sleepiness. It is an offence to fall asleep at the wheel of a car and custodial sentences can be imposed. Patients with OSA can present reporting daytime sleepiness, but can also present with non-specific symptoms such as irritability and poor concentration. The Epworth questionnaire has been used in patients with suspected OSA to measure pre-treatment sleepiness. Moderate-to-severe OSA is treated with nasal CPAP; weight loss should be encouraged in all patients. Patients should not drive if they report daytime sleepiness. Once diagnosed, patients should be told verbally and in writing that they must inform the DVLA. Those working with machinery or driving should be referred to a sleep centre for assessment.

17.5   C: Organise an urgent chest X-ray

The NICE guidelines for the diagnosis and management of suspected lung cancer suggest urgent referral for a chest X-ray in smokers and ex-smokers over the age of 40 with:

- Haemoptysis
- Persistent or unexplained (>3 weeks):
    - cough
    - chest/shoulder pain
    - weight loss
    - dyspnoea
    - chest signs
    - clubbing
    - hoarseness
    - cervical/supraclavicular lymphadenopathy
    - signs of metastatic disease.

17.6   D: Give salbutamol nebuliser and prednisolone 40 mg orally; arrange hospital assessment

The patient has features of acute severe asthma and warrants referral. Features of acute severe asthma include:

- Respiratory rate >25/min
- Inability to complete a sentence in one breath
- Pulse >110 beats/min
- Peak flow 33–50% of best or predicted.

High-flow oxygen should be administered if available. Salbutamol or terbutaline can be administered by spacer or nebuliser as available, with oxygen-driven nebuliser the preferred method. D was the best option out of those given.

17.7   C: Administer oxygen and give 1 in 1000 adrenaline, 0.5 ml intramuscularly

Gastrointestinal manifestations of anaphylaxis include abdominal pain and vomiting, and are more common in cases of food allergy. This child has signs of respiratory compromise and should be given intramuscular adrenaline and oxygen while an ambulance is called. An inhaled β_2 agonist might help if the bronchospasm does not respond to your initial treatment.

17.8   C: Long-acting bronchodilator (β agonist or anticholinergic)

NICE guidelines suggest that patients who are not controlled with a single short-acting bronchodilator can be started on a combination of two short-acting bronchodilators or a single long-acting bronchodilator. Mucolytic therapy is used in patients with chronic cough productive of sputum. Oxygen therapy, inhaled steroids and theophylline are all considered, but as later more invasive treatments.

17.9   B: Pneumonia

The X-ray shows consolidation within the right middle lobe and some patchy airspace consolidation adjacent to the horizontal fissure. The patient needs to be assessed using the CR B-65 scoring system and then treated at home or in hospital as appropriate.

17.10   C: 15 hours

This patient is receiving long-term oxygen therapy (LTOT) from an oxygen concentrator. NICE guidelines state that mortality is reduced in COPD patients with severe hypoxaemia (PaO_2 <7.3 kPa) who receive LTOT (evidence level A). Patients with a PaO_2 between 7.3 kPa and 8.0 kPa and one other risk factor are also likely to benefit from LTOT (evidence level D). Treatment with LTOT needs to be given for at least 15 hours each day to significantly reduce the mortality rate.

17.11   D: Pulmonary fibrosis

Lung involvement in scleroderma is common and ultimately up to 80% of patients with the condition will develop abnormal pulmonary function tests. The spirometry measurements show a restrictive pattern (FVC and FEV_1 spirometry measurements are reduced and the FEV_1:FVC ratio is normal).

17.12   D: 4, 1, 2, 3

Rank ordering: 4 Bronchodilator as needed; 1 Addition of inhaled corticosteroid; 2 Addition of long-acting β agonist; 3 Addition of regular oral steroids.

The stepwise approach for chronic asthma involves starting with bronchodilators as required, and then adding to that sequentially until control is established, with regular reviews and stepping down according to symptoms.

EXTENDED MATCHING ANSWERS

Shortness of breath

17.13   A: Bronchial carcinoma

The patient has shortness of breath, haemoptysis and early finger clubbing. Non-small-cell carcinoma presents with finger clubbing more often than small-cell carcinoma. He needs to be referred as an urgent outpatient.

17.14   F: Pneumonia

This 55-year-old has signs and symptoms consistent with right-sided pneumonia. His examination findings show that he should be managed in the community. He does not need further investigations such as a chest X-ray at present. A course of amoxicillin should be provided as long as he is not allergic to penicillins. The patient should be advised to rest and drink plenty of fluids.

17.15   **J:**   **Upper respiratory tract infection**

The patient's chest is clear and her respiratory examination shows only injection of her oropharynx, which is often present during upper respiratory infections. Her upper respiratory tract infection requires only symptomatic relief but she should have her BP rechecked and should be encouraged to attend smoking cessation services.

17.16   **C:**   **COPD**

This patient needs full investigation and management as he probably has COPD. If COPD is confirmed on further testing, he should stop smoking and is likely to need regular treatment to control his current symptoms.

17.17   **B:**   **Bronchiolitis**

Bronchiolitis affects babies aged <12 months. Infection with RSV is the most common cause. It classically presents with coryzal symptoms, increased work of breathing, cough and reduced feeding. Infants aged <2 months can present with a history of apnoeic episodes. Treatment is supportive; referral is required if fluid intake is reduced to less than two-thirds of normal or if the child is showing signs of respiratory distress.

Assessment of airflow obstruction in COPD

17.18   **C:**   **50–80% predicted**
17.19   **E:**   **33-49% predicted**
17.20   **G:**   **<33% predicted**
17.21   **A:**   **Cough and sputum production common**
17.22   **I:**   **Severe dyspnoea on minimal exertion**

Patients with COPD should undergo spirometry testing as part of their diagnosis and also on at least an annual basis. Mild COPD usually causes minimal symptoms, but progression to moderate and severe COPD markedly affects symptomatology. Continuing to smoke is the major cause of disease progression; patients should stop smoking to limit disease progression as soon as possible.

Management of asthma

17.23	**F:**	**Short-acting β₂ agonist as needed**
17.24	**A:**	**Inhaled steroid 200–800 μg/day**
17.25	**D:**	**Long-acting β₂ agonist**
17.26	**C:**	**Leukotriene receptor antagonist**
17.27	**G:**	**Sustained-release theophylline**
17.28	**B:**	**Inhaled steroid up to 2000 μg/day**
17.29	**E:**	**Refer for specialist opinion**

Step 1	Intermittent mild symptoms	Short-acting β_2 agonist as needed
Step 2	Regular preventive treatment	Add inhaled steroid 200–800 μg/day
Step 3	Add on treatment	Consider adding long-acting β_2 agonist, if no improvement after 12-week trial of leukotriene receptor antagonist
Step 4	Failure to control at step 3	Trial of sustained-release theophylline; if no improvement after 12 weeks, increase inhaled steroid up to 2000 μg/day
Step 5	Regular use of rescue oral steroids despite step 4	Refer for specialist opinion

Chapter 18
Therapeutic indications and adverse reactions

SINGLE BEST ANSWER QUESTIONS

18.1 Antidepressant safety
A 48-year-old man who has been taking citalopram for 18 months comes to see you concerned about media reports re the safety of this drug. Which one of the following statements is true with regard to the safety of this drug?

○ A Citalopram has been shown to cause hepatic impairment

○ B Citalopram has been shown to cause renal impairment

○ C Citalopram is associated with increased risk of suicide compared with other SSRIs

○ D Citalopram is associated with prolonged QT interval at higher doses

○ E Citalopram should not be used in patients aged >65

18.2 Constipation in palliative care
A 74-year-old woman currently in the local cottage hospital is taking morphine orally for bone pain from her myeloma. She has been constipated for 1 week despite enemas, Movicol and bisacodyl. She is in a great deal of discomfort. On examination she is constipated but there are no signs of bowel obstruction. Which one of the following would be appropriate in this situation?

○ A Change morphine to oxycodone/naloxone

○ B Fybogel

○ C Lactulose

○ D Methylnaltrexone

○ E Sodium picosulfate

18.3   Prescribing for children
With regard to the prescribing of medications to children, which one of the following statements is true?

○   A   Intramuscular injections are preferable to intravenous injections in small children because of the difficulty in achieving adequate cannulation

○   B   Quantities of medicine of <5 ml should be given by syringe rather than by spoon

○   C   The small quantity of sugar in medicine is unlikely to cause tooth decay

○   D   The use of unlicensed medications in children is strictly forbidden

○   E   To ensure compliance with unpalatable medicines, these should be mixed in with food (eg mashed potato)

18.4   Drug treatment of osteoporosis
With regard to drug treatments for osteoporosis, which one of the following statements is true?

○   A   Bisphosphonates can only be given either daily or weekly

○   B   Calcitonin is taken orally

○   C   Patients with poor dental hygiene should see their dentist before starting bisphosphonate therapy

○   D   Strontium is taken as a once-weekly preparation

○   E   Teriparatide can be used to prevent osteoporosis in those at high risk

18.5   Rash

A 78-year-old woman with dementia is brought to see you by her carer after he noticed a rash on her back. He thinks that she is on some medication for her dementia but is not sure what this is. The rash is shown below.

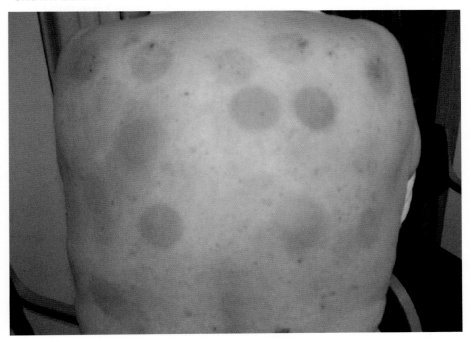

What is the most likely cause of her rash?

○   A   Contact dermatitis

○   B   Erythema multiforme

○   C   Erythema nodosum

○   D   Non-accidental injury

○   E   Shingles

18.6 Interpretation of lithium levels

A 67-year-old woman who suffers from bipolar disorder has been taking lithium for 6 months. She attends for routine blood tests and the following results are obtained:

Lithium	1.6 mmol/l (normal range 0.4–1.0 mmol/l)
Creatinine	112 μmol/l (normal range 60–110 μmol/l)
eGFR	57 ml/min per 1.73m²
TSH	5.3 mU/l (normal range 0.5–4.5 mU/l)
FT4	13 pmol/l (normal range 10–24 pmol/l)

What action should be taken?

○   A   Check compliance

○   B   Increase dose of lithium

○   C   Reduce dose of lithium

○   D   Start an ACE inhibitor for chronic renal impairment

○   E   Start levothyroxine 50 μg/day and repeat thyroid function in 3 months

18.7 Drug treatment of eczema

Select the rank order of the options (1–4) that best fulfils the requirements given in the question.
The following is a list of eczema treatment options:

○   1   Beclomethasone cream

○   2   Clobetasol cream

○   3   Hydrocortisone cream

○   4   Mometasone cream

The responses (A–E) rank the treatment options in various orders. Select the response that places the treatment options (1–4) in the order of potency, with the **weakest** cream first to the **strongest** cream last.

Select one rank order only.

○   A: 2, 3, 1, 4

○   B: 3, 1, 4, 2

○   C: 3, 1, 2, 4

○   D: 1, 3, 4, 2

○   E: 1, 3, 2, 4

EXTENDED MATCHING QUESTIONS

Side effects of antidepressants

Options

A   Citalopram
B   Duloxetine
C   Fluoxetine
D   Mirtazapine
E   Paroxetine
F   Sertraline
G   Venlafaxine
H   All of the above

For each of the statements below, select the most appropriate option from the list above. Each option may be used once, more than once or not at all.

18.8   Associated with the lowest incidence of sexual dysfunction.
18.9   Can cause severe discontinuation reactions.
18.10   Frequently causes sedation.
18.11   Associated with reduced risk of suicide in the over-25 age group.

Adverse drug reactions

Options

A Amiloride
B Amiodarone
C Azithromycin
D Bendroflumethiazide
E Colchicine
F Diclofenac
G Indometacin
H Methotrexate
I Prednisolone
J Sulfasalazine

For each of the scenarios described below, select the drug most likely to be responsible from the list above. Each option can be used once, more than once or not at all.

18.12 **A man who has inflammatory arthritis starts a new medication, but it has to be withdrawn promptly by the specialist when the patient develops a dry cough, fever and breathlessness.**

18.13 **A woman with rheumatoid arthritis starts taking a new daily medication but has to stop it after developing neutropenia.**

18.14 **A woman develops dizziness after starting a medication prescribed by her GP for an acutely swollen and painful metatarsophalangeal joint.**

18.15 **A patient develops severe diarrhoea after starting a medication prescribed for an acutely swollen and painful metatarsophalangeal joint.**

18.16 **A patient develops hypothyroidism 6 months after starting this new medication.**

Suspected adverse reaction

18.17–18.21

Options

A Black triangle drug
B Consider reporting
C No
D Paediatric drug
E Report under yellow card scheme
F Serious reaction
G Yes

The following flow chart illustrates the hierarchy of actions that should be taken in the event of a suspected adverse drug reaction.

For each of the numbered spaces in the flow chart, select the most appropriate option from the list above. Each option can be used once, more than once or not at all.

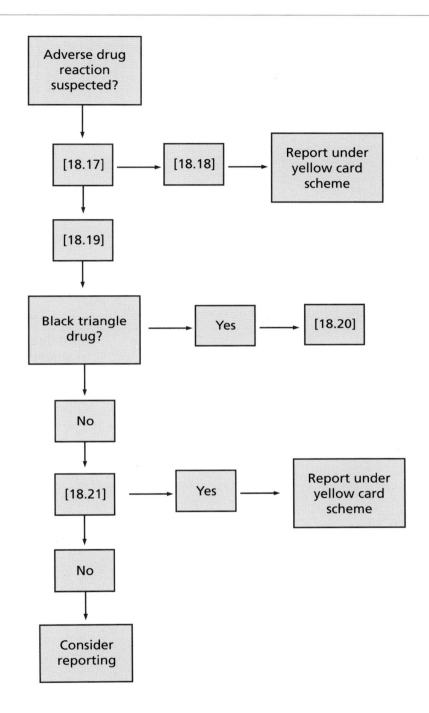

Management of diabetic neuropathy

18.22–18.26

Options

A   Amitriptyline
B   Carbamazepine
C   Duloxetine
D   Fentanyl
E   Gabapentin
F   Morphine
G   Pregabalin
H   Topical lidocaine
I   Tramadol
J   None of the above

Complete the table below describing the stepwise approach to the management of painful diabetic neuropathy, using the list of option above. Each option may be used once, more than once or not at all.

	First-line treatment	Second-line treatment	Third-line treatment
No contraindications	18.22	18.24	18.25
Alternative if contraindications	18.23		18.26

FREE TEXT QUESTIONS

18.27 Analgesic doses

A 76-year-old woman with chronic backache has been using Oramorph regularly but wishes to convert to a regular dose to minimise exacerbations of pain. She has in the past found that sustained-release morphine and oxycodone have made her nauseous. You decide to prescribe a fentanyl patch. What strength patch, in micrograms per hour, would be appropriate to use if her daily Oramorph consumption is 40 mg over 24 hours? Write your answer in the box below.

18.28 Travel advice

A 19-year-old man with no previous history of note comes to see you for advice about his forthcoming gap year trip. He is planning to trek to Everest base camp in Nepal and would like to take prophylaxis against altitude sickness. Which drug would you recommend? Write your answer in the box below.

18.29 Collapse

A 23-year-old temporary resident is brought to your local minor injury unit by a friend who tells you that he has stopped breathing. He does not give any more information, and quickly leaves. On examination the patient has pinpoint pupils, is unrousable and has a respiratory rate of 4. You cannot see any sign of a head injury but there are bruises in his right antecubital fossa. What drug would be appropriate to administer at this stage? Write your answer in the box below.

SINGLE BEST ANSWER

18.1   D: Citalopram is associated with prolonged QT interval at higher doses

Citalopram has a dose-dependent effect on QT interval and should not be used in patients taking other drugs that have the same effect, such as amiodarone. The maximum dose in those >65 or those with pre-existing heart disease is 20 mg (10 mg for escitalopram) and 40 mg for those <65 without heart disease. Patients with a history of heart disease should have an ECG and blood tests before starting treatment.

18.2   D: Methylnaltrexone

For severe opioid-induced constipation not responding to oral or rectal treatment, an injection of methylnaltrexone is often helpful. This is a peripherally acting opioid antagonist that reverses constipation without causing withdrawal or loss of analgesic affect. It is given parenterally and works within 30 minutes. Once the acute constipation has been dealt with, changing to oxycodone/naloxone might be effective in preventing recurrence but this can take 1–2 weeks for the bowels to return to normal. Co-prescription of Fybogel, lactulose and Movicol is often helpful in patients who wish to stay on morphine.

18.3   B: Quantities of medicine <5 ml should be given by syringe rather than by spoon

The *BNF for children* has a wealth of advice on prescribing for children. Unpalatable medicines can be mixed with small quantities of food but not with a large amount because of the risk of not taking the full dose, and the risk of developing an aversion to the food if there is an unpalatable taste. There is a risk of dental caries if frequent medication needs to be taken and sugar-free preparations should be used wherever possible. Many common medicines are unlicensed in children, but their use is acceptable where there is a body of evidence that it is appropriate to do so and the prescriber accepts the professional responsibility and potential liability.

18.4   C: Patients with poor dental hygiene should see their dentist before starting bisphosphonate therapy

Strontium is taken as an oral suspension, 2 g/day. It is useful in those who cannot tolerate bisphosphonates and promotes new bone growth as well as reducing resorption. Bisphosphonates are associated with osteonecrosis of the mandible and patients should have regular dental follow-up. Ibandronic acid is given monthly as an oral tablet or 3-monthly by intravenous infusion. Teriparatide is initiated by specialists and only in patients who are intolerant of bisphosphonates, or where these have failed to prevent a fracture and the patient has either extremely low bone mineral density or very low bone density, and has had fractures and risk factors such as low BMI. Calcitonin is taken as either an injection or a nasal spray.

18.5   A: Contact dermatitis

This woman is using rivastigmine patches and has had a reaction to the adhesive in the patch. This is a common side effect of patches and can be reduced by rotation of sites but, as shown here, this does not always prove effective. Changing the patient to oral treatment results in resolution. Patients should be warned about this side effect. With some drugs (eg transdermal buprenorphine) co-prescription of antihistamines is recommended initially.

18.6   C: Reduce dose of lithium

These blood tests show stage 3 chronic kidney disease and subclinical hypothyroidism with elevated lithium levels. Lithium is toxic to the thyroid and kidneys, and at higher dose causes increasing confusion, disorientation, hyperreflexia, and eventually convulsions and death. Regular monitoring of renal and thyroid function, together with lithium levels, is necessary in all patients.

18.7   B: 3, 1, 4, 2

Rank ordering: 3 Hydrocortisone cream; 1 Beclomethasone cream; 4 Mometasone cream; 2 Clobetasol cream

Eczema should be treated with the mildest treatment possible, to avoid steroid-related side effects. Treatment with potent and very potent steroids should be for short periods of 1–2 weeks at a time. Where this fails to control symptoms referral for systemic immunosuppressants should be considered.

EXTENDED MATCHING ANSWERS

Side effects of antidepressants

18.8   D: Mirtazapine

Mirtazapine is reported to cause sexual dysfunction in only 24% of patients, compared with 70–80% for selective serotonin reuptake inhibitors (SSRIs) and venlafaxine. Duloxetine is better than other SSRIs and serotonin and noradrenaline reuptake inhibitors (SNRIs), but still causes this side effect in 42% of patients.

18.9   E: Paroxetine

Antidepressants with a short half-life cause the most marked discontinuation effects. Typically these are venlafaxine and paroxetine, but paroxetine seems to be more commonly associated with this side effect, although it is possible with all of these medications.

18.10   D: Mirtazapine

Mirtazapine commonly causes sedation and weight gain, and can be helpful in patients with disturbed sleep.

18.11   H: All of the above

SSRIs and SNRIs increase the risk of suicide or attempted suicide in adolescents and young adults (relative risk, RR = 1.92) but reduce the risk in adults (RR = 0.57).

Adverse drug reactions

18.12   H: Methotrexate

Methotrexate can cause pneumonitis. This can be fatal and methotrexate needs to be withdrawn and corticosteroids administered under specialist supervision in hospital. Other side effects of methotrexate include pulmonary fibrosis and blood dyscrasias.

18.13   J: Sulfasalazine

Sulfasalazine is known to cause blood dyscrasias, including neutropenia, particularly in patients with rheumatoid arthritis. Methotrexate is also used in rheumatoid arthritis and can cause neutropenia, but is given weekly rather than daily.

18.14   G: Indometacin

This patient has arthritis affecting her metatarsophalangeal joint, the classic joint affected by gout. NSAIDs are used in the treatment of gout. Indometacin can cause dizziness as a side effect and the *BNF* recommends that patients are warned that this can affect the performance of skilled tasks (eg driving).

18.15   E: Colchicine

Colchicine is used in the treatment and prevention of gout. Nausea and vomiting and profuse diarrhoea are well-recognised side effects.

18.16   B: Amiodarone

Both hypo- and hyperthyroidism are recognised adverse effects of amiodarone treatment. Thyroid function tests should be performed before commencing treatment and after 6 months.

Suspected adverse reaction

18.17   F: Serious reaction

18.18   G: Yes

18.19   C: No

18.20   E: Report under yellow card scheme

18.21   D: Paediatric drug

Management of diabetic neuropathy

18.22	C:	Duloxetine
18.23	A:	Amitriptyline
18.24	G:	Pregabalin
18.25	I:	Tramadol
18.26	H:	Topical lidocaine

	First-line treatment	Second-line treatment	Third-line treatment
No contraindications Alternative if contraindications	Duloxetine Amitriptyline	Pregabalin	Tramadol Topical lidocaine

NICE guidance (CG96) on managing painful diabetic neuropathy suggests duloxetine as first line, unless contraindicated, in which case amitriptyline should be used. Second-line treatment should involve addition of pregabalin on its own or in combination with the first-line treatment. Failure to improve on maximally tolerated doses is usually an indication for specialist referral, but tramadol or topical lidocaine may be useful while specialist review is awaited. The guidelines suggest that strong opioids should not be used.

FREE TEXT ANSWERS

18.27   12 µg/h

When converting oral morphine to transdermal fentanyl the conversion rate is 45 mg oral morphine over 24 hours to 12 µg/h transdermal fentanyl. Transdermal fentanyl should never be used in opioid-naive patients due to risk of respiratory depression.

18.28   Acetazolamide

Acetazolamide 250 mg/day in divided doses is recommended for prophylaxis of acute mountain sickness, whereas a dose of 250 mg twice daily is used for treatment. An alternative where rapid ascent is needed and acetazolamide is not appropriate (eg sulphonamide allergy) would be dexamethasone, but the side-effect profile of dexamethasone makes it unsuitable for routine use.

18.29   Naloxone

This patient has symptoms and signs consistent with heroin overdose. Naloxone will bring about a rapid reversal if this is the case, but he should be observed for some time after giving it due to tendency to wear off and early relapse.

Chapter 19
Critical appraisal

SINGLE BEST ANSWER QUESTIONS

19.1 Statistical definitions
Which one of the following best describes the term 'external validity'?

○ A The agreement between two raters using the same test at the same time

○ B The consistency of a measure used on two separate occasions

○ C The extent to which one can appropriately apply the results to other populations

○ D The level of agreement between two or more raters using the same test on two or more separate occasions

○ E The level of consistency between two separate halves of the same test

19.2 Study design

You attend a lunchtime meeting sponsored by a drug company at which the drug company representative presents a novel treatment that has just been licensed for the treatment of osteoarthritis. He presents the following data comparing the new treatment (drug X) with standard treatment:

One hundred patients with rheumatoid arthritis were randomised to receive either drug X 400 mg once daily or ibuprofen 800 mg three times a day for a 4-week period. They were instructed to stop their existing treatment 3 weeks before the trial to allow for an adequate washout period. To avoid bias, the patients were not told whether they were taking ibuprofen or the new drug. Each group was given a questionnaire to fill in weekly regarding side effects and symptom control. In addition, the patients in the ibuprofen group were given a supplementary questionnaire on gastrointestinal side effects. The questionnaires were administered by a trained nurse to standardise responses.

Which one of the following statements is true with regard to this trial?

A   The study design is not blinded, so the results are not valid

B   The study population was appropriate for the drug's indication

C   The trial was a randomised, double-blind, placebo-controlled trial

D   The use of a trained nurse to administer the questionnaires in this way excluded reporting bias

E   This study supports the use of drug X in the management of osteoarthritis

19.3 Cohort study
Which one of the following study designs most accurately describes a cohort study?

A   A study that aims to establish the normal height of 4-year-old children by measuring heights at school entry

B   A study that compares a group of children whose heights are below the 10th centile with a group of matched controls of normal height, aiming to identify possible causative factors

C   A study that compares two groups of 4-year-olds with similar characteristics: one group is given a drug and the other a placebo, and the growth of each group is measured after this intervention

D   A study that compares the height of a group of 4-year-olds living near a nuclear plant with the height of a group of 4-year-olds who live elsewhere

E   A study that looks at all children born at one hospital in 1 year and measures their height at intervals up to 4 years of age

19.4 Critical appraisal

One of the doctors in your practice is an enthusiastic supporter of acupuncture for the treatment of chronic pain and wishes to introduce an acupuncture service into the practice. Unfortunately, however, the senior partner is of the opinion that this is mere quackery. After a search of the available information on the internet, a meta-analysis of acupuncture trials is identified to support the argument. The paper was published in the *Chinese Medical Journal* in 1997. It included all 256 trials that were published in peer-reviewed, Chinese-language journals between 1976 and 1996, and included trials of treatment for nausea, backache, migraine, abdominal pain and depression. Which one of the following statements is true with regard to the interpretation of this paper?

- A Meta-analysis of this type can be considered the gold standard of evidence-based medicine
- B The methodology of this paper is prone to bias
- C These results have been the subject of peer review and so can be assumed to be valid
- D This paper has followed the Cochrane Collaboration guidelines for meta-analysis
- E This paper includes a large number of trials and the findings therefore have high validity

19.5 Morbidity and mortality

You attend a presentation by the local public health team at which the data are presented on the top three causes of child deaths in your locality over the last 30 years. The data are presented below, with the most common cause of death first.

	1989	1999	2009
First	Trauma	Trauma	Neoplasm
Second	Infection	Neoplasm	Trauma
Third	Neoplasm	Infection	Infection

Which one of the following statements is correct with regard to these data?

- A No conclusions can be drawn on changes in incidence
- B The data confirm that child mortality is falling
- C The data suggest that the incidence of childhood cancer is increasing
- D The data suggest that the incidence of serious accidents is falling
- E The decrease in mortality from infection reflects increased immunisation coverage

19.6 Alcohol and mortality

Consider the graph below, which shows alcohol consumption and all-cause mortality.

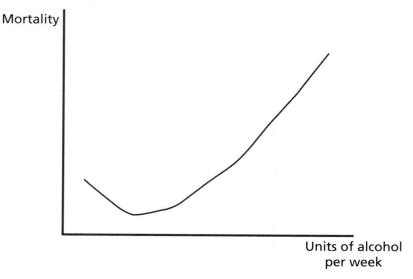

Which one of the following is a correct interpretation of this graph?

- ○ A Alcohol in moderate doses is beneficial to health
- ○ B Avoidance of alcohol is more dangerous than moderate consumption
- ○ C Heavy drinkers who reduce their alcohol consumption can reduce their risk of dying
- ○ D There is no question that high levels of alcohol consumption increase mortality
- ○ E These data demonstrate an association rather than a causal relationship

19.7 **Epidemiology**

The graph below shows the standardised (for age, sex and ethnic group) incidence ratios of three different cancers in patients followed up for 10 years after exposure to a potential carcinogen.

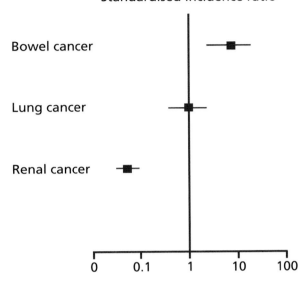

Standardised incidence ratio

Which one of the following statements is correct with regard to interpretation of these data?

- A The confidence intervals for all three cancers are wide so there might not be a true increase in incidence

- B The incidence of all three cancers is increased

- C The incidence of bowel cancer is increased, whereas the incidence of renal cancer is reduced

- D The incidence of renal cancer is increased, whereas the incidence of bowel cancer is reduced in this cohort of patients

- E These data confirm that the chemical causes cancer

19.8 Interpretation of symptom scores

After a 6-month pilot project to assess the impact of a nurse practitioner on the management of prostatic symptoms in primary care, the following results for cost and impact on mean symptom score are presented:

	Cost per patient (£)			Symptom score		
	Nurse practitioner care	Standard care	Difference	Intervention	Standard care	Difference
Baseline	0	0	0	5	5	0
6 months	200	100	100	1	3	−2

Which of the following is correct with regard to the cost-effectiveness of this service compared with standard care? Select one option only.

A The additional cost per unit change in symptom score is £200

B The additional cost per unit change in symptom score is £100

C The additional cost per unit change in symptom score is £50

D The data suggest that the intervention is cost-effective

E There is a net reduction in costs

19.9 Drug safety data

A study is carried out into drug use in the 3 months before an admission with acute upper gastrointestinal bleeding. The results of this are shown below.

	Drug A	Drug B	Ulcer-healing drugs
Incidence of gastrointestinal bleeding (odds ratio)	2.1	1.9	3.4

Based on these data, which of the following are valid conclusions? Select one option only.

A Drug A is more likely to cause gastrointestinal bleeding than drug B

B Drug B is more likely to cause gastrointestinal bleeding than drug A

C These results are not statistically significant

D The use of ulcer-healing drugs is likely to be a confounding variable

E Ulcer-healing drugs are a proven cause of gastrointestinal bleeding

19.10 ACCORD study

Consider the following data from the ACCORD study (*British Medical Journal* 2009;339:b4909) with regard to the association between symptomatic severe hypoglycaemia and annualised mortality in type 2 diabetes:

Therapy	Mortality rate per annum (%)		Adjusted hazard ratio for no previous events versus at least one previous event (95% CI)
	No previous events	At least one previous event	
Intensive	1.2	2.8	1.41 (1.03–1.93)
Standard	1.0	3.7	2.30 (1.46–3.65)

Which one of the following conclusions is correct with regard to these data?

- A A history of previous symptomatic severe hypoglycaemia is associated with increased mortality in both treatment arms

- B Intensive treatment is more hazardous than standard treatment

- C Lack of previous symptomatic severe hypoglycaemia is associated with increased mortality in both treatment arms

- D The data do not show a statistically significant difference between the two treatment arms

- E These data suggest an increased mortality in patients on insulin therapy

19.11 Fracture prevention

Your practice is reviewing the prescribing of calcium and vitamin D in patients at risk of fracture. You decide to look into the data on fracture prevention with different preparations and come across the following data from the DIPART group (*British Medical Journal* 2010;340:b5463).

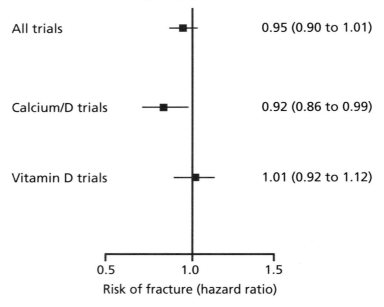

All trials	0.95 (0.90 to 1.01)
Calcium/D trials	0.92 (0.86 to 0.99)
Vitamin D trials	1.01 (0.92 to 1.12)

0.5   1.0   1.5

Risk of fracture (hazard ratio)

Which one of the following is a correct interpretation of these results?

A   Calcium alone will lead to a statistically significant reduction in fractures

B   Co-administration of calcium and vitamin D is necessary to prevent fractures

C   Meta-analysis of all trials of calcium and vitamin D confirm efficacy in preventing fractures

D   Vitamin D alone will prevent fractures

E   Vitamin D use is associated with a statistically significant increase in the risk of fracture

19.12 Mortality in diabetes

Consider the following data from a study of mortality and mean HbA1c levels:

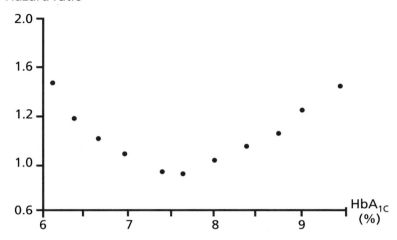

Hazard ratio

Which one of the following is a correct interpretation of these data?

○ A An HbA1c of 7.5% is associated with the highest mortality

○ B An HbA1c of 7.5% is associated with the lowest mortality

○ C Intensive glycaemic control is associated with lower mortality

○ D Intensive glycaemic control is associated with lower morbidity

○ E There is a direct relationship between glycaemic control and mortality

19.13 Diet treatment in sleep apnoea

A trial carried out to assess the impact of a very-low-energy diet on moderate and severe sleep apnoea in obese men (*British Medical Journal* 2009;339:b4609) gives the results below after a 9-week period:

	Intervention	Control	Mean difference	P
Apnoea:hypopnoea index (AHI)	−25	−2	−23 (−30 to −15)	<0.001
Weight (kg)	−18.7	1.1	−19.8 (−21.4 to −18.2)	<0.001

Which one of the following statements about these data is correct?

○ A The intervention improved daytime symptoms

○ B The intervention improved night-time symptoms

○ C The results suggest that weight loss is an effective treatment for snoring

○ D Weight loss provides lasting relief of symptoms

○ E Weight loss reduces long-term complications of sleep apnoea

19.14 Qualitative research

Your commissioning group decides to audit its nurse-led, walk-in centre. It carries this out by doing semi-structured interviews with a nurse practitioner who works in the clinic. She selects 50 patients over a 4-week period and assesses their satisfaction with various aspects of their care. The results are shown below:

Number of patients completing the interview = 50
Number of patients expressing overall satisfaction = 49
Number of patients who found that the visit satisfied their needs = 49
Number of patients who, when asked, felt that their visit was superior to normal GP care = 44

The group announce that on the basis of these results they will introduce more walk-in centres. Which one of the following statements is true with regard to the validity of this study?

○ A Extremely high satisfaction rates suggest inclusion bias

○ B This methodology is a bias-free method of collecting data

○ C The data confirm that nurse-led care is superior to GP care

○ D The methodology is designed to ensure a representative range of participants

○ E This study is a quantitative study

19.15 Drug treatment in arthritis

The results of a trial of treatment for arthritis with drug X compared with ibuprofen are shown below (CI = confidence interval; WOMAC = Western Ontario and McMaster Universities Index of Osteoarthritis):

Mean reduction in WOMAC score after 4 weeks:
Patients taking drug X = 2.4 (95% CI 1.7–2.6, $P = 0.66$)
Patients taking ibuprofen = 1.8 (95% CI 1.6–2.2, $P = 0.57$)
Cumulative incidence of gastrointestinal side effects after 4 weeks:
Patients taking drug X = 6% (95% CI 3.0–8.4%, $P = 0.04$)
Patients taking ibuprofen = 4% (95% CI 2.2–5.4%, $P = 0.05$)

Which one of the following statements about these data is true?

A   Drug X has a significantly greater anti-inflammatory effect than ibuprofen

B   Drug X has a superior long- and short-term safety profile

C   Drug X improves quality of life to a much greater extent than ibuprofen

D   Drug X is significantly safer than ibuprofen

E   The reductions in WOMAC scores are not statistically significant

19.16 Screening tests

A new test to screen for cystic fibrosis carriers is being considered. Preliminary results for the test in 100 children, in comparison with the gold standard of chromosome analysis, are shown below.

	Gold standard	
	Positive chromosome analysis	Negative chromosome analysis
New test positive	4	8
New test negative	1	87

Based on this information, which one of the following claims about the new test is correct?

A   The accuracy of the test is 91%

B   The new test is better than the gold standard test

C   The positive predictive value is 80%

D   The sensitivity is 96%

E   The specificity is 87%

19.17 Population studies

Consider the graph below, which summarises the relative risk of macrosomia for pregnant diabetic mothers according to the 20-week fasting glucose levels:

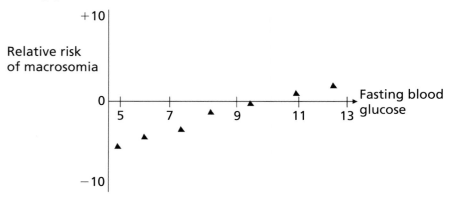

Which one of the following statements is true with regard to the interpretation of these data?

A   Caesarean section is significantly more likely in diabetic women

B   Gestational diabetes is becoming more common with time

C   Glucose levels <10 mmol/l are never associated with macrosomia

D   Low blood sugar levels are associated with small babies, ie intrauterine growth retardation

E   Tight control of blood sugar reduces the risk of macrosomia

19.18 Treatment efficacy

A new statin has just been launched with the following advertisement:

'Lowers death rate from myocardial infarction by 33%'

Closer inspection of the original paper reveals the following data:

Number of patients in treatment arm = 200
Number of patients in control arm = 200
Number of patients experiencing MI in treatment arm = 6
Number of patient experiencing MI in the control arm = 7
Number of patients who die as a result of MI in the treatment arm = 4
Number of patients who die as a result of MI in the control arm = 6

Which one of the following statements about these data is true?

A   The absolute risk reduction for death by MI is 33%

B   The number needed to harm with the new drug is 100

○   C   The number needed to treat (NNT) with the new drug to prevent one death from MI is 3

○   D   The NNT with the new drug to prevent one MI is 200

○   E   The relative risk reduction for MI is 33%

19.19 Diagnostic tests

A trial is conducted to determine which symptoms and signs have the most impact on the diagnosis of pneumonia in patients with respiratory symptoms presenting in primary care. The results are presented below:

Symptom/sign	Likelihood ratio for diagnosis
Fever	0.94
Cough	1.00
Abnormal chest examination	1.25
Tachypnoea	1.34
Otalgia	0.07

Which of the following statements with regard to these results is true? Select one option only.

○   A   An abnormal chest examination increases the probability that a patient has pneumonia by 25%

○   B   Tachypnoea has a negative association with the diagnosis of pneumonia

○   C   The presence of cough increases the likelihood that a patient has pneumonia by 100%

○   D   The presence of fever makes the diagnosis of pneumonia more likely in patients with respiratory disease

○   E   These results allow the diagnosis of pneumonia to be made without examining the patient

19.20 Homeopathic studies

A trial is conducted of blood pressure treatment with homeopathic remedies. One group of patients is treated with homeopathic treatment whereas the other group has no treatment. Both groups are monitored by a nurse for BP and side effects at monthly intervals. The data are shown below:

	Number of patients with raised BP in the homeopathy group	Number of patients with raised BP in the control group
Baseline	100	100
1 month	75	85
3 months	74	83
6 months	72	84
12 months	75	87

Which one of the following statements is a correct interpretation of these results?

A   Homeopathy has a statistically significant effect on BP

B   Homeopathy is well tolerated

C   The results in the control group are due to the Hawthorne effect

D   These data suggest that the effect of homeopathy on BP is purely a placebo effect

E   This trial is a randomised, double-blind, controlled trial and the results are therefore 'gold standard'

19.21 Survival data

Consider the Kaplan–Meier survival plot below, taken from a paper comparing the use of a novel treatment for osteoarthritis with conventional treatment. The end-point in the trial was the need for joint replacement.

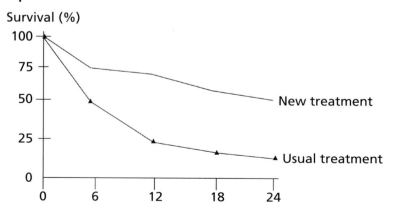

Which one of the following statements about these data is true?

○ A At 12 months 75% of the usual treatment group have died

○ B At 6 months 50% of the new treatment group have had joint surgery

○ C At 12 months a patient receiving the usual treatment is three times as likely to have had surgery as a patient on the new treatment

○ D The flattening off of the curves in later months shows that the effects of the treatments wear off with time

○ E The new treatment is better tolerated than the usual treatment

19.22 Meta-analysis
The results of a meta-analysis comparing drug A with drug B are shown below:

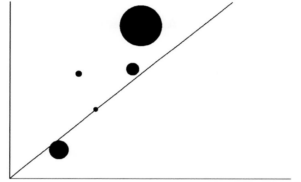

Favours
drug A

Favours
drug B

Which one of the following statements about these data is true?

○ A As some of trial data cross the line of no effect, larger trials are needed to determine the true effect

○ B The majority of the trials suggest that drug B is favourable

○ C There is no difference between drug A and drug B

○ D The results unequivocally support drug A

○ E The size of the circles represents the size of individual trials

19.23 Relative risk

A study compares the suicide risk in adolescents and adults who are taking two different classes of antidepressants. The standardised incidence of suicide is shown in the table below:

	Number of suicides in patients on drug A	Number of suicides in patients on drug B
Adolescents	150	100
Adults	50	100

Which one of the following statements with regard to these data is correct?

A   The relative risk (RR) of suicide for drug A in adolescents compared with drug B is 1.5

B   The RR of suicide for drug A in adolescents compared with drug B is 3

C   The RR of suicide for drug A compared with drug B in adults is 2

D   The RR of suicide for drug A compared with drug B is higher for adults than for adolescents

E   The results show a clear association with suicide for both drugs

19.24 Literature review

A review of published papers for a new drug contains the figure shown below:

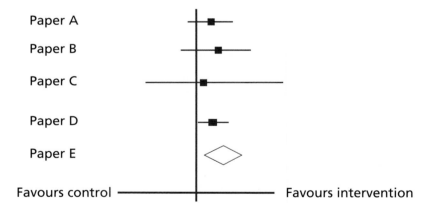

Which one of the following statements about these data is correct?

A   None of the papers shows a statistically significant effect

B   Paper E is a randomised controlled trial

C   Pooling results from individual papers gives a statistically significant result

○   D   The individual studies are too small to give statistically significant results

○   E   The published papers all confirm that the drug is effective

19.25 Screening

A study looks at the association between certain symptoms and a disease to see if any of these are useful as a screening tool. The following results are obtained:

	Number with symptom	Number without symptom
Patients with disease	60	40
Patients without disease	40	60

What is the likelihood ratio that a patient with the symptom will have the disease? Select one option only.

○   A   0.66

○   B   1.5

○   C   40%

○   D   60%

○   E   100%

19.26 Mortality in the UK

Select the rank order of the options (1–4) that best fulfils the requirements given in the question. The following is a list of causes of death in the UK (options 1–4):

1   Cancer
2   Circulatory disease
3   Mental and behavioural illness
4   Respiratory disease

The responses (A–E) rank the causes of death options in various orders. Select the response that places the options (1–4) in the order of **least** common cause of death first to the **most** common cause of death last. Select one rank order only.

○   A: 2, 4, 3, 1

○   B: 2, 3, 1, 4

○   C: 3, 4, 2, 1

○   D: 3, 2, 4, 1

○   E: 3, 1, 2, 4

EXTENDED MATCHING QUESTIONS

Study types

Options

A   Case–control study
B   Case report
C   Cohort study
D   Double-blinded, randomised, placebo-controlled trial
E   Meta-analysis
F   Qualitative study
G   Single-blinded, randomised, placebo-controlled trial

For each of the trials described below, select the option from the list above that most correctly describes the trial. Each option can be used once, more than once or not at all.

19.27   The Framingham Heart Study
19.28   The Cochrane Collaboration
19.29   A study of patients' experiences of bereavement

FREE TEXT QUESTIONS

19.30 Meta-analysis

The graph below shows the results of a meta-analysis of studies of a putative risk factor for stroke.

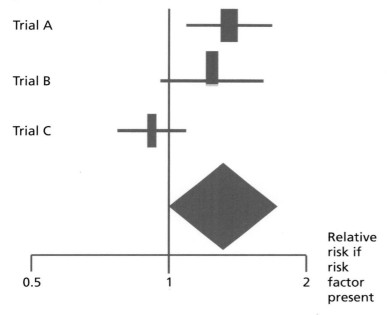

In the box below, write a best estimate for the relative risk of stroke for patients with the risk factor.

19.31 & 19.32

A new drug to prevent stroke is trialled in 100 patients at high risk of a stroke, compared with 100 matched controls. The results are shown in the table below:

	No. of patients who have a stroke	No. of patients with GI bleeding
Intervention group	46	20
Control group	50	10

19.31 Risk reduction

What is the absolute risk reduction for patients treated with the new drug?

Write the answer in the box below as a percentage

19.32 Numbers needed to harm

What is the number needed to harm for the new drug?

Write the answer in the box below

SINGLE BEST ANSWER

19.1   **C:**   **The extent to which one can appropriately apply the results to other populations**

Answer B describes test–retest reliability, answer E is split-half reliability, answer A is inter-rater reliability and answer D describes intra-rater reliability.

19.2   **A:**   **The study design is not blinded, so the results are not valid**

This study fails at a number of levels. Neither patients nor researchers are blinded as a result of both the different dosage regimen and the supplementary questionnaire, which reveal the ibuprofen group. It is therefore prone to reporting bias by the nurse and the patients. It is randomised but not placebo controlled. It is testing patients with rheumatoid arthritis, which is a different disease from osteoarthritis, and the findings are therefore not relevant for the licensed indication. Furthermore, it uses a very high dose of ibuprofen, which would be expected to cause significant gastrointestinal side effects, resulting in unfavourable comparisons with the new drug.

19.3   **C:**   **A study that compares two groups of 4-year-olds with similar characteristics: one group is given a drug and the other a placebo, and the growth of each group is measured after this intervention**

Study A is a cross-sectional study, study B is a case–control study, study C is a cohort study, study D is a controlled trial and study E is a longitudinal study.

19.4   **B:**   **The methodology of this paper is prone to bias**

This paper is prone to bias on a number of levels. The first is publication bias: papers published only in Chinese journals are significantly more likely to be both submitted and published if they report positive results for acupuncture, a treatment deeply rooted in Chinese society. Papers with negative findings are therefore significantly less likely to be published than papers with positive findings. Second, the inclusion of all studies published in Chinese-language journals results in inclusion bias, because negative studies are far more likely to be undertaken and published in western journals. The inclusion of all studies published over a set time period also results in potential inclusion of poorly conducted trials, which could therefore influence the overall findings significantly. The validity of data is increased with bigger data-sets, but only once poorly conducted and biased trials have been removed. The inclusion of non-peer-reviewed data in the trial also means that further publication of data in a peer-reviewed journal as part of a meta-analysis might give false credence to the data. The Cochrane Collaboration has extensive rules for the conduct of meta-analyses and these should be followed where possible.

19.5   A: No conclusions can be drawn on changes in incidence

The table shows relative incidence only, rather than absolute incidence. The decrease of trauma from first place in 1999 to second place in 2009 could be due to a fall in absolute incidence of trauma, but could also represent an increase in the incidence of neoplasms.

19.6   E: These data demonstrate an association rather than a causal relationship

These data appear to suggest that there is an association between mortality and alcohol consumption. It is not possible to say, however, that this is a causal relationship because of the need to remove confounding variables. Alcohol consumption could be a cause of increased mortality but it could equally be a surrogate marker for an unhealthy lifestyle. Drinkers are more likely to be obese and smokers, and take little exercise. There is also a possible confounding effect of class because alcohol consumption varies with social class. The graph is a population survey and does not give information on longitudinal outcomes, so conclusions cannot be made on the effects of changing consumption for individuals.

19.7   C: The incidence of bowel cancer is increased, whereas the incidence of renal cancer is reduced

Standardised incidence ratios (SIRs) compare the incidence of a condition in a patient under study with that of 'equivalent' patients. An SIR of 1.0 suggests that the incidence is the same as in an unexposed population. An SIR >1.0 suggests an increased risk, whereas an SIR <1.0 suggests a reduced risk. The results of studies like this suggest association rather than confirm causation.

19.8   C: The additional cost per unit change in symptom score is £50

The intervention produces a reduction in average symptom score of 4 points, whereas standard care reduces the symptom score by 2 points, a difference of 2. The intervention cost, however, is £100 more per patient, making the cost per additional point reduction £50. These data cannot be used alone to judge the cost-effectiveness of an intervention because this requires agreement of an acceptable cost per improvement in symptom control, which commissioners and patients would need to agree. There is a net increase in costs.

19.9   D: The use of ulcer-healing drugs is likely to be a confounding variable

Patients at high risk of upper gastrointestinal bleeding will often use ulcer-healing drugs because of previous bleeding or the development of new symptoms. The finding that the use of these drugs is three times more common in those admitted with an acute gastrointestinal bleed is therefore not unexpected, and use of ulcer-healing drugs is likely to be a confounding variable. There is unlikely to be a significant difference between drug A and drug B, although no comment can be made without information on confidence intervals and *P* values.

19.10   A: A history of previous symptomatic severe hypoglycaemia is associated with increased mortality in both treatment arms

These data suggest that increased mortality is seen in both intensive and standard treatment for patients with a history of severe, symptomatic hypoglycaemia. Furthermore they also suggest that the risk of death is lower in the intensive treatment arm in this subset of patients. There is no information on drug management and, although it could be surmised that hypoglycaemia is more common in patients on insulin, this might also be seen with sulphonylureas. Lack of a previous hypoglycaemic attack is less harmful, but is still associated with a mortality rate of 1.0–1.2% a year. The confidence intervals suggest that this is a true effect, because neither group has confidence intervals that cross 1.0.

19.11   B: Co-administration of calcium and vitamin D is necessary to prevent fractures

The data suggest that trials of vitamin D alone show a non-significant increase in the risk of fracture, whereas calcium and vitamin D in combination will reduce fractures and this finding is statistically significant. There are no trials of calcium alone in the data so conclusions cannot be drawn about this. Meta-analysis of all trials shows a non-significant reduction in fracture rate.

19.12   B: An HbA1c of 7.5% is associated with the lowest mortality

These data show a U-shaped association between HbA1c levels and mortality, with the lowest mortality associated with an HbA1c around 7.5%, whereas higher mortality is associated with very low and very high HbA1c levels. Hazard ratios are higher in patients at higher risk of an outcome, in this case mortality, so the lowest mortality is associated with the lowest point on the graph. These data apply only to mortality, so conclusions on morbidity cannot be made. Again, conclusions on causation of this effect cannot be made because these data reflect all-cause mortality and this could include death from hypoglycaemic attack as well as from diabetic ketoacidosis.

19.13   B: The intervention improved night-time symptoms

Obstructive sleep apnoea causes night-time symptoms of apnoea and wakening, which can be quantified with the apnoea:hypopnoea index (AHI), and daytime fatigue, which is assessed with the Epworth score. This study measured effect of a very-low-energy diet on the AHI rather than on the Epworth score. It is assumed that daytime symptoms correlate with night-time symptom severity, and it could therefore be assumed that daytime symptoms are improved, but that has not been measured as an outcome in this trial. The data are measured only after 9 weeks and no long-term conclusions can be drawn. Snoring is a clinical entity that is distinct from sleep apnoea and it is not possible to draw conclusions on the effects of this intervention on snoring on the basis of these data. There are no outcome measures relating to complications in this study.

19.14   A: Extremely high satisfaction rates suggest inclusion bias

Qualitative studies are fraught with methodological difficulties and should be used only in appropriate studies, eg when canvassing opinions that cannot be quantified as hard data. Semi-structured interviews are frequently used but the study needs to be well designed to avoid reporting bias or leading questions. Patients should, however, still be selected on a structured basis to ensure that participants are representative of the wider population and not selected on a whim, resulting in inclusion bias. A suitable model might be to enrol every third patient. Ideally, the people working in the clinic should not be aware that they are being audited to avoid 'playing up' to the study. The opinions of patients with regard to their experience of care cannot be extrapolated to determine whether one form of care is superior to another because this was not studied.

19.15   E: The reductions in WOMAC scores are not statistically significant

The reductions in WOMAC scores (a quantitative assessment of symptoms and handicap) show a benefit for drug X but the 95% confidence interval is wide and the limits overlap those of ibuprofen, with P values >0.05, meaning that the results do not achieve statistical significance. The results for gastrointestinal side effects also overlap but P for drug X is 0.04 (ie the true result is likely to lie in the range 3.0–8.4); again, these 95% CIs overlap those of ibuprofen and it cannot be said that there is a true difference between the two groups. A larger study would have greater power to detect these small differences. No long-term safety data are presented here, so no conclusions can be drawn in this area.

19.16   A: The accuracy of the test is 91%

	Gold standard	
	Positive	Negative
New test positive	a	b
New test negative	c	d

Accuracy is the proportion of tests that have given the correct result, ie

$(a + d)/(a + b + c + d)$, so $91/100 = 91\%$.

Sensitivity is the true-positive rate, ie

$a/(a + c)$, so $4/5 = 80\%$.

Specificity is the true-negative rate, ie

$d/(b + d)$, so $87/95 = 92\%$.

Positive predictive value is the probability of having the condition, once the test is positive, ie

$a/(a + b)$, so $4/12 = 33\%$.

Negative predictive value is the probability of not having the condition, once the test is negative, ie

$d/(c + d)$, so $87/88 = 99\%$.

19.17   E: Tight control of blood sugar reduces the risk of macrosomia

These data support a link between the risk of large babies and fasting blood glucose levels. Large babies are associated with difficult labour and probably with increased caesarean section rates, but that observation cannot be confirmed from these data. Similarly, a low risk of macrosomia is not the same as a high risk of intrauterine growth retardation, because this would be based on an assumption that the same disease mechanisms apply to both clinical situations. These data do suggest an association between fasting glucose at 20 weeks and macrosomia, so it is reasonable to conclude that tight control of sugar will reduce macrosomia. These data do not provide any time frame, however, so no conclusions on incidence can be made.

19.18   D: The NNT with the new drug to prevent one MI is 200

The absolute risk reduction (ARR) is the event rate in the control group minus the event rate in intervention group. The relative risk reduction (RRR) is (the event rate in the control group minus the event rate in treatment group) $\div$ (the event rate in control group). The number needed to treat is 1/ARR. The number needed to harm cannot be calculated from these data as no adverse outcome data are presented. The results are therefore:

ARR for death by MI $= 3\% - 2\% = 1\%$
ARR for all MI $= 3.5\% - 3\% = 0.5\%$
NNT for prevention of death by MI $= 1/0.01 = 100$
NNT for all MI $= 1/0.005 = 200$
RRR for death by MI $= 1/3 = 33\%$

19.19   A: An abnormal chest examination increases the probability that a patient has pneumonia by 25%

Likelihood ratios are used to determine the impact of a finding on the outcome. The results are expressed as a ratio: a score of 1 makes both outcomes (presence or absence of disease) equally likely, whereas a likelihood ratio >1 makes the diagnosis more likely and a likelihood ratio <1 makes the diagnosis less likely. In these results the presence of otalgia and fever have likelihood ratios of <1, making them unhelpful in differentiating pneumonia from other chest infections, but the presence of tachypnoea and abnormal chest examination have likelihood ratios of >1, making a diagnosis of pneumonia more likely. Cough alone has a likelihood ratio of 1.00, making a diagnosis neither more nor less likely, meaning that it is unhelpful in excluding or confirming a diagnosis.

19.20   C: The results in the control group are due to the Hawthorne effect

The control group have no treatment but are monitored. The phenomenon whereby observed outcomes improve merely as a result of being observed is called the 'Hawthorne effect' and is a form of placebo effect. The data presented do not provide any indication of statistical significance or tolerability. This trial is not blinded in any way.

19.21　　**C:**　　**At 12 months a patient receiving the usual treatment is three times as likely to have had surgery as a patient on the new treatment**

The Kaplan–Meier curves demonstrate the proportion of patients who have not met the endpoint, meaning survival without treatment rather than true survival. The rate of decline in the new treatment group is slower than in the usual treatment group, implying that this treatment protects patients from reaching the end-point of joint replacement. The flattening of the curves later on in the trial suggests that those patients who need surgery will have it early on. The study does not measure side effects, so no comment can be made on tolerability. At 12 months, 25% of the new treatment group have had surgery, compared with 75% of the usual treatment group.

19.22　　**E:**　　**The size of the circles represents the size of individual trials**

This is a L'Abbé plot. Each circle represents a trial and the size of each circle represents the size of the trial. The line bisecting the plot is the 'line of no effect'. Data to the right favour drug B and to the left favour drug A. The further away from the line the more significant the effect, so circles crossing the line do not show a net effect.

19.23　　**A:**　　**The relative risk (RR) of suicide for drug A in adolescents compared with drug B is 1.5**

The relative risk is the number of events in the treatment group divided by the number of events in the control group. In this example drug A has a higher RR of suicide in adolescents than drug B but in adults the RR is lower (1.5 in adolescents versus 0.5 in adults). No inference can be made as to causation because there is no true control group in this study, ie the rate in a control group might be higher than both groups if both drugs reduce suicide but by differing degrees.

19.24　　**C:**　　**Pooling results from individual papers gives a statistically significant result**

This figure shows results from four individual studies and also a Forest plot of pooled data, as would be found with a meta-analysis. This increases the statistical power of an analysis but also introduces potential bias because all the individual component studies might not be equivalent, in terms of either patient selection or follow-up measures. Papers A, B and C show a positive result but with wide confidence intervals that cross zero, whereas paper D shows a positive effect with confidence intervals that favour intervention, but only marginally.

19.25　　**B:**　　**1.5**

The likelihood ratio is the ratio of the probability that an individual with the target condition has a specified symptom (or test result) to the probability that an individual without the target condition has the same specified symptom. It is used to determine the validity of association between symptoms or tests and disease, eg headache and brain tumour. In this example the probability that the individual with the symptom has the condition is 60%, whereas the probability that a patient with the symptom does not have the condition is 40%. The likelihood ratio is therefore 60/40 or 1.5.

19.26   C: 3, 4, 2, 1

Rank ordering: 3 Mental and behavioural illness; 4 Respiratory disease; 2 Circulatory disease; 1 Cancer

The Office for National Statistics records data on causes of death in the UK. Cancer is the leading cause, with circulatory disease a close second.

EXTENDED MATCHING ANSWERS

Study types

19.27   C: Cohort study

The Framingham Study was a cohort study that looked at a population living in the town of Framingham and provided much of our understanding of cardiovascular risk factors.

19.28   E: Meta-analysis

The Cochrane Collaboration is a network of researchers who use the strictest criteria for carrying out meta-analysis, excluding any trials that are prone to bias. It is therefore the purest form of meta-analysis.

19.29   F: Qualitative study

This is a qualitative study. These studies are prone to different forms of bias and need to be interpreted accordingly.

FREE TEXT ANSWERS

19.30   1.4

The pooled studies shown in the lozenge give a peak risk at around 1.4, ie patients with the risk factor are 1.4 times as likely to have a stroke as patients without the risk factor. The individual studies give inconclusive results but the pooled studies give a positive result with the lower 95% CI >1, suggesting a true-positive result.

19.31   4%

The event rate in the control group is 50%, but in the intervention group it is 46%, ie. an absolute risk reduction of 4%.

19.32   10

The absolute risk increase for side effects is 10%, hence the number needed to harm is 1/10%, or 10.

Chapter 20
Administration

SINGLE BEST ANSWER QUESTIONS

20.1 Read codes
Which one of the following statements is correct with regard to the Read codes in general practice?

○   A   Read codes are based on the ICD-10 database

○   B   Read codes are used for diagnoses only

○   C   Read codes are used to encrypt data

○   D   Read codes should be accompanied by free text

○   E   Use of the Read codes is mandatory in the UK

20.2 Caldicott principles
Which one of the following statements about the Caldicott principles is true?

○   A   The Caldicott principles apply only to clinicians

○   B   The Caldicott principles apply only where data are passed outside the NHS (eg insurance reports)

○   C   Every practice must have its own Caldicott guardian

○   D   Every primary care organisation must have a Caldicott guardian

○   E   The Caldicott principles are part of the Data Protection Act

20.3   Freedom of Information Act
Which one of the following statements about the Freedom of Information Act is correct?

○   A   General practices are covered by the Data Protection Act, so they are specifically excluded from the Freedom of Information Act

○   B   Individuals can seek information on individual salaries of doctors working in the practice

○   C   Practices are able to question the motive for a request before deciding whether to comply with a request

○   D   Practices have 20 working days to respond to a request

○   E   The Freedom of Information Act allows patients to gain access to their medical records

20.4   Exception reporting in QOF
Which of the following situations with regard to the use of exception codes for the QOF would be appropriate? Select one option only.

○   A   A 23-year-old woman with epilepsy has frequent fits despite apparently taking her medication. She is removed from the practice register as 'unsuitable'

○   B   An 84-year-old woman with diabetes is housebound. She does not respond to three letters asking her to come into the surgery for a diabetic check. She is removed from the register as 'patient unsuitable'

○   C   A 24-year-old woman with asthma has received three letters from the practice asking her to come in for an asthma check. She telephones the practice to say that she does not wish to be seen in the clinic. She is coded as 'informed dissent'

○   D   A 73-year-old man with stable ischaemic heart disease cannot take aspirin. He is coded as 'patient unsuitable' for the ischaemic heart disease register

○   E   A 79-year-old man with ischaemic heart disease is on warfarin for atrial fibrillation. To avoid adversely affecting the QOF performance for antiplatelet drugs, he is coded as 'H/O aspirin allergy'

20.5 Healthcare spending in the UK

Select the rank order of the options (1–4) that best fulfils the requirements given in the question. The following is a list of NHS areas of expenditure (options 1–4):

1   **Community care**
2   **Elective hospital care**
3   **Mental health**
4   **Non-elective hospital care**

The responses (A–E) rank the expenditure area options in various orders. Select the response that places the options (1–4) in the order of expense, with the **lowest** NHS expenditure first to the **highest** NHS expenditure last.

Select one rank order only.

○   A   1, 3, 2, 4

○   B   1, 3, 4, 3

○   C   3, 1, 2, 4

○   D   2, 1, 3, 4

○   E   3, 2, 4, 1

EXTENDED MATCHING QUESTIONS

Decision support tools

Options

A   Apache score
B   CHADS$_2$ score
C   Frax score
D   Gleason's score
E   Marburg's score
F   QRISK2
G   QCancer
H   Rosier's scale
I   Townsend's score
J   Well's score

For each of the conditions below, select the single most appropriate decision support tool from the list above. Each option may be used once, more than once or not at all.

20.6   **Osteoporosis**
20.7   **Stroke**
20.8   **Atrial fibrillation**
20.9   **Deep vein thrombosis**
20.10   **Deprivation**

Legislation affecting general practice

Options

A   Data Protection Act
B   Disability Discrimination Act
C   Employment Equality (Age) Regulations 2006
D   Equality Act
E   Freedom of Information Act
F   Human Rights Act
G   Mental Capacity Act 2005
H   Race Relations Act (RRA) 1976
I   Sex Discrimination (Amendment of Legislation) Regulations 2008
J   None of the above

For each of the statements below, select the most relevant piece of legislation from the list above. Each option can be used once, more than once or not at all.

20.11   **Outlaws discrimination on the basis of sexual orientation.**
20.12   **Allows adults to make decisions on behalf of learning disabled children.**
20.13   **Prevents discrimination on the basis of pregnancy.**
20.14   **Allows access to medical reports.**

Sickness certification

Options

A	Cannot issue certificate
B	Fit Note
C	Med 10
D	Private sick certificate
E	SC2

For each of the following patients select the most appropriate certificate from above. Each option can be used once, more than once or not at all.

20.15 A 36-year-old man has been off work for 3 months with a stress related illness. He now feels ready to start back at work but requests shortened hours initially.

20.16 A 9 year old boy has been off school for one day with vomiting. He has now completely recovered but his mother telephones the surgery and asks for a sick note for school, since he has an unacceptably high unauthorized absence rate. The family did not seek medical attention when he was unwell.

20.17 Mr West has not been to work today (Monday). He has been unwell since Friday evening and you diagnose viral gastroenteritis and recommend that he does not return to work until 48 hours after he is better. In the past his employer has not been happy with absences for sickness so Mr West requests a certificate.

20.18 Mrs Shand is currently an inpatient having been admitted 2 weeks ago with an exacerbation of her Crohn's disease. Her husband phones you and asks for a sick note to cover this period.

20.19 Mrs Ward is going through a relationship break-up and has financial problems. She is low and tearful and not coping at work. You decide that she would benefit from 2 weeks off work.

Revalidation

20.20–20.24

Options

A   3 years
B   5 years
C   Appraisee
D   Appraiser
E   Clinical commissioning group
F   General Medical Council
G   Local medical committee
H   Primary care trust
I   Responsible officer
J   None of the above

Complete the algorithm below describing the process of revalidation for general practitioners from the list of options above. Each option may be used once, more than once or not at all.

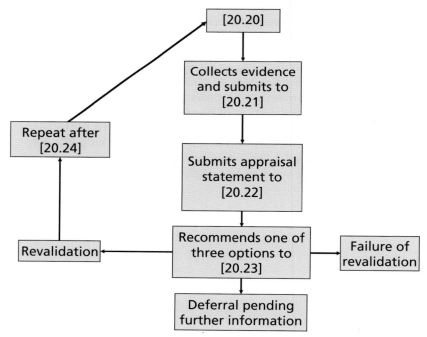

SINGLE BEST ANSWER

20.1   D: Read codes should be accompanied by free text

Read codes were developed to facilitate data collection. They are a parallel system to ICD-10 but the Read code system includes all ICD-10 codes. There are Read codes for diagnoses, symptoms, procedures and occupations, and they should be supported by free text to ensure an accurate clinical record. The use of these is not mandatory, although payment for the QOF is based on computer-generated audits of a standard battery of Read codes.

20.2   D: Every primary care organisation must have a Caldicott guardian

The Caldicott principles suggest the following: all uses of patient data should be justified; identifiable data should be used only when absolutely necessary, including when data are sent between different parts of the NHS; and each practice should have a responsible individual who ensures compliance with good practice and the law, including the Data Protection Act.

20.3   D: Practices have 20 working days to respond to a request

The Freedom of Information Act specifically includes general practices, which are expected to maintain a publication scheme containing policies and practice income. However, individual salaries are covered by the Data Protection Act. Practices cannot question motives, but a charge can be made. Failure to comply with a request will result in the practice being held in contempt of court.

20.4   C: A 24-year-old woman with asthma has received three letters from the practice asking her to come in for an asthma check. She telephones the practice to say that she does not wish to be seen in the clinic. She is coded as 'informed dissent'

The use of exception codes is an area of misreporting in many areas and is one that PCTs are keen to investigate at annual QOF visits. Valid reasons for exception reporting include informed dissent or inappropriateness (eg people who are terminally ill), but being housebound or poorly controlled is not generally seen to be a valid reason. Caution should be taken when choosing the code to make sure that these are accurate. Individual indicator exception codes should be used wherever possible, rather than exclusion from the whole disease area.

20.5   C: 3, 1, 2, 4
3 Mental health; 1 Community care; 2 Elective hospital care;
4 Non-elective hospital care

Mental health accounts for 10%, community care 12.5%, and inpatient elective and non-elective care for 17.5% and 27.5%, respectively. Primary care and prescribing each account for 10% of funds.

EXTENDED MATCHING ANSWERS

Decision support tools

20.6	C:	Frax score
20.7	H:	Rosier's scale
20.8	B:	CHADS$_2$ score
20.9	J:	Well's score
20.10	I:	Townsend's score

Apache scores are used in critical care to assess disease severity. CHADS$_2$ assesses the risk of stroke in atrial fibrillation, whereas Well's scores for DVT and PE can be used to guide decisions on whether scanning is appropriate. Gleason's score is a grading system for prostate cancer whereas Marburg's score is used in assessing chest pain for possible cardiac origin. Rosier's scale is used in accident and emergency departments to assist diagnosis of stroke whereas QRISK2 and QCancer will calculate risk of heart disease and cancer respectively. Townsend's scores are epidemiological markers of deprivation. Frax is used to determine fracture risk.

Legislation affecting general practice

20.11   D: Equality Act

Since 2007 the Equality Act outlaws discrimination on the basis of sexual orientation.

20.12   G: Mental Capacity Act 2005

The Mental Capacity Act governs decision-making on behalf of adults, where either they lose mental capacity at some point in their lives or the incapacitating condition has been present since birth.

20.13   I: Sex Discrimination (Amendment of Legislation) Regulations 2008

This amendment prevents direct or indirect discrimination on the basis of pregnancy now or in the last 26 weeks.

20.14   J: None of the above

The Access to Medical Reports Act allows access for patients to medical reports about them.

Certification

20.15   B: Fit Note.

Since 2010 sick notes have been replaced with Fit Notes, which place much greater emphasis on rehabilitation and amended duties/hours. GPs are encouraged to consider adaptations that would allow a patient to return to work. These can be specified in the sick note and also a time scale.

20.16   A: Cannot issue certificate.

Sick notes should not be issued when there is no evidence from a healthcare professional that a patient has been unwell. Sick certification is a legal process and rules must be complied with.

20.17   D: Private sick certificate.

Fit notes should not be issued for periods of illness of less than 7 days, and there is no statutory duty to issue certificates for periods less than 7 days. This patient should be encouraged to self certificate using form SC2. If they do not wish to they may have a private sick certificate.

20.18   C: Med10.

These are still in use for inpatient stays, and should be supplied by the treating clinician.

20.19   B: Fit Note.

If someone is unfit for work and the period is likely to last more than 7 days, a Fit note should be issued. If the patient is unfit for work the box should be ticked indicating this.

Revalidation

20.20	C:	Appraisee
20.21	D:	Appraiser
20.22	I:	Responsible officer
20.23	F:	General Medical Council
20.24	B:	5 years

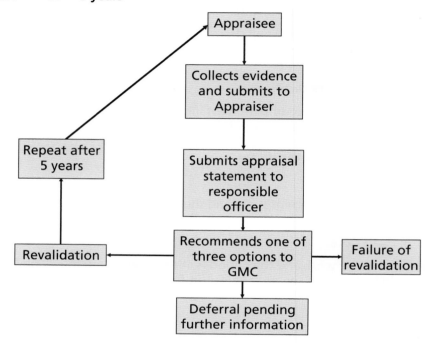

Paper 1 Questions

Total time allowed is three hours.

P1.1 Shoulder problems
Which one of the following statements regarding frozen shoulder is correct?

○ A Ninety per cent of patients make a complete recovery

○ B Frozen shoulder is more common in patients with diabetes mellitus

○ C Frozen shoulder is usually directly attributable to injury

○ D The mean age of onset is 20–30 years

○ E X-rays are necessary to make a diagnosis

P1.2 Contraception
A 22-year-old woman is going travelling around the world for 18 months and comes to see you to discuss using implants for contraception. Which one of the following statements about this contraceptive method is true?

○ A Progestogen implants cause weight gain in 50% of patients

○ B Progestogen implants are intrauterine contraceptive devices that release progesterone into the lining of the womb

○ C Progestogen implants need to be changed every 5 years

○ D Irregular bleeding is the most common side effect of progestogen implants

○ E Normal fertility returns in 3–6 months in 90% of women after removal of progestogen implants

Trials in atrial fibrillation

Options

A   AFFIRM (Atrial Fibrillation Follow-up Investigation of Rhythm Management) trial
B   ARISTOTLE (Apixaban for Reduction in Stroke and Other Thromboembolic Events in Atrial Fibrillation) trial
C   BAFTA (Birmingham Atrial Fibrillation Treatment of the Aged) trial
D   PIAF (Pharmacological Intervention in Atrial Fibrillation) trial
E   RELY (Randomized Evaluation of Long-Term Anticoagulation Therapy) trial
F   ROCKET-AF (Rivaroxaban Once Daily Oral Direct Factor Xa Inhibition Compared with Vitamin K Antagonism for Prevention of Stroke and Embolism Trial in Atrial Fibrillation) trial
G   None of the above

For each of the statements below, select the single most likely option from the list above. Each option may be used once, more than once or not at all.

P1.3   Suggested that all patients over the age of 75 with atrial fibrillation should be considered for anticoagulation.
P1.4   Showed that rate control was superior to rhythm control.
P1.5   Found a lower incidence of intracranial bleeds and disabling stroke for dagibatran compared with warfarin.
P1.6   Demonstrated a statistically significant reduction in overall mortality for patients taking apixaban compared with warfarin.

P1.7   Skin ulcer
A 91-year-old man who lives alone is brought to see you by his daughter who is visiting from Australia. She is concerned about the skin lesion shown below, which he says has been there for some time.

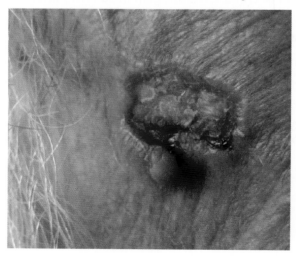

What is the single most likely diagnosis?

○   A   Actinic keratosis

○   B   Basal cell carcinoma

○   C   Dermatitis artefacta

○   D   Malignant melanoma

○   E   Squamous cell carcinoma

P1.8   **Blood pressure measurement**
A 67-year-old man complains of pains in his legs when walking. You ask the nurses to do ankle and brachial blood pressures. These results are shown below:

Right brachial systolic pressure 150 mmHg
Left brachial systolic pressure 150 mmHg
Right dorsalis pedis systolic pressure 120 mmHg
Left dorsalis pedis systolic pressure 150 mmHg

Which one of the following statements is correct regarding this patient?

○   A   The readings are inaccurate and should be repeated

○   B   The readings show an ankle–brachial pressure index (ABPI) of 0.8 on the left side

○   C   The readings show an ABPI of 1.25 on the right side

○   D   The readings suggest the presence of significant peripheral vascular disease affecting the left side only

○   E   The readings suggest the presence of significant peripheral vascular disease affecting the right side only

P1.9   **Neuralgia**
Which one of the following statements regarding post-herpetic neuralgia is correct?

○   A   No treatments have been shown to be effective in preventing post-herpetic neuralgia

○   B   Pregabalin has been shown to be the most effective treatment for post-herpetic neuralgia

○   C   Prodromal dermatomal pain is a risk factor for post-herpetic neuralgia

○   D   The presence of paraesthesia suggests an alternative diagnosis

○   E   The side-effect profile of amitriptyline outweighs its benefits

P1.10   Abdominal swelling

A 15-month-old girl is brought in by her father, who has noticed that her umbilicus looks 'lumpy'. He tells you that it gets bigger when she cries or strains and is smaller when she is asleep. Her abdomen is shown below.

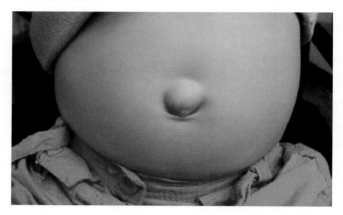

What is the single most appropriate management at this stage?

○   A   Admit under the on-call surgeons

○   B   Refer urgently to surgical outpatients

○   C   Reassure the parents that it will usually resolve spontaneously in time

○   D   Reassurance that this is normal at her age

○   E   Treat with a surgical support

Drug management of asthma

Options

A   Combination of inhaled corticosteroid and long-acting β_2 agonist
B   Inhaled anticholinergic
C   Inhaled β_2 agonist
D   Inhaled long-acting β_2 agonist
E   Inhaled low-dose corticosteroid
F   Oral β_2 agonist
G   Oral corticosteroids
H   Oral leukotriene receptor antagonist
I   Oral theophylline

For each of the statements below regarding the drug management of asthma, select the most appropriate option from the list above. Each option may be used once, more than once or not at all.

P1.11 Indicated for the maintenance of asthma and relief of seasonal allergic symptoms.

P1.12 The SMART regimen allows patients to safely tailor their treatment with these drugs according to their symptoms.

P1.13 This drug has a narrow therapeutic window and toxicity is increased by concurrent use of erythromycin, quinolones and cimetidine.

P1.14 Inhibits bronchoconstriction and reduces mucus secretion in the lungs.

P1.15 If used for more than 10 days consideration should be given to co-prescription of bisphosphonates.

P1.16 Knee pain
A 28-year-old man complains of knee pain after being hit below the knee by an outstretched boot in a football match. On examination there is a small effusion but no laceration and the knee is fully mobile but seems to have excessive backward movement on pushing the lower leg back. What is the single most likely diagnosis?

○   A   Anterior cruciate tear

○   B   Medial collateral tear

○   C   Meniscal tear

○   D   Patellar tendon tear

○   E   Posterior cruciate tear

P1.17 Neck lumps

You see an 82-year-old woman for a medication review and notice the appearance of her neck, shown below. She tells you it has been like that for many years. The lump moves on swallowing and is asymmetrical. You check her thyroid function and both TSH and T$_4$ are reported as normal.

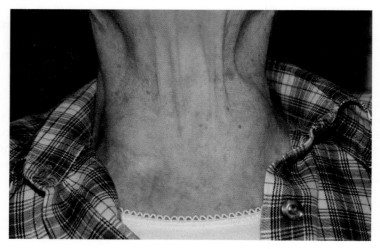

What is the single most likely diagnosis?

○ A Endemic goitre

○ B Multinodular goitre

○ C Thyroid cancer

○ D Thyrotoxicosis

○ E None of the above

P1.18 Lipid management

Which one of the following statements is correct regarding current NICE guidelines on lipid levels?

○ A Ezetemibe/simvastatin combination therapy should be used first line for patients with acute coronary syndromes

○ B All patients at risk of ischaemic heart disease should be treated with 40 mg simvastatin and do not require follow-up cholesterol tests

○ C Patients with acute coronary syndromes should be treated with 40 mg simvastatin

○ D Patients with diabetes mellitus should have a total cholesterol of ⩽5.0 mmol/l and an LDL level of <3.0 mmol/l

○ E Patients with diabetes mellitus should have a total cholesterol of ⩽4.0 mmol/l and an LDL of <2.0 mmol/l

P1.19 Catheter care

An elderly man living in a nursing home has had a catheter fitted for the last 5 weeks. One of the staff in the home has sent a routine urine specimen, which has been reported as showing a pure growth of *Proteus* sp. sensitive to trimethoprim and ciprofloxacin. He is afebrile, with no urinary symptoms. Which one of the following would be the most appropriate management of this patient?

○　　A　Flush the catheter with citrate solution

○　　B　No action required

○　　C　Prescribe ciprofloxacin for 5 days

○　　D　Prescribe trimethoprim for 3 days

○　　E　Replace the catheter

Death certification

Options

A　Contact the police
B　Discuss the case with a doctor from a neighbouring practice
C　Discuss the case with the coroner
D　Discuss the case with the crematorium referee
E　Issue Certificate of Stillbirth
F　Issue Medical Certificate of Cause of Death
G　Issue Neonatal Death Certificate
H　None of the above

For each of the situations below select the single most appropriate action from the list of options above. Each option may be used once, more than once, or not at all.

P1.20　A 78-year-old woman diagnosed with untreatable metastatic bowel cancer 3 months ago is found dead in bed by her daughter. She was last seen by you 16 days ago.

P1.21　An 83-year-old man who has not seen a doctor for 7 years is found dead in an armchair at home. He has no medical history of note and seems to have died in his sleep.

P1.22　A 69-year-old former boiler-maker dies after a long illness with mesothelioma. You saw him the day before he died.

P1.23　A 57-year-old woman with a long history of mental illness commits suicide 2 days after a review by her consultant psychiatrist. She was last seen by you 10 days ago.

P1.24　A 37-year-old woman living on a remote farm who is 22 weeks pregnant goes into premature labour and rapidly delivers a baby at home, before the paramedics can arrive. The baby did not show any sign of life and was not successfully resuscitated. You attend the woman before admission to hospital and are asked to certify the death of the baby.

P1.25 A 93-year-old woman dies of heart failure in a nursing home. She was seen the day before death by you but was confirmed dead by the out-of-hours service and has been taken to an undertaker 30 miles away. The family have made an appointment to register the death this afternoon and have asked you to issue a certificate.

P1.26 Panic attacks
A 17-year-old student requests a note for school regarding her absences from lectures. She tells you that for several months she has been finding it increasingly difficult to cope with being in public places. She admits to having been shy since childhood but is now increasingly panicky in groups and feels inadequate around others, although she copes at home. Things have escalated to the point where she has vomited on several occasions. She has no other symptoms of note. Which of the following statements regarding her management is correct?

○ A Cognitive–behavioural therapy is ineffective

○ B Reassurance that there is no organic disease is usually sufficient

○ C She should be treated with lithium

○ D She should be treated with olanzapine

○ E SSRIs should be used as first-line treatment

P1.27 Diarrhoea
A 4-year-old girl who returned from a camping holiday at a farm in Wales 2 days ago is brought in by her parents complaining of abdominal pain, vomiting and diarrhoea. This has been going on for 3 days but the diarrhoea has now become bloody. On examination she looks listless and has a capillary refill time of 3 seconds, a temperature of 37.6°C and generalised abdominal tenderness but no peritonism. A urine specimen shows microscopic haematuria. What is the single most appropriate management of this patient?

○ A Admit under paediatrics

○ B Advise parents regarding oral rehydration and review if no better

○ C Send urine for culture and treat if positive

○ D Send stool for culture and review with results

○ E Treat with oral trimethoprim and review in 3 days

P1.28 Chronic fatigue
Which one of the following statements regarding chronic fatigue syndrome is correct?

○ A Cognitive difficulties are unusual

○   B   Exacerbations of fatigue are triggered by exertion and usually start during exertion, forcing patients to abandon the activity

○   C   NICE guidelines suggest that the diagnosis should be considered in patients with unexplained fatigue of more than 6 weeks' duration

○   D   The presence of chronic pain suggests an alternative diagnosis

○   E   Cognitive–behavioural therapy (CBT) should be offered to all patients with this condition

P1.29   **Eye pain**
A 35-year-old man complains of a tender lump on the side of his eyeball. He says that it has been there for several days and came on acutely. He has no other symptoms and his vision is normal. On examination his cornea looks clear, with a reactive pupil and no conjunctival injection. There is no foreign body and no fluorescein staining, but he has an injected nodular area close to the corneal limbus on the white of the eye. The eyeball is tender over the nodule but otherwise is soft. What is the single most likely diagnosis?

○   A   Acute angle-closure glaucoma

○   B   Episcleritis

○   C   Herpes simplex keratitis

○   D   Iritis

○   E   Scleritis

P1.30   **Genetic counselling**
A 34-year-old woman comes to see you for advice on genetic testing. Her mother and aunt have both had breast cancer in the late 40s and her mother has just told her that she has tested positive for the *BRCA-1* gene. She asks what her risk of inheriting the gene is. What is the risk in per cent? Type your answer in the box.

Childhood infections

Options

A   Group A streptococci
B   *Escherichia coli* O157
C   *Mycoplasma pneumoniae*
D   Parainfluenza virus
E   Paramyxovirus
F   Parvovirus B19
G   Poxvirus
H   Respiratory syncytial virus (RSV)
I   Rotavirus
J   Rubella
K   *Staphylococcus aureus*
L   Varicella

For each of the statements below, select the most appropriate option from the list above. Each option may be used once, more than once or not at all.

P1.31   Causes crops of pinky-white shiny papules with a central pit.

P1.32   Causes epidemics of respiratory illness in approximately 3-year cycles, often associated with target-like skin lesions.

P1.33   After a prodromal fever this causes a macular rash to appear on the cheek that spreads to the trunk over several days.

P1.34   Around 24 hours after the development of tonsillitis this causes a macular rash to appear over the whole body; 2–3 days later the skin is shed, particularly on the hands and soles.

P1.35   After an incubation period of 14 days crops of vesicular lesions appear over the body. These heal over 2–3 days with new lesions appearing for 7–10 days.

P1.36   **Bloody diarrhoea**
A 27-year-old man complains of 3 weeks of diarrhoea and abdominal pain, with weight loss and fever. The stools are bloody on occasion. He has no recent history of travel and takes no regular medications. He reports recently being under a great deal of stress at work. On examination he is tender in the left iliac fossa with no peritonism and no perineal abnormalities. A stool sample is sent which is reported as negative for viral, bacterial and parasitic infections. What is the single most likely diagnosis?

    ○   A   *Campylobacter* sp.

    ○   B   Crohn's disease

    ○   C   Diverticulitis

    ○   D   Irritable bowel syndrome

    ○   E   Ulcerative colitis

P1.37 Unwanted pregnancy
Which one of the following statements regarding termination of pregnancy is correct?

○   A   Girls under the age of 16 cannot have a termination without the consent of their parents

○   B   Medical termination is only suitable in patients up to 9 weeks' gestation

○   C   RU-486 (mifepristone) is safe to use in patients who are not fit for general anaesthesia

○   D   Suction termination can be carried out under local anaesthesia

○   E   The legal limit for abortion is 22 weeks

Personality disorders

Options

A   Anankastic personality disorder
B   Antisocial personality disorder
C   Borderline personality disorder
D   Histrionic personality disorder
E   Hyperthymic personality disorder
F   Narcissistic personality disorder
G   Paranoid personality disorder
H   Schizoid personality disorder

For each of the descriptions below, select the most appropriate option from the list above. Each option may be used once, more than once or not at all.

P1.38   **Always happy and optimistic, but tend to make rash decisions without fully considering the consequences.**

P1.39   **Characterised by impulsivity, outbursts of anger and unpredictable behaviour, often with episodes of deliberate self-harm or violence.**

P1.40   **A lack of adaptability to new situations, eg failing to take advantage of new opportunities, disabling perfectionism in even the most mundane tasks and lack of imagination.**

P1.41   **Typified by an excessive sense of self-importance and power without warmth or empathy.**

P1.42   **Solitary, humourless people who tend to avoid situations where they will have to socialise.**

P1.43 Bladder problems

A 76-year-old man who is currently awaiting investigation for alternating diarrhoea and constipation presents with an episode of frank haematuria. He presents you with a specimen that is heavily blood stained with some sediment. On closer questioning he reports passing small lumps and bubbles in his urine. What is the single most likely diagnosis?

- A Bladder cancer
- B Glomerulonephritis
- C Renal calculus
- D Urinary tract infection
- E Vesicocolic fistula

P1.44 Swollen arm

A 53-year-old man had a pacemaker fitted for heart block last week. He complains that his left arm is swollen. On examination the left arm is red and swollen from the humerus down, with engorged veins that do not empty on elevating the arm. He is afebrile. What is the single most likely diagnosis?

- A Cellulitis
- B Compartment syndrome
- C Deep vein thrombosis
- D Postoperative wound infection
- E Subclavian arterial embolism

P1.45 Haemochromatosis

Mrs Jones comes to see you after her brother, who lives in New Zealand, is diagnosed with haemochromatosis. She asks for a screening test to see if she has the disease. She does not have any additional information about his diagnosis. You do some routine blood tests, including iron studies. Which one of the following is most indicative of haemochromatosis in this situation?

- A Raised mean corpuscular haemoglobin and raised mean corpuscular volume
- B Raised serum ferritin and raised total iron-binding capacity
- C Raised serum ferritin with reduced total iron-binding capacity
- D Reduced mean corpuscular haemoglobin and reduced mean corpuscular volume
- E Reduced serum ferritin with raised total iron-binding capacity

P1.46 Cough

A 23-year-old man complains that for the last 7 weeks he has had outbreaks of violent coughing, which last for minutes at a time, during which he feels he cannot breathe. He feels relatively well in between attacks. He has no previous medical history of note and takes no regular medications. He has been seen in accident and emergency twice and in the practice twice with no adverse findings. Which one of the following is the single most likely diagnosis?

○ A Asthma

○ B Diphtheria

○ C *Mycoplasma pneumoniae* infection

○ D Pertussis

○ E Pneumococcal chest infection

Biological therapies

Options

A Infliximab (Remicade)
B Natalizumab (Tysabri)
C Omalizumab (Xolair)
D Ranibizumab (Lucentis)
E Rituximab (Rituxan)
F Trastuzumab (Herceptin)

For each of the diseases below, select the most appropriate treatment agent from the list above. Each option may be used once, more than once or not at all.

P1.47 Allergy-mediated asthma
P1.48 Multiple sclerosis
P1.49 Severe psoriasis resistant to PUVA and standard systemic treatment
P1.50 Breast cancer
P1.51 Macular degeneration

P1.52 Indigestion

A 39-year-old man with longstanding gastro-oesophageal reflux comes to see you about his condition. In spite of treatment with high-dose proton-pump inhibitors and alginates he is troubled by symptoms on a daily basis. He has tried lifestyle measures but feels that he cannot go on. He begs you to refer him for surgery. Which one of the following statements is true regarding this treatment option?

○ A Nissen fundoplication requires a laparotomy

○ B Patients who have had a fundoplication have a reduced gastric capacity and have to eat regular small meals

○ C Surgery is indicated in patients who do not wish to take long-term medication

○ D Surgery is suitable only for patients with a sliding hiatus hernia

○ E Surgery will control symptoms and eliminate the need for maintenance medication

P1.53 Backache

A 27-year-old man asks for stronger painkillers for his back. He has always had backache, but is now finding it increasingly difficult to work. He is particularly stiff in the morning, although finds this improves somewhat during the day, and has been present for several years. He also suffers from intermittent iritis, but is on no regular medication. He frequently wakes in the early hours and on examination he has limited flexion and extension in his back. What is the most likely diagnosis?

○ A Ankylosing spondylitis

○ B Mechanical backache

○ C Polymyalgia rheumatica

○ D Prolapsed intervertebral disc

○ E Spinal stenosis

P1.54 Management of arthritis

A 36-year-old woman with severe rheumatoid arthritis has been advised to start methotrexate by her rheumatologist. She comes to see you to discuss this, having read about this treatment on the internet. Which one of the following statements regarding this treatment is correct?

○ A If a full blood count is normal initially and 1 month after starting treatment, no further testing is required

○ B If LFTs increase by 10% after starting treatment the drug should be stopped

○ C Methotrexate can be safely used in pregnancy

○ D Methotrexate frequently causes menstrual disturbances

○ E Methotrexate should not be used in patients taking folic acid supplements

P1.55 **Behavioural problems**

A 7-year-old boy is brought in to see you by his parents at the request of his schoolteachers. He has no friends in his class, is aloof and seems to find it very difficult to interact with others. He likes to play on his own and seldom shares his experiences in the classroom. His only interest is in Thomas the Tank Engine and he plays with these toys in a repetitive manner. He also flaps his hands many times through the day. He was born at term after an uneventful delivery and showed normal speech and language development up to the age of 3 years. What is the single most likely diagnosis?

- A Asperger syndrome
- B Attention deficit hyperactivity disorder
- C Cerebral palsy
- D Normal variant
- E Temporal lobe epilepsy

Sleep disturbance

P1.56–1.59

Options

A   Bed-time restriction
B   Cognitive–behavioural therapy
C   Intermittent short-term hypnotics
D   Light therapy
E   Melatonin
F   Mirtazapine
G   Regular hypnotics
H   Tricyclic antidepressant

Complete the algorithm below detailing the management of sleep disturbance in primary care from the list of options above. Each option may be used once, more than once or not at all.

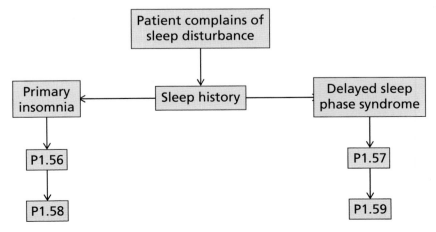

P1.60   Fibroids
A 38-year-old woman with a history of heavy periods has tried using the combined oral contraceptive pill, anti-inflammatories, progesterone-only pill and tranexamic acid without success. She has an ultrasound scan which confirms large fibroids. You refer her for a specialist opinion and she is listed for surgery, but asks if there is anything that she can try in the meantime as her daughter is getting married next month and she is worried about flooding. Which one of the following would be the most appropriate management option?

○   A   Cerazette

○   B   Danazol

○   C   Hormone replacement therapy

○   D   Mefenamic acid

○   E   Ulipristal acetate

P1.61   Sea sickness
A 67-year-old woman, who is about to embark on a cruise, requests a prescription for some sea-sickness tablets. Which one of the following statements is correct regarding this condition?

○   A   Cinnarazine is an effective treatment

○   B   Drug treatment has a placebo effect only

○   C   Hyoscine should not be used because it exacerbates motion sickness

○   D   Patients suffering sea-sickness should be advised to avoid standing on deck because the view of the moving sea can exacerbate symptoms

○   E   Promethazine is effective, with minimal side effects, making it the first-line treatment for most patients

P1.62   Tuberculosis
One of your patients has recently been diagnosed with tuberculosis. He has spent several weeks in the last 3 months in a community hospital and was a frequent visitor to the surgery. You attend a public health meeting to discuss contact tracing. Which one of the following statements regarding contact tracing is correct?

○   A   All contacts should be removed from patient care until they have been screened

○   B   Heaf testing has high sensitivity and specificity

○   C   Presence of a BCG scar implies immunity and these patients do not need to be screened

○   D   Quantiferon testing is the investigation of choice in screening contacts

○   E   An X-ray is the most appropriate investigation in TB outbreaks

P1.63 **Sore eyes**
A 39-year-old man with no history of note complains that his eyes are constantly sore. He has been seen several times both in the surgery and by his optician and has been found to have blepharitis. In spite of good eyelid hygiene and short courses of topical antibiotics he still has daily troublesome symptoms. Which one of the following would be an appropriate management option at this stage?

○ A Encourage to persevere with lid cleaning

○ B Oral doxycycline 100 mg once daily for 6 weeks

○ C Prednisolone eye drops for 1 week

○ D Refer to outpatients

○ E Topical Fucithalmic for 6 weeks

P1.64 **Ankle pain**
A 27-year-old man complains of pain above his right ankle after a dry ski slope session in preparation for his skiing holiday. He reports falling awkwardly and was unable to continue, but he can weight bear. On examination he has tenderness and bruising 4 inches (10 cm) above his lateral malleolus, with numbness over the lateral border of the foot. What is the single most appropriate management?

○ A Advise him to return if he is still in pain when the swelling has subsided

○ B Advise rest, ice, compression and elevation (RICE)

○ C Apply a backslab cast for support

○ D Reassure him that he can weight bear, making a fracture unlikely

○ E Refer immediately to the emergency department for X-ray

Abdominal pain

Options

A   Abdominal aortic aneurysm
B   Acute appendicitis
C   Acute cholecystitis
D   Acute pancreatitis
E   Crohn's disease
F   Colonic carcinoma
G   Diverticulitis
H   Gastric carcinoma
I   Irritable bowel syndrome
J   Peptic ulcer
K   Renal colic
L   Ruptured ectopic pregnancy

For each of the clinical scenarios described below, select the most appropriate diagnosis from the list of options above. Each option may be used once, more than once or not at all.

P1.65 **A 76-year-old man complains of recurrent attacks of colicky left iliac fossa pain. On examination he has left iliac fossa tenderness but no peritonism.**

P1.66 **A 39-year-old man complains of acute colicky pains radiating from his back to his groin and coming in waves.**

P1.67 **A 33-year-old woman complains of 3 months of diarrhoea, weight loss and abdominal pain. On examination she has a right iliac fossa swelling and fleshy skin tags around her anus.**

P1.68 **A 44-year-old woman complains of fever, vomiting and pain in her shoulder. On examination she is tender in the right upper quadrant.**

P1.69 **A 67-year-old man complains of several weeks of dysphagia, weight loss and, more recently, epigastric pain. On examination he is cachectic with generalised abdominal tenderness.**

P1.70 **Drug side effects**
A 56-year-old diabetic woman who takes simvastatin has come to see you after reading an article in her daily newspaper about the dangers of taking statins. She would like your advice on whether to continue. Which one of the following statements about the side effects of cholesterol-lowering treatment is true?

○   A   Ezetimibe has been reported to be associated with an increased risk of cancer

○   B   Patients with familial hypercholesterolaemia should all be treated with 40 mg simvastatin

○   C   Patients with mixed hyperlipidaemias should be treated with a statin and a fibrate

○   D   Simvastatin is the only statin that interacts significantly with other drugs

○   E   Sleep disturbance is rare

P1.71   **Hair problems**

A 7-year-old girl is brought to see you by her mother who has noticed that her hairs have the appearance below. Examination of her hair is otherwise normal, although there are several other similar hairs. Her mother admits to having treated her for nits some months ago.

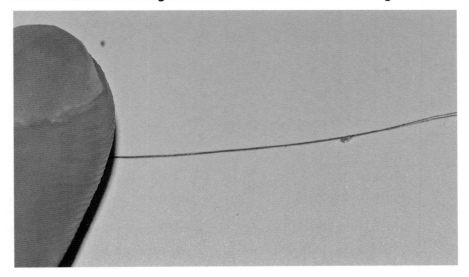

Which one of the following would be appropriate management in this situation?

○   A   Malathion used twice 7 days apart

○   B   Permethrin used twice 7 days apart

○   C   Simethicone used twice 7 days apart

○   D   Wet combing with conditioner

○   E   No treatment needed

P1.72 **Data interpretation**
The figures below show changes in the incidence of prostate cancer
and death rates over the last 10 years.

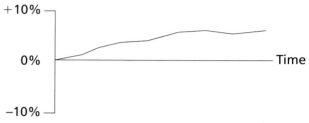

Figure (a) Percentage change in new cases of prostate cancer diagnosed
per year.

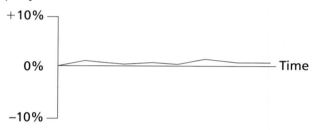

Figure (b) Percentage change in deaths from prostate cancer per year.

Which one of the following is the most likely explanation for these data?

A   Advances in treatment have led to improved survival rates

B   Changes in lifestyle have increased the risk of developing cancer

C   Clinically asymptomatic cancers are being diagnosed earlier

D   New cases are being diagnosed at the same rate but survival is
increasing

E   Newer treatments do not improve life expectancy

P1.73 **Lipid therapy**
Which one of the following statements regarding the ASCOT (Anglo-
Scandinavian Cardiac Outcomes Trial) study is correct?

A   It demonstrated significant benefits in treating hypertensive
patients with calcium antagonists and ACE inhibitors compared with
β blockers and thiazides

B   There was found to be an increased risk of diabetes in the calcium
antagonist arm compared with the thiazide arm

C   It showed no difference in cardiac disease in the three treatment
arms of thiazides, calcium antagonists and ACE inhibitors

D   The trial compared aggressive treatment of hypertension with
watchful waiting

E   This was a secondary prevention study

P1.74 **Throat pain**
A 47-year-old man complains of recurrent episodes of fleeting pain radiating from his tonsils to his right ear. He describes the pain as like an electric shock, typically lasting a few seconds. The only obvious trigger that he can identify is eating certain foods. Examination of the head and neck is unremarkable, with no skin lesions or lymphadenopathy. He has no associated vertigo, deafness or tinnitus. What is the single most likely diagnosis?

- ○ A Glossopharyngeal neuralgia
- ○ B Ménière syndrome
- ○ C Ramsay Hunt syndrome
- ○ D Tonsillar carcinoma
- ○ E Trigeminal neuralgia

P1.75 **Pain control in palliative care**
A 39-year-old woman being treated for cervical cancer is getting breakthrough pain on her current medication. You decide to start her on a strong opioid. Which one of the following statements is true regarding these drugs?

- ○ A Constipation is less common with sustained-release opioids
- ○ B Constipation should be treated on an as needed basis
- ○ C Morphine is safe in renal impairment
- ○ D Sedation is usually transient
- ○ E Visual analogue scales are the best way of assessing pain in adults

P1.76 **Epidemiology**
Comparing retrospective with prospective studies, which one of the following statements is true?

- ○ A Retrospective studies are less prone to bias than prospective studies
- ○ B Retrospective studies are more expensive to conduct than prospective studies
- ○ C Retrospective studies are quicker to conduct than prospective studies
- ○ D Results from retrospective studies carry more statistical significance than prospective studies
- ○ E Prospective studies are designed to detect differences in populations and therefore always produce statistically significant data

Skin lesions

Options

A   Actinic keratosis
B   Basal cell carcinoma
C   Keratoacanthoma
D   Malignant melanoma
E   Pyogenic granuloma
F   Seborrhoeic keratosis
G   None of the above

For each of the lesions shown below, select the most likely diagnosis from the list of options above, each option may be used once, more than once or not at all.

P1.77   **P1.78**

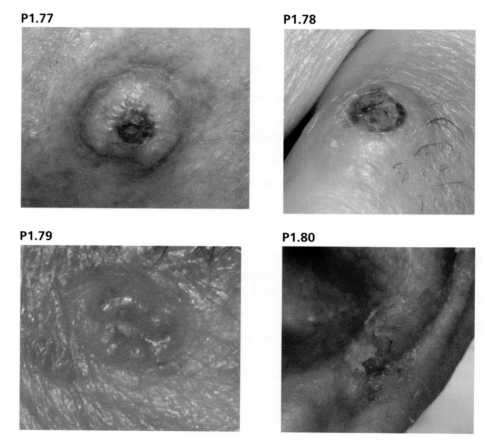

P1.79   **P1.80**

P1.81 Management of eczema

A 35-year-old businessman has been treated unsuccessfully for a flare of his eczema with emollients and Betnovate. He has avoided all soaps and cannot identify any other obvious triggers. Which one of the following would be an appropriate treatment at this stage?

○ A Azathioprine

○ B Ciclosporin

○ C Dermovate

○ D Prednisolone

○ E PUVA

P1.82 Antenatal care

A 33-year-old woman who is 33 weeks into her second pregnancy presents with reduced fetal movements. She has no abdominal pain or bleeding but has not felt the baby move since the previous evening. On examination her abdomen is soft, with fundal height consistent with dates. Which one of the following is the single most appropriate management of this situation?

○ A Admit under on-call obstetric team

○ B Ask her to contact the midwife if she has not felt 10 movements by 17:00 the following day

○ C Do cervical examination to assess for pre-term labour

○ D Reassure her that this is normal in the last trimester

○ E Refer directly to the antenatal unit for biophysical profile

P1.83 Agoraphobia

You are asked to visit a 20-year-old man at home. His mother is at the end of her tether, and tells you that he has not left the house for 3 years. He reports feelings of panic, dizziness and depersonalisation at the thought of going out, which get much worse when he is out. He presents as a rather shy, introvert character but denies any other symptoms of mental illness. Which one of the following is the most appropriate management for this patient?

○ A Diazepam used as needed

○ B Fluoxetine

○ C Hypnotherapy

○ D Risperidone

○ E Systematic desensitisation therapy

P1.84 Nail changes

A 27-year-old marketing executive asks for advice about her nails. She has recently been through a stressful relationship break-up and is applying for new jobs. She is self-conscious about the appearance of her thumbnails, shown below.

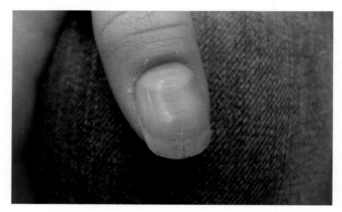

Which one of the following would be the most appropriate management of this condition?

- A Amorolfine nail lacquer
- B Avoidance of nail rubbing
- C Calcium supplementation
- D Reassurance
- E Terbinafine tablets

P1.85 Swollen arm

A 56-year-old woman who had a wide local excision of a breast cancer and axillary clearance 5 years ago presents with a 6-month history of an increasingly swollen arm on the side of her previous surgery. On examination the oedema is non-pitting, with no erythema and minimal tenderness. Which one of the following is the single most likely diagnosis?

- A Cellulitis
- B Deep vein thrombosis
- C Lymphoma
- D Lymphoedema
- E Recurrent breast cancer

P1.86 **Data Interpretation**

A 56-year-old man attends for routine blood tests in the surgery. He has a history of chronic obstructive pulmonary disease (COPD), with an FEV$_1$ of 75% predicted, and also suffers from essential hypertension. Unfortunately he continues to smoke 10–20 cigarettes a day. A full blood count is taken and the results are shown below.

Haemoglobin	19.6 g/dl (NR 13.5–18.0 mg/dl)
WCC	6.7 × 10^9/l (4.0–11.0 × 10^9/l)
Platelets	276 × 10^9/l (150–400 × 10^9/l)

What would be the single most appropriate initial management step in this case?

A   Prescribe aspirin 300 mg once daily

B   Reassure him that these results are normal

C   Refer under 2-week rule to haematology

D   Start a smoking cessation programme and repeat the blood tests in 4 weeks

E   Venesect until the haemoglobin is in the normal range

P1.87 **Moles**

While visiting your parents your mother asks you if you can have a look at a mole that she is worried about. She tells you that she doesn't particularly like her own GP due to his rudeness and is too busy to see one of the other doctors at the surgery. Which one of the following would be the most appropriate response in this situation, according to General Medical Council guidelines?

A   Encourage her to complain to the practice manager about the doctor's rudeness

B   Examine the mole and advise her on management accordingly

C   Suggest that she sees another doctor at the practice

D   Refer her to a local dermatologist

E   Telephone her GP and explain the situation

Upper gastrointestinal disorders

Options

A Achalasia
B Barrett's oesophagus
C Coeliac disease
D Hiatus hernia
E MALToma
F Oesophageal cancer
G Oesophageal dysmotility
H Oesophageal stricture
I Plummer–Vinson syndrome
J Reflux oesophagitis

For each of the statements below, select the option from the list above that is most appropriate. Each option may be used once, more than once or not at all.

P1.88 Associated with *Helicobacter pylori* infection.
P1.89 Causes a slowly progressive, intermittent dysphagia, often causing chest infections.
P1.90 Associated with a 1% annual risk of developing oesophageal cancer.
P1.91 Usually presents with bolus obstruction.
P1.92 Causes dysphagia in association with glossitis, koilonychia and angular stomatitis.

P1.93 **PSA screening**
A 44-year-old man asks for a PSA test to make sure that he doesn't have prostate cancer. He has no urinary symptoms and no family history of note. Which of the following statements is true regarding screening for prostate cancer?

- A PSA screening has been shown to increase diagnosis of early prostate cancer
- B PSA screening has been shown to increase quality of life
- C PSA screening has been shown to reduce mortality
- D PSA screening is cost-effective
- E Surgical treatment of asymptomatic prostate cancer detected on routine screening improves long-term morbidity and mortality

P1.94 **Genetic disease**

A 43-year-old man has recently discovered that his father has Huntington's disease. He has been tested and does not have the disease. He has two small children and would like to know their risk of developing the disease. There is no family history of Huntington's disease in the mother's pedigree. Which one of the following statements is true regarding this situation?

    A   Each child has a 25% chance of being affected

    B   Each child has a 25% chance of being a carrier

    C   Each child has a 0% chance of being affected

    D   He has a 25% chance of being a carrier

    E   He has a 50% chance of being a carrier

P1.95 **Cold sores**

A 29-year-old woman comes to see you for advice. She is due to get married in 3 weeks and is concerned that she will have a flare of her cold sores, which always seems to occur when she is stressed. She asks if anything can be done to prevent this. Which one of the following statements is correct regarding this scenario?

    A   Cold sores are caused by infection with *Staphylococcus aureus* and using flucloxacillin will usually prevent an exacerbation

    B   Cold sores are caused by primary infection with herpes simplex virus and can be prevented by taking oral aciclovir

    C   Exacerbations are more common in the winter

    D   Topical aciclovir is an effective prophylactic treatment

    E   Ultraviolet light used at the onset of symptoms may abort the attack

P1.96 **Wrist pain**

A 45-year-old woman complains of pain on the radial side of her wrist, which came on after a weekend trimming flowers for a wedding display. On examination she has tenderness and swelling along the radial border of the thumb, with maximal tenderness over the head of the radius. Resisted abduction exacerbates the pain. What is the single most likely diagnosis?

    A   Carpal tunnel syndrome

    B   De Quervain's tenosynovitis

    C   Lateral epicondylitis

    D   Medial epicondylitis

    E   Osteoarthritis of the first metacarpophalangeal joint

P1.97 **Renal problems**

A 34-year-old man has a renal ultrasound scan carried out to investigate renal colic. He is shocked to be told he that has a duplex ureter on the right and comes to see you to discuss the significance of this. Which one of the following statements about this condition is true?

- A   Duplex ureters are of no clinical significance
- B   Pelviureteric junction (PUJ) obstruction is more common in patients with duplex ureters
- C   Surgery is indicated in all cases
- D   This condition is extremely rare
- E   Treatment with an ACE inhibitor is indicated to prevent nephropathy

P1.98 **Squint**

A 2-year-old boy is brought to see you by his mother, who is concerned that he is developing a squint. On examination he appears to have a right-sided squint, and also when you look at his eyes with an ophthalmoscope you see that he has a white pupillary reflex on that side. He was adopted at birth and his parents have no knowledge of his family or antenatal history. Which one of the following would be the most appropriate management for this child?

- A   Reassure the mother and arrange to review him in 4 weeks
- B   Refer to ophthalmology for assessment of vision
- C   Refer to optician for glasses
- D   Refer to the orthoptic department for patching
- E   Refer under the 2-week rule

P1.99 **Weight gain**

A 53-year-old woman complains of increasing difficulties with her figure. She tells you that she has always had a slim figure but that over the last 6 months she has noticed that her waist is getting bigger in spite of regular exercise and dieting. She also reports new onset of urinary frequency and constipation. On examination she has some dullness in her flanks but no other obvious abnormalities on abdominal palpation. Which one of the following would be the most appropriate next step in her assessment?

- A   Bimanual examination
- B   Check thyroid function
- C   Refer for colonoscopy in view of change in bowel habit
- D   Refer for ultrasound scan
- E   Trial of anticholinergic

P1.100 Haematuria

A 9-year-old boy is brought into the surgery by his mother after an episode of frank haematuria. This seems to have started after a viral infection and he has complained of loin pain over the last 24 hours. On examination he appears well with no fever or oedema and no masses in his abdomen. Urinalysis is positive for blood but negative for nitrites and leukocytes, with protein 1+. Reviewing his notes you discover that he was treated last year for a suspected urinary tract infection by a locum after presenting with macroscopic haematuria. What is the single most likely diagnosis?

- ○   A   Beetroot consumption
- ○   B   IgA nephropathy
- ○   C   Polycystic kidneys
- ○   D   Urinary tract infection
- ○   E   Wilms' tumour

P1.101 Rash

A 44-year-old man attends for a routine insurance medical. While taking his blood pressure you notice an unusual area of skin on his elbow. He does not have any patches elsewhere apart from his other elbow, and is otherwise well. He has mild hypertension treated with ramipril and suffered from eczema when he was younger, but takes no other medication. A photograph of his arm is shown below.

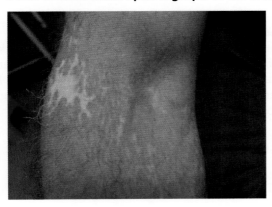

What is the most likely cause of this appearance?

- ○   A   Drug reaction
- ○   B   Lichenification
- ○   C   Tinea
- ○   D   Traumatic depigmentation
- ○   E   Vitiligo

P1.102 Child health surveillance

Which one of the following should be part of a routine 8-week check for newborn infants?

- ○ A Coordination
- ○ B Cover test for squint
- ○ C The Guthrie test
- ○ D Hearing
- ○ E Presence of cataracts

P1.103 Visual loss

A 41-year-old woman complains of sudden onset of visual loss in her right eye, which she noticed on waking. She also complains of discomfort in the eye, which is worse when looking upwards. On examination she has a central defect on field testing and a relative afferent pupillary defect, although her fundus looks normal. The contralateral eye is normal. What is the single most likely diagnosis?

- ○ A Acute glaucoma
- ○ B Amaurosis fugax
- ○ C Central retinal vein occlusion (CRVO)
- ○ D Optic neuritis
- ○ E Papilloedema

P1.104 Levothyroxine treatment

You meet a new patient for the first time at his new patient check. He had a thyroidectomy for thyroid cancer 25 years ago and has been taking levothyroxine ever since. He tells you that he has not had his thyroid function tested for some time so you send him for a blood test. Which one of the following statements is correct regarding this situation?

- ○ A He should stay on his current dose and does not need thyroid function tests
- ○ B He should have a TSH level within the normal range
- ○ C His T_4 level should be within the normal range
- ○ D His T_3 level should be within the normal range
- ○ E His TSH should be <0.01 μU/l

Statistical terms

Options

A False positive
B False negative
C Incidence
D Odds ratio
E The *p* value
F Prevalence
G Sensitivity
H Specificity
I Standard deviation
J Standard error of the mean
K Standardised mortality rate
L True positive
M True negative

For each of the statements below, select the most appropriate term from the list above. Each option may be used once, more than once or not at all.

P1.105 **Quantifies the spread of the distribution of data within a series; it is equal to the square root of the variance.**

P1.106 **An estimate of risk used in case–control studies.**

P1.107 **An estimate of statistical significance.**

P1.108 **The proportion of new cases of a disease diagnosed within a specified time period.**

P1.109 **The proportion of people without a condition diagnosed as being disease free with a particular screening test.**

P1.110 **Barrett's oesophagus**
One of your patients has recently had an upper gastrointestinal endoscopy that has shown Barrett's oesophagus. He is concerned that this means that he will get cancer and comes to see you to discuss this diagnosis. Which one of the following statements regarding this condition is true?

○ A Barrett's oesophagus is a benign condition with no long-term complications

○ B Barrett's oesophagus will often resolve if *Helicobacter pylori* infection is treated

○ C Patients with Barrett's oesophagus should be referred for oesophagectomy

○ D There is a 1% annual risk of developing malignancy in patients with Barrett's oesophagus

○ E There is no treatment for Barrett's oesophagus other than surveillance

P1.111 Chronic obstructive pulmonary disease
Which one of the following statements is correct regarding current management of COPD?

○   A   β Blockers are contraindicated in COPD

○   B   Long-acting β agonists need to be given twice daily in patients with COPD

○   C   Patients who wish to fly should be reassured that, if their oxygen saturation at rest is >90%, they can fly without supplemental oxygen

○   D   Self-management of COPD has been shown to significantly reduce hospital admission

○   E   Tiotropium should be considered at step 2 in COPD management

P1.112 Headache
A 47-year-old woman with a history of focal migraine comes to you with 3-hour history of severe headache centred around her right eye, with loss of vision in that eye and nausea and vomiting. On examination her conjunctiva is injected and her pupil does not constrict to light. What is the single most likely diagnosis?

○   A   Acute angle-closure glaucoma

○   B   Cluster headache

○   C   Giant-cell arteritis

○   D   Focal migraine

○   E   Subarachnoid haemorrhage

P1.113 Data interpretation
The local prescribing officer has generated the Cates' plot below to help explain to patients the benefits of an exercise programme for osteoarthritis, as part of a drive for greater patient involvement in clinical decisions.

Which one of the following statements is correct regarding interpretation of this data?

○ A Although there are no side effects from the intervention, 30% of patients will not benefit from the intervention

○ B Each patient has a 70% chance of improving after the intervention

○ C Individual patients will experience an average improvement of 70% in their symptom score

○ D The intervention is as likely to produce harm as benefit

○ E The intervention is cost-effective

P1.114 Ankle pain

A 52-year-old woman who enjoys recreational jogging is diagnosed with a chest infection and treated with levofloxacin. One week later she complains of pain in both ankles, with stiffness in her Achilles tendon, worse on waking. On examination there is diffuse tenderness but no palpable defect and she is able to plantarflex her feet against resistance. What is the single most likely diagnosis?

○ A Achilles tendon rupture

○ B Achilles tendinopathy

○ C Overuse injury

○ D Polymyalgia rheumatica

○ E Rhabdomyolysis

P1.115 Chest symptoms

A 33-year-old farm labourer complains that he has developed a cough, chest tightness and breathlessness, with myalgia. He has had this in the past and has been treated with a salbutamol inhaler with slight benefit. He is well most of the year but reports getting these symptoms at certain times of the year when he is working indoors. On examination he is afebrile and has a respiratory rate of 30/min with fine crepitations in both lung fields. He has no wheeze or finger clubbing. Which one of the following is the most likely diagnosis?

○ A Asthma

○ B Atypical pneumonia

○ C Bronchiectasis

○ D Extrinsic allergic alveolitis

○ E Pulmonary fibrosis

P1.116 Period pains
Which one of the following statements regarding evidence-based management of dysmenorrhoea is correct?

○   A   Aspirin is the most effective NSAID in the management of primary dysmenorrhoea

○   B   The combined oral contraceptive has a number needed to treat of 5 for management of primary dysmenorrhoea

○   C   COX-2 inhibitors have been shown to have no additional efficacy compared with placebo

○   D   Paracetamol is as effective as ibuprofen, with fewer side effects

○   E   Spinal manipulation has been proved to be of benefit in primary dysmenorrhoea

P1.117 Partnership agreements
Which one of the following statements regarding partnership agreements is correct?

○   A   A partnership agreement does not need to be updated to reflect partnership changes, as long as new partners agree to the terms of the old agreement

○   B   A partnership without a formal partnership agreement is not considered to be a legal partnership

○   C   Only qualified general practitioners can legally be partners in a medical practice

○   D   Under the Partnership Act 1890 all financial decisions made by a partnership must be unanimous

○   E   Where a partnership agreement does not exist, the partnership can be terminated at any time by one of the partners

Learning and teaching methods

Options

A   Cathartic
B   Counselling
C   Didactic
D   Heuristic
E   Reflective
F   Socratic

For each of the descriptions of teaching methods below, select the most appropriate option from the list above. Each option may be used once, more than once or not at all.

P1.118 Facilitates learning through awareness-raising questions.

P1.119 Explores feelings and assumptions.

P1.120 Promotes learner autonomy and self-directed learning.

P1.121 A formal lecture style.

P1.122 Toe pain

A 23-year-old keen runner comes to see you a few hours after completing a fell running competition complaining of pain in his toes. The appearance is shown below.

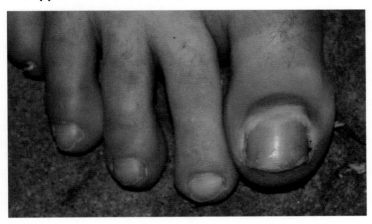

In the box below, write the most appropriate intervention if any, for this condition.

| |
| |
| |

P1.123 Contraceptive choices

A 23-year-old woman comes to see you for her 6-week check after delivering a boy by caesarean section. She is breastfeeding and has not had a period yet, but would like to discuss contraception. Which one of the following statements is true?

- ○ A A negative pregnancy test is required before starting the contraceptive pill if periods have not yet returned

- ○ B A combined oral contraceptive pill (COCP) can be started at any time from 1 week after the birth onwards

- ○ C The earliest possible fertile ovulation is around 28 days postpartum

- ○ D Ovulation does not occur until after the return of periods

- ○ E Progesterone-only pills interfere with breastfeeding and should be avoided in lactating mothers

Management of back pain

P1.24–1.28

Options

A Discharge
B GP management
C NSAIDs
D Physiotherapy
E Red flag symptoms
F Refer to back school
G Refer to secondary care
H Review in 2 weeks
I Review in 4 weeks
J Strong opioids

Your local physiotherapy department have developed a new spinal triage system to simplify the management of mechanical back pain. They wish to simplify this with a flowchart. Complete the figure below from the list of options above. Each option may be used once, more than once or not at all.

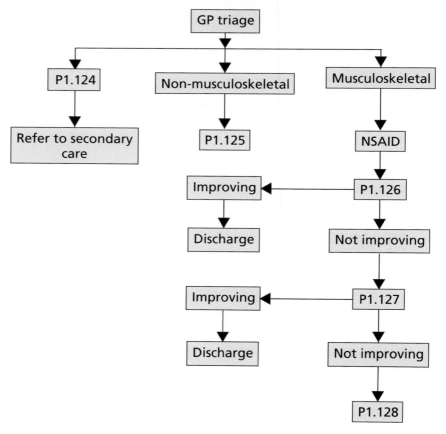

P1.129 MMR vaccination

You receive a telephone call from a concerned mother. Her 17-month-old son had his MMR vaccination at 14 months. There have been six confirmed cases of measles at her son's crèche and she asks your advice as to what precautions she should take. Which one of the following is the most appropriate advice in this case?

- A He should have a MMR booster at $4\frac{1}{2}$ years of age
- B He should have a measles booster vaccine
- C He should have an MMR booster immediately
- D He should have blood sent to assess if he is immune
- E She should be reassured that no further vaccinations are required

P1.130 Heart murmurs

A 35-year-old woman is diagnosed with a heart murmur at a routine employment medical. A subsequent echocardiogram shows mitral valve prolapse. She comes to see you to discuss the implications of this. Which one of the following statements is correct regarding this condition?

- A All patients should be referred for valve replacement
- B It commonly causes congestive cardiac failure
- C It is usually caused by streptococcal infection
- D It can be associated with palpitations
- E Patients should be anticoagulated with warfarin

P1.131 Loss of smell

A 48-year-old man complains of 6 months of loss of smell and reduced taste. He reports that his symptoms are constant and seemed to have started for no obvious reason. He is a lifelong hayfever sufferer but says he can breathe through his nose. You do not have a Thudichum's nasal speculum in the surgery but limited examination of the nose with an otoscope does not show any obvious pathology. Which one of the following is the most likely diagnosis?

- A Deviated nasal septum
- B Frontal lobe tumour
- C Head injury
- D Nasal polyps
- E Overuse of decongestant

Causes of pneumonia

Options

A	Aspergillosis
B	Actinomycosis
C	*Coxiella burnetii* pneumonia
D	Cytomelagovirus
E	Legionnaires' disease
F	Measles
G	*Mycoplasma pneumoniae*
H	*Pneumocystis jiroveci* pneumonia
I	Psittacosis
J	Q fever
K	Tuberculosis
L	Varicella

For each of the descriptions below, select the most appropriate option from the list above. Each option may be used once, more than once or not at all.

P1.132 Epidemics occur in 3- to 4-year cycles, predominantly affecting children.

P1.133 Causes a prodromal illness with fever, coryza, conjunctivitis and cough, followed by the development of a rash starting on the neck.

P1.134 Affects immunocompromised individuals, causing a suppurative pneumonia; it has a poor prognosis.

P1.135 Causes a primary viral pneumonia in adults.

P1.136 Causes a prodromal illness with fever, diarrhoea, headache and myalgia, followed by the development of respiratory symptoms; hyponatraemia is often found.

P1.137 Rash

A 65-year-old woman develops a painful rash on her back. On examination she has numerous circular target lesions over her back and torso. These have a central blister. Which one of the following statements is correct regarding this scenario?

○ A   These lesions are never seen in the mouth

○ B   This condition is always iatrogenic and a full drug history should be taken

○ C   This condition often has an infectious cause

○ D   This condition usually resolves spontaneously in 3–5 days

○ E   This patient has erythema nodosum and should have a chest X-ray to exclude sarcoidosis

P1.138 Neck lumps

A 48-year-old woman complains of a sore throat. While talking to her you notice that she has a swollen neck and on examination she has a smooth swelling, more pronounced on the right side, which moves with swallowing. She thinks that this has been present for a number of years. There are no palpable lymph nodes. She is otherwise well. Blood tests reveal a normal full blood count, normal renal and liver function, and normal thyroid function. Which one of the following statements regarding her management is correct?

A   She should have a blood sent for thyroid autoantibodies and if these are normal she should be reassured

B   She should be prescribed levothyroxine 100 μg once a day initially

C   She should be reassured

D   She should be referred for an ultrasound examination

E   She should be referred under the 2-week rule

P1.139 Palpitations

A 78-year-old man is thought to have an irregular heartbeat at a blood pressure check. The nurse who sees him takes an electrocardiogram, which is shown below.

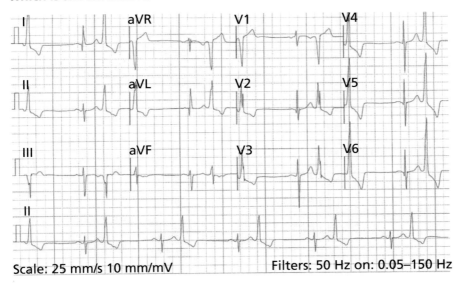

Scale: 25 mm/s 10 mm/mV   Filters: 50 Hz on: 0.05–150 Hz

Which one of the following is the correct diagnosis of this ECG trace?

A   Atrioventricular dissociation

B   Paroxysmal atrial fibrillation

C   Ventricular bigeminy

D   Wenckebach's phenomenon

E   2:1 heart block

P1.140 Ear lesions

A 79-year-old man complains of deafness. On examining his ears you find wax impaction on both sides but also note the lesion below, in front of his ear. He reports that this has been present for a number of years and sometimes bleeds.

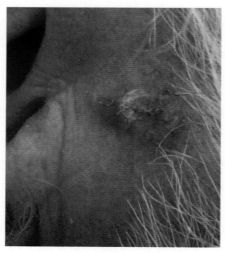

What is the single most likely diagnosis?

○ A Actinic keratosis

○ B Basal cell carcinoma (BCC)

○ C Chondrodermatitis nodularis helicis

○ D Keratoacanthoma

○ E Squamous cell carcinoma (SCC)

Difficult patients

Options

A Dependent clingers
B Entitled demanders
C Frequent attenders
D Heartsink patient
E Manipulative help rejector
F Self-destructive denier
G None of the above

For each of the descriptions below, select the most appropriate option from the list above. Each option may be used once, more than once or not at all.

P1.141 Often try to take control of the doctor–patient relationship.
P1.142 More commonly identified by male rather than by female GPs.
P1.143 Unconsciously engages in behaviour that is likely to be detrimental to the patient's own health.

P1.144 Seem to derive satisfaction from the physician's inability to treat their symptoms.

P1.145 An objective description that is medicolegally appropriate.

P1.146 Eye symptoms

A 39-year-old schoolteacher complains that her right eye seems to be protruding more than the left. She has no visual symptoms or pain. Previous history is unremarkable other than chronic rhinosinusitis, for which she takes nasal steroids. On examination she does appear to have some asymmetry and proptosis. She saw her optician before this visit and has normal visual acuity, colour vision, fundoscopy and visual fields. She has no headache or any symptoms of hypothyroidism or hyperthyroidism. Blood tests, including thyroid function, are normal. What is the single most appropriate next step in her management?

- A   Check thyroid autoantibodies
- B   Check for anti-acetylcholine receptor antibodies
- C   Reassure her that this is normal
- D   Refer under the 2-week rule for suspected brain tumour
- E   Treat with broad-spectrum antibiotics

P1.147 Water-borne disease

Your local water supply has been temporarily suspended due to the discovery of *Cryptosporidium* sp. in a reservoir. A number of your patients have come to see you, concerned that they might have been exposed before the shutdown. Which one of the following statements is true with regard to this situation?

- A   Cryptosporidia affect all age groups, causing severe diarrhoea and vomiting
- B   Cryptosporidia can be resistant to chlorination of water
- C   Cryptosporidia in children cause a mild diarrhoea that lasts less than 48 hours
- D   Cryptosporidia can cause haemoytic uraemic syndrome
- E   Humans are a secondary host and do not transmit the infection to others

Hypertension trials

Options

A   4S
B   ALLHAT
C   CAMBO
D   DASH
E   GREACE
F   HOPE
G   HOT
H   HYVET
I   STOP

For each of the statements below, select the single most appropriate hypertension study from the list above. Each option may be used once, more than once or not at all.

P1.148 Demonstrated an increase in cerebrovascular disease and heart failure with doxazosin.

P1.149 Showed that dietary modification could reduce blood pressure by 11.4/5.5 mmHg.

P1.150 Demonstrated the importance of value hypertension in elderly people.

P1.151 Found no difference among ACE inhibitors, calcium antagonists or β blockers in morbidity and mortality.

P1.152 Found that automated clinic blood pressure readings eliminated the white coat effect.

P1.153 Cardiomyopathy
Which one of the following statements with regard to hypertrophic obstructive cardiomyopathy (HOCM) is true?

A   The cause is usually viral

B   It is a cause of sudden death in young athletes

C   It is a benign condition

D   Treatment with β blockers will increase life expectancy

E   It usually presents with signs of congestive cardiac failure

P1.154 Drug side effects
Which of the following statements about the side effects of painkillers is true?

A   Buprenorphine cannot be taken with other opioids

B   Co-proxamol is toxic and is no longer available

C   Tramadol is not an opioid and is not associated with nausea or constipation

○   D   Transdermal fentanyl patches are not associated with constipation

○   E   Transdermal opioid patches do not reach steady-state analgesic levels for 24 hours

P1.155 Irregular bleeding

A 25-year-old nulliparous woman complains of breakthrough bleeding most months on her 30-µg COCP. She has been taking this for 12 months now, takes no other medications and does not miss pills. Examination is unremarkable and she recently had a cervical smear that was reported as negative. She does not get any post-coital bleeding and high vaginal swabs and chlamydial swabs were recently negative. Which one of the following is the most appropriate management?

○   A   Advise her to take two pills a day

○   B   Change to a triphasic pill

○   C   Change to the mini-pill for better cycle control

○   D   Suggest a Mirena intrauterine system (IUS)

○   E   Reassure her that this is normal and no action is needed

P1.156 Problem drinking

Which one of the following statements about the management of problem drinking is true?

○   A   Acamprosate reduces the desire to drink

○   B   Antabuse (disulfiram) is safe to use in the community

○   C   Non-specialist interventions do not lead to statistically significant reductions in alcohol use

○   D   Only 10% of problem drinkers are abstinent at 1 year

○   E   The aim in managing problem drinking should always be abstinence

Treatment of prostate cancer

Options

A   Brachytherapy
B   Cryotherapy
C   Cyproterone acetate
D   Docetaxel
E   External-beam radiotherapy
F   LHRH analogue
G   Orchidectomy
H   Radical prostatectomy
I   Watchful waiting

For each of the statements below regarding the management of prostate cancer, select the most appropriate option from the list above. Each option may be used once, more than once or not at all.

P1.157 Associated with a >10% risk of proctitis.
P1.158 Shown in the Scandinavian Prostate Cancer Group Study to be as effective as radical prostatectomy in terms of its effect on overall mortality.
P1.159 Indicated for non-hormone-sensitive recurrent disease in patients who have previously been treated with radiotherapy.
P1.160 Useful in patients with metastatic disease who cannot tolerate LHRH agonist treatment.
P1.161 Causes an initial increase in testosterone production.

P1.162 Gout
Which one of the following statements about gout is true?

○   A   Colchicine should be prescribed as one tablet every hour until the pain resolves or diarrhoea develops

○   B   Dietary factors are the most common triggers for an acute attack of gout

○   C   Joint aspiration typically reveals cloudy fluid and this is diagnostic in larger joints

○   D   Normal serum uric acid during an acute attack of arthritis excludes gout

○   E   Patients who are intolerant of colchicine or NSAIDs should be treated with prednisolone

P1.163 Skin disease
A 63-year-old woman has noticed an itchy rash in her cleavage.

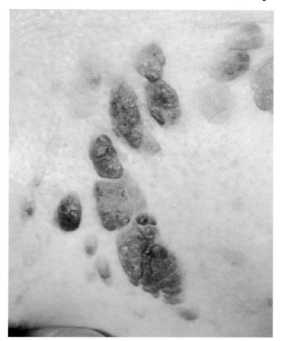

What is the single most likely diagnosis? Select one option only.

○   A   Basal cell carcinoma

○   B   Dermatofibroma

○   C   Malignant melanoma

○   D   Seborrhoeic keratosis

○   E   Viral wart

P1.164 Vaginal discharge
Regarding vaginal infections, which one of the following statements is true?

○   A   A fishy smell suggests candidal infection

○   B   Bacterial vaginosis is always symptomatic

○   C   Candidal infection is more common in pregnancy

○   D   *Trichomonas* sp. does not cause disease in men

○   E   Where bacterial vaginosis is confirmed, the partner must also be treated to prevent re-infection

P1.165 Data interpretation

A pilot weight-loss clinic has been running for 12 months and the primary care trust would like to extend the service based on its results. The results are shown below (BMI, body mass index; CI, confidence interval; N/A, not applicable).

Time since start (months)	No. patients	Mean weight change (kg)	95% CI	Mean BMI (kg/m^2)
0	1500	N/A	N/A	32
1	1200	−2.6	−4.1 to +1.3	31
2	1000	−3.1	−3.9 to +0.5	29
3	900	−3.3	−3.4 to −1.8	28
6	600	−3.4	−3.6 to −2.5	28
12	300	−2.9	−3.2 to −2.6	29

Which one of the following statements about these data is correct?

- A On an intention-to-treat basis the data show a mean weight loss of −2.9 kg at 12 months
- B The data show a statistically significant weight loss at 3 months
- C The data show high levels of concordance
- D Most patients who complete 12 months' treatment achieve a normal BMI
- E Weight loss is maintained at 12 months in most patients

Viral infections

Options

A Adenovirus
B Coxsackievirus
C Epstein–Barr virus
D Herpes simplex
E Human papillomavirus
F Hepatitis D
G Influenza A
H Norovirus
I Parvovirus B19

For each of the diseases below, select the single most likely causative agent from the list above. Each option may be used once, more than once or not at all.

P1.166 Oropharyngeal cancer
P1.167 Gastroenteritis
P1.168 Slapped cheek syndrome
P1.169 Hand, foot and mouth disease
P1.170 Burkitt's lymphoma

P1.171 Groin pain

A 6-year-old girl comes to see you with her mother. She has been complaining of 6 months of intermittent pain in the right side of her groin and she has a persistent limp. She is otherwise well but seems to be limping most of the time. On examination she has a full range of movement on the left side of her hip but movements on the right side are limited in all directions. Examination of the groin reveals no hernia and no lymphadenopathy. Blood tests are taken, which are normal. **What is the single most likely diagnosis?**

- A   Congenital dislocation of the hip
- B   Irritable hip
- C   Perthes' disease
- D   Septic arthritis
- E   Slipped upper femoral epiphysis

P1.172 Bone health

Which one of the following statements with regard to the management of osteopenia and osteoporosis is correct?

- A   Bisphosphonates are available only in oral formulation
- B   Bisphosphonates have been shown to increase bone density but not to reduce fractures
- C   Patients diagnosed with osteoporosis should be investigated for coeliac disease
- D   Patients diagnosed with postmenopausal osteoporosis should be treated with bisphosphonates for life
- E   A T score <1.5 is diagnostic of osteoporosis

P1.173 Knee pain

A 67-year-old man complains of increasing frequency of pain in both knees, worse on the right. He has is slightly overweight with a body mass index of 27 but has no previous medical history of note and takes no regular medication. Clinical examination reveals a mild varus deformity, some crepitus on both sides on flexion, but no erythema or effusion. **Which one of the following statements regarding management is correct?**

- A   All patients should be advised to exercise regularly
- B   All patients should have an initial X ray
- C   Referral to an orthopaedic surgeon is indicated if symptoms cannot be controlled with oral analgesia
- D   Weight-bearing exercise is contraindicated
- E   Weight loss is unlikely to be helpful in patients with a BMI <30

P1.174 Headache

A 34-year-old woman in week 12 of her first pregnancy complains of several weeks of increasing headaches. These are present mostly in the mornings and late at night, and seem to resolve once she gets up. She has no other previous history of note. Examination reveals a blood pressure of 128/72 mmHg, negative urinalysis and a BMI of 34. Her pupils are equal and reactive and she has no ophthalmoplegia or obvious visual field loss. Fundoscopy shows a hyperaemic disc with loss of cupping. What is the single most likely diagnosis?

○ A Acute glaucoma

○ B Benign intracranial hypertension

○ C Brain tumour

○ D Malignant hypertension

○ E Pre-eclampsia

Management of abnormal smears

Options

A   Refer for colposcopy
B   Refer under 2-week rule
C   Repeat in 1 month
D   Repeat in 6 months
E   Repeat in 1 year
F   Repeat in 3 years
G   Repeat in 5 years
H   Smear no longer necessary

Regarding the management of cervical smear results, for each of the situations described below select the most appropriate management option from the list above. Each option may be used once, more than once or not at all.

P1.175 A 34-year-old woman has had a smear reported as 'borderline, with endocervical changes'. She has not previously had abnormal smears.

P1.176 A 27-year-old woman with a history of previous chlamydial infection has had two consecutive inadequate smears.

P1.177 A 63-year-old woman who has not had any previous abnormal smears has a normal smear. She enquires about follow-up smears.

P1.178 A 36-year-old woman with no history of abnormal smears has a smear reported as showing mild dyskariosis.

P1.179 A 31-year-old woman has a smear that shows suspected carcinoma *in situ*.

P1.180 Rashes

A 24-year-old girl attends for a new patient check. She asks if there is anything else that she can use for the rash on her arms. She has had this for most of her life and uses regular moisturisers, otherwise the skin becomes dry. She also reports that the rash improves when she is away from the stress of the office on holiday. The rash is shown below.

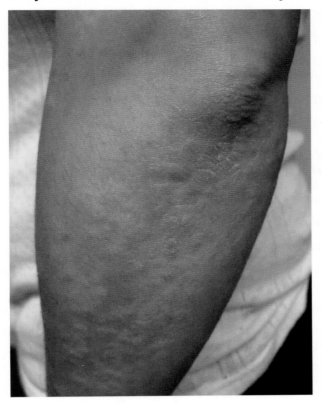

What would the single most appropriate management be in this instance?

○ A Prescribe topical steroids

○ B Prescribe topical tacrolimus

○ C Prescribe vitamin D analogues

○ D Refer for PUVA therapy

○ E Treat with antifungal treatment

P1.181 Eye symptoms

A 17-year-old girl has a lump in her lower eyelid, which has been present for 9 months and is slowly enlarging. She reports that this started after she developed a stye, but she is becoming increasingly self-conscious and would like your advice on management. Which one of the following is the single most appropriate action?

○   A   She should be offered incision and curettage

○   B   She should be told that it is unlikely to resolve spontaneously

○   C   She should be referred immediately to ophthalmology outpatients for excision

○   D   She should be treated with antibiotic ointment

○   E   She should be treated with cryotherapy

P1.182 Pre-pregnancy care

You see a 31-year-old woman who is planning to start a family soon. Which one of the following statements is correct regarding pre-pregnancy counselling?

○   A   All pregnant women should take vitamin D supplements

○   B   Nicotine replacement therapy is contraindicated in pregnancy

○   C   Patients should be advised to drink no more than 14 units of alcohol a week

○   D   Patients taking anticonvulsants should take 400 µg folic acid a day

○   E   Patients with pre-existing hypertension should be switched to an ACE inhibitor pre-conception

P1.183 Diarrhoea

A 36-year-old woman with no previous history of note complains of nausea and vomiting with fever, followed by watery diarrhoea and abdominal pain, which started 12 hours after attending a wedding with a buffet reception. Which one of the following is the most likely organism responsible?

○   A   *Campylobacter* sp.

○   B   Cryptosporidia

○   C   *Salmonella* sp.

○   D   *Shigella* sp.

○   E   Typhoid

P1.184 Eye problems

A 52-year-old man attends his optician for a routine eye test. His optician asks him to make an appointment to see you, and the letter from the optician states that he has normal intraocular pressure but has cupped discs. Which one of the following statements is correct regarding this situation?

- A   Annual follow-up is indicated with onward referral if intraocular pressures exceed 21 mmHg

- B   Cupping of the disc indicates damage to the eye despite normal intraocular pressure

- C   Laser iridotomy is indicated to reverse the cupping

- D   No action is required at this time but he should be asked to report any change in his vision

- E   No further action is needed

P1.185 Backache

A 78-year-old man complains of mid-thoracic backache for the last 3 months. He looks pale and has lost weight. On examination he has some tenderness over his eighth thoracic vertebra, but there are no other obvious signs. You arrange for some blood tests, which show raised plasma viscosity, a normochromic/normocytic anaemia with normal WCC and platelets, a raised calcium and an eGFR of 42 ml/min. What is the single most likely diagnosis?

- A   Chronic lymphocytic leukaemia (CLL)

- B   Lung cancer

- C   Multiple myeloma

- D   Prostate cancer

- E   Sarcoma

P1.186 Molar pregnancy

A 32-year-old woman has recently been discharged from hospital after having a molar pregnancy. She comes to see you to discuss the implications of this diagnosis. Which one of the following statements is true?

- A   Ninety per cent of patients with a molar pregnancy will go on to develop neoplastic disease within 2 years

- B   Prognosis is poor in patients who develop neoplastic disease

- C   Patients should be monitored with regular βhCG levels for 2 years

- D   Recurrence risk is high and patients should be advised to undergo sterilisation

- E   The COCP is suitable contraception in the βhCG monitoring phase

The Mental Health Act

Options

A   Section 2
B   Section 3
C   Section 4
D   Section 7
E   Section 12
F   Section 17
G   Section 135
H   Section 136
I   None of the above

For each of the situations described below, select the single most appropriate option from the list above. Each option may be used once, more than once or not at all.

P1.187 A 23-year-old man who has been living with his mother has developed an addiction to heroin. He refuses treatment but his mother asks you to have him sectioned so that he can be treated.

P1.188 A 77-year-old man is found confused and wearing only his pyjamas in the street in the middle of the night in early February. He is unable to give his name to the police or explain why he is there, but refuses to go with them. They feel that he is at risk and would like to take him to a safe place.

P1.189 A 31-year-old paranoid schizophrenic has stopped taking his medication and is refusing to leave the house where he lives with his mother. He has started to self-harm and will not see his doctor, who he believes is the devil.

P1.190 A 52-year-old man with severe learning disabilities due to Down syndrome can no longer be looked after by his elderly mother, but refuses to go into a residential home. Social services have requested that he be admitted to one under the provisions of the Mental Health Act.

P1.191 The 31-year-old paranoid schizophrenic has been assessed and treated in hospital and it is felt that he needs a further period of supervised patient treatment, but that this can be given in the community. He has a history of non-compliance and subsequent relapse.

Management of heavy menstrual bleeding

P1.192–1.196

Options

A   Contraceptive pill
B   Danazol
C   Fibroids present on ultrasound
D   Luteal phase progestogens
E   Mirena
F   Normal ultrasound
G   Refer routinely
H   Refer under the 2-week rule
I   Tranexamic acid

The algorithm below describes the management of women with heavy menstrual bleeding. From the list of options above, select the most appropriate management for each missing step. Each option may be used once, more than once or not at all.

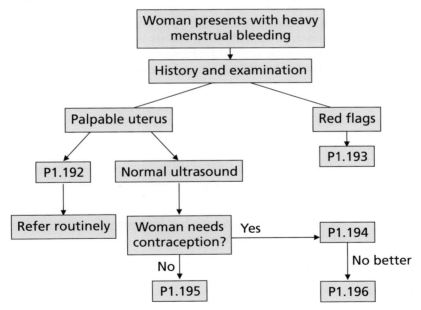

P1.197 Snoring

A 37-year-old man comes to see you with his new wife. They have been married for only 3 months but already she has had to resort to sleeping in the spare room because of his snoring. He has no symptoms or signs of sleep apnoea, and is otherwise well. On examination he has a collar size of 15 inches, a BMI of 27 kg/m^2, and examination of his nose and throat are normal. Which one of the following is the most appropriate action in this situation?

○   A   Advise the patient that his snoring is harmless and no treatment is needed

○   B   Check thyroid function

○   C   Prescribe sedatives for his wife

○   D   Refer for continuous positive airway pressure (CPAP) treatment

○   E   Refer for uvulopalatoplasty (UVPP)

P1.198 Hepatitis

Following a needlestick injury to one of your practice nurses and the subsequent significant-event audit, your practice decides to undertake an active approach to identifying patients who might have hepatitis C. This would have the benefit of treating early infection and reducing the risk of transmission. Which one of the following patients are at risk and would benefit from screening?

○   A   A 56-year-old man who worked as an oil worker in West Africa for many years

○   B   A 23-year-old man who has recently returned from a year travelling in south-east Asia with a new tattoo

○   C   A 38-year-old woman who had a 4 unit blood transfusion following a postpartum haemorrhage in 1988

○   D   A 31-year-old businessman who has had extensive dental treatment in a dental facility in Singapore

○   E   A 56-year-old man with a persistently raised GGT on his blood results

P1.199 Down syndrome

Your practice covers a local home for patients with learning disability. A number of the residents have Down syndrome, and you are asked by your colleagues to develop a template to standardise the routine health monitoring of these patients. Which of the following statements is true regarding health problems in these patients?

○   A   Depression is uncommon in patients with Down syndrome

○   B   Down syndrome is associated with glue ear in childhood, but the risk of hearing impairment in adults is similar to unaffected patients

○   C   Gait changes and disturbed bladder and bowel function are a sign of early onset dementia in these patients

○   D   Routine blood tests should be avoided due to the stress that they cause

○   E   Women with Down syndrome should be screened for premature menopause

P1.200 Depression

A 26-year-old woman is brought in by her mother concerned about her low mood. She has been unhappy for several months without any obvious triggers. A PHQ-9 questionnaire is completed and the result is 13. Which one of the following is a correct interpretation of this result?

○   A   Normal

○   B   Mild depression

○   C   Moderate depression

○   D   Moderately severe depression

○   E   Severe depression

Paper 1
Answers

P1.1 **B:** **Frozen shoulder is more common in patients with diabetes mellitus**

Long-term studies suggest that only 39% of patients make a full recovery, although another 54% have no functional limitation despite a small reduction in mobility. Secondary frozen shoulder is generally rare, but diabetes increases the risk with prevalence up to 36% in this group. Mean age of onset is 40–60 years. The diagnosis is essentially a clinical one, although X-rays or blood tests might be necessary to exclude other pathology if clinically suspected.

P1.2 **D:** **Irregular bleeding is the most common side effect of progestogen implant**

Implanon capsules are inserted in the skin above the elbow and consist of a single capsule changed every 3 years, unlike Norplant, which consisted of five rods that were changed every 5 years. Irregular bleeding is common in Implanon users, and can be treated with the combined contraceptive pill or tranexamic acid in the first 6 months, after which it usually settles down. Acne is common, but there is no evidence of an effect on mood, weight or libido. Around 50% of women become amenorrhoeic on Implanon. After removal, blood levels of etonogestrel are undetectable within 1 week and ovulation occurs in 90% of women within 3 weeks. The implants are changed after 3 years and the pregnancy rate in users is <0.1 in 100 women over 3 years.

Trials in atrial fibrillation

P1.3 **C:** **BAFTA**

The BAFTA trial found that risk predictors such as $CHADS_2$ do not predict risk well in the over-75 age group and that all patients aged >75 with atrial fibrillation should be considered for anticoagulation.

P1.4 **A:** **AFFIRM trial**

The AFFIRM trial showed that rhythm-control strategy offers no survival advantage over the rate-control strategy, whereas rate control had a lower risk of adverse drug effects.

P1.5 **E:** **RELY trial**

Dagibatran was superior to warfarin in controlling strokes, reducing complications and reducing all-cause mortality.

P1.6   B: ARISTOTLE

The ARISTOTLE trial showed an annual mortality rate of 2.13% with apixaban compared with 3.09% for warfarin, superior to dagibatran and rivaroxaban in meta-analyses.

P1.7   B: Basal cell carcinoma

This lesion is superficial with a rolled edge and central ulceration, suggestive of a basal cell carcinoma. Biopsy may be necessary to exclude a squamous cell carcinoma. Dermatitis artefacta is usually an unusual appearance not fitting any diagnostic pattern, usually seen in patients with psychological problems. Malignant melanoma would usually have areas of pigmentation. Actinic keratosis is characterised by red scaly lesions on the forehead or scalp.

P1.8   E: The readings suggest the presence of significant peripheral vascular disease affecting the right side only

The ABPI is 0.8 on the right side and 1.0 on the left. An ABPI <0.9 suggests the presence of significant peripheral vascular disease, whereas an ABPI <0.8 suggests a risk of ulceration. Once the ABPI is <0.5 this indicates critical ischaemia. ABPI readings >1.0 can be seen where the patient is not supine or where there is reduced arterial compliance, as in atherosclerosis.

P1.9   C: Prodromal dermatomal pain is a risk factor for post-herpetic neuralgia

Risk factors for severe post-herpetic neuralgia include age >50, prodromal pain, and severe pain and rash during the attack. Prompt use of antivirals reduces the incidence of post-herpetic neuralgia by up to 50%. Systematic review suggests the best evidence is for tricyclic antidepressants, although there is also evidence for anticonvulsants, 5% lidocaine plasters, opiates and capsaicin. Severe intractable pain might be helped by ketamine injections.

P1.10   C: Reassure the parents that it will usually resolve spontaneously in time

This is a paraumbilical hernia. Spontaneous closure is the norm and surgery is indicated only if closure fails to occur. Such hernias are more common in African–Caribbean children and occur twice as commonly in boys as girls. Incarceration is uncommon below the age of 3 years, so there is usually no indication for surgical treatment below this age, and 93% close without any intervention. Some surgeons advocate taping the skin over the hernia to bring the edges of the hernia together in an attempt to hasten closure, but this is not usually necessary.

Drug management of asthma

P1.11   H: Oral leukotriene receptor antagonist

Leukotriene receptor antagonists are of no value in acute asthma but have a role in the maintenance treatment of asthma. They also have some benefits in allergic rhinitis. They are licensed in children and can be useful as a steroid-sparing agent.

P1.12   A: Combination of inhaled corticosteroid and long-acting β_2 agonist

The SMART (Symbicort as maintenance and reliever therapy) approach allows patients to self-manage their asthma according to their symptoms. It has been shown to reduce the use of oral steroids and the number of doctor consultations.

P1.13   I: Oral theophylline

Theophylline is rarely used due to the risk of adverse effects, including arrhythmias, nausea and diarrhoea. Particular care should be taken to ensure that patients are not using inhaled theophylline before starting oral treatment due to the risk of toxicity.

P1.14   B: Inhaled anticholinergic

Inhaled anticholinergics reduce vagal tone and have the benefit of reducing mucus secretion, which makes them useful in patients with chronic obstructive pulmonary disease.

P1.15   G: Oral corticosteroids

Long-term (>3 months) oral steroids at a dose >5 mg/day should prompt the use of bisphosphonates to prevent osteoporosis. The Royal College of Physicians further recommends that three separate short courses over a 12-month period should be considered to be equivalent to 3 months' prescribing.

P1.16   E: Posterior cruciate tear

The positive posterior draw test indicates a posterior cruciate tear. This injury is typically seen in patients who have received a blow to the proximal tibia with the knee flexed, eg in a road traffic accident or by falling on to a flexed knee. Management involves a splint initially, followed by physiotherapy. Anterior cruciate tears are associated with a positive anterior draw test. In younger patients, surgery is usually necessary, particularly in sportsmen and -women. Patellar tendon tears result in an inability to extend the knee. Medial and lateral collateral tears are associated with laxity when the knee is stressed laterally or medially.

P1.17   B: Multinodular goitre

This is a multinodular goitre. It may be associated with thyrotoxicosis or hypothyroidism. Multinodular goitre with abnormal thyroid function tests should be referred to endocrinology, whereas new presentations of non-toxic goitre should be referred to ENT for investigation to exclude a dominant nodule, associated with increased risk of malignancy. The overall rate of malignant transformation in a multinodular goitre is 5%.

P1.18   E: Patients with diabetes mellitus should have a total cholesterol of ≤4.0 mmol/l and an LDL of <2.0 mmol/l

Recent NICE guidance suggested that patients with diabetes mellitus should be treated to a target of 4/2. In the Heart Protection Study all patients were treated with 40 mg simvastatin with no further testing, but the NICE guidance recommends treating to target. Patients with acute coronary syndromes should be treated with a high-intensity statin such as atorvastatin. Inegy, a combination of simvastatin and ezetimibe, has been associated with increased risk of cancer in some studies. It is recommended for patients who cannot tolerate a sufficient dose of simvastatin to reach target levels.

P1.19   B: No action required

The presence of asymptomatic bacteriuria is common in catheterised patients and no action is necessary unless they are unwell. *Proteus* sp. is often associated with urinary stones or foreign bodies. Replacing the catheter would increase the risks of infection by causing local trauma, and irrigation would simply flush bacteria into the bladder.

Death certification

P1.20   C: Discuss the case with the coroner

Where a patient has not been seen in the last 14 days you cannot issue a death certificate without discussing the case with the coroner. In a situation such as this the coroner will often allow a death certificate to be issued.

P1.21   A: Contact the police

Sudden deaths should be referred to the police who will arrange appropriate investigation and a postmortem examination. You cannot issue a death certificate in this situation.

P1.22   C: Discuss the case with the coroner

Where industrial disease is implicated the employment box should be ticked on the death certificate and the coroner informed.

P1.23   C: Discuss the case with the coroner

Unnatural deaths should always be referred to the coroner.

P1.24   H: None of the above

A stillborn baby can be certified on a Certificate of Stillbirth only after 24 weeks of pregnancy. If the baby does breathe after birth, no matter what gestation, a neonatal death form should be used. This case should be referred to the obstetrics and gynaecology department to arrange investigation and appropriate counselling, and to liaise with the coroner.

P1.25   F: Issue Medical Certificate of Cause of Death

Death certificates do not require the doctor to have seen the body after death, as long as another medical practitioner has seen the body and confirmed death.

P1.26 E: SSRIs should be used as first-line treatment

Social phobia has a lifetime risk of 13% and is particularly common in women from lower social classes. Affected people experience feelings of panic in public situations and nausea and vomiting are common. Management comprises CBT where available and SSRIs in the short term. Benzodiazepines or β blockers can also help with crises.

P1.27 A: Admit under paediatrics

This patient has haemolytic uraemic syndrome, which may follow *Escherichia coli* O157 infection. Risk factors include extremes of age. Clinical suspicion should be raised in children with bloody diarrhoea. Oliguria and dehydration are common and thrombocytopenic purpura can be seen. Treatment is supportive, although some patients need short-term dialysis.

P1.28 E: CBT should be offered to all patients with chronic fatigue syndrome

The diagnosis of chronic fatigue syndrome should be considered in patients with unexplained fatigue lasting more than 3 months in a child or 4 months in an adult. Chronic pain, sleep disturbance and cognitive difficulties are common. Exacerbations usually start 24–48 hours after exertion. The treatment of this condition involves graded exercise and CBT. The prognosis is extremely variable, with some patients making a quick recovery and others developing chronic disease. The disease has been reported to follow infection with a number of viruses, and it is estimated that 10% of patients with clinical Epstein–Barr virus infection will develop chronic fatigue syndrome.

P1.29 B: Episcleritis

Episcleritis is a localised, self-limiting condition affecting the sclera. Iritis can be excluded on examination and scleritis is usually a severe boring pain rather than a dull ache. Scleritis is usually bilateral and associated with connective tissue disease. The inflammation in episcleritis is usually limited to a small sector and typically settles over 7–10 days. Topical non-steroidal drops might accelerate this process and steroid drops are also helpful, but should be given only after expert assessment to exclude keratitis. Keratitis is usually obvious on fluorescein staining but a slit lamp should be used. Acute angle-closure glaucoma usually causes stony-hard eyes and vomiting with severe pain.

P1.30 50%

The *BRCA-1* and *BRCA-2* genes are inherited as autosomal dominants with incomplete penetration, ie can be inherited from either father or mother. The risk of carrying the gene if you have a carrier parent is 50%. Carriers of the *BRCA-1* gene have lifetime risk of breast cancer of 80% and of ovarian cancer of 40–60% whereas *BRCA-2* has a lower rate of ovarian cancer, of 20–30%. Patients testing positive can be offered prophylactic surgery, although those with a carrier in the family who do not choose to be tested are offered annual mammograms from age 40.

Childhood infections

P1.31   G: Poxvirus

Molluscum contagiosum causes crops to appear and spread through autoinoculation. They are typically seen in the pre-school age group and individual lesions can last from 2–3 weeks to several months. No specific treatment is needed and they regress spontaneously.

P1.32   C: *Mycoplasma pneumoniae*

Mycoplasma pneumoniae causes respiratory symptoms in young children and can be associated with erythema multiforme. These patients usually respond to oral macrolides, eg erythromycin.

P1.33   F: Parvovirus B19

Parvovirus B19 (also called erythrovirus B19) causes a mild, self-limiting disease in children but unexposed pregnant women can develop fetal hydrops as a result of this infection.

P1.34   A: Group A streptococci

Scarlet fever follows infection with β-haemolytic streptococci and can cause rheumatic fever or glomerulonephritis. Children should be treated with at least 10 days of phenoxymethylpenicillin and excluded from school until the antibiotics are started.

P1.35   L: Varicella

Varicella need be treated only in adults, neonates or immunocompromised individuals.

P1.36   E: Ulcerative colitis

Ulcerative colitis often presents as an isolated proctitis and attacks can start after periods of stress. The diagnosis is usually made at proctoscopy, where a typical granular and ulcerated appearance is seen. Crohn's disease is the major differential in this age group but is often associated with piles or fistulae, and tends to cause more systemic features. Management usually consists of rectal steroids or aminosalicylates; loperamide should not be used because it does not work and can increase the risk of toxic megacolon. Long-term management is usually with aminosalicylates. Patients with ulcerative colitis are at increased risk of colorectal cancer and should be screened regularly.

P1.37   D: Suction termination can be carried out under local anaesthesia

Mifepristone can be used for late abortions (>15 weeks) with prostaglandin pessaries and is an alternative to surgical termination. It cannot be used in women with a history of cardiac or respiratory disease. Two doctors must sign the certificate before a termination can take place; if they feel that a patient is Gillick competent the parents need not be informed. The legal limit for termination is 24 weeks but there is some debate about lowering this to 22 weeks. At present <1% of abortions take place after 20 weeks.

Personality disorders

P1.38   E: Hyperthymic personality disorder

Hyperthymic personality is characterised by persistent enthusiasm and optimism which is associated with rash judgements (eg poor financial investments).

P1.39   C: Borderline personality disorder

Borderline personality disorders are typified by young men who frequently get drunk and are involved in fights or acts of vandalism. They are often lonely and crave company, but are unable to develop rewarding relationships.

P1.40   A: Anankastic personality disorder

Anankastic personality disorders show considerable overlap with obsessional neurosis, and these people are often ill at ease in company and very sensitive to criticism.

P1.41   F: Narcissistic personality disorder

Narcissistic personality types are also very sensitive to criticism, but are easily bored and have difficulty forming emotional attachments to others.

P1.42   H: Schizoid personality disorder

Schizoid personality types are typically seen as aloof or boring, and are happiest in their own company.

P1.43   E: Vesicocolic fistula

Recurrent or refractory symptoms of UTI with pneumaturia or faecaluria are hallmarks of vesicocolic fistula. These affect men more than women in the ratio 3:1 and are the most common of the abdominal fistulae. Diverticulosis is the most common cause, although bowel and bladder cancer should be excluded. Crohn's disease may also present as a vesicocolic fistula. Approximately 50% of fistulae close spontaneously once the underlying cause has been treated, but where they don't surgery is indicated

P1.44   C: Deep vein thrombosis

DVT is a complication of pacemaker placement and should be treated with low molecular weight heparin and warfarinisation, as for other thromboembolic disease. Cellulitis or wound infection should be considered in the differential but would be unusual in the absence of fever. Arterial embolism would normally cause pain, pulselessness and pallor.

P1.45   C: Raised serum ferritin with reduced total iron-binding capacity

Haemochromatosis is due to iron overload and commonly damages the heart, liver, pancreas and pituitary. It may be hereditary or acquired. Hereditary cases can be investigated with genotyping if this has been done on the index case. Siblings should be screened, and the characteristic findings on iron studies are raised ferritin with reduced total iron-binding capacity and raised iron-binding saturation. If liver function is abnormal a biopsy should be considered. Raised MCV and MCH are suggestive of vitamin B_{12}/folate deficiency whereas reduced MCV and MCH are suggestive of iron deficiency.

P1.46   D: Pertussis

Pertussis causes a prolonged cough characterised by paroxysms lasting minutes, during which the patient may feel unable to breathe. It lasts 4–8 weeks and can be associated with loud whoops at the end of the spasm of coughing. Antibiotics such as azithromycin will reduce infectivity but not shorten the duration of illness. Vaccination programmes offer 95% coverage but cases in children and adults do occur, with significant morbidity and mortality for infants.

Biological therapies

P1.47   C: Omalizumab (Xolair)

Omalizumab is useful in allergy-mediated asthma. Patients need to have elevated IgE levels, and it is not suitable for other forms of asthma. It is given by regular injection.

P1.48   B: Natalizumab (Tysabri)

Natalizumab acts on T cells to reduce severity of symptoms in multiple sclerosis. It is licensed as monotherapy for relapsing MS and is given by injection. It can reduce the frequency of attacks and slow down the accumulation of disability. It might also be helpful in Crohn's disease.

P1.49   A: Infliximab (Remicade)

NICE guidance recommends the use of infliximab for severe psoriasis (a psoriasis area severity index >20) in patients not responding to or not suitable for PUVA or ciclosporin and other systemic treatments. It also has a role in acute Crohn's disease and rheumatoid arthritis.

P1.50   F: Trastuzumab (Herceptin)

Trastuzumab acts on the HER2 receptors on malignant cells, and is accordingly licensed for HER2-positive patients. It reduces the risk of early recurrence by 50%. NICE recommends its use after surgery, chemotherapy and radiotherapy if appropriate. It can cause congestive cardiac failure and cardiac work-up is required.

P1.51   D: Ranibizumab (Lucentis)

Ranibizumab is licensed for wet macular degeneration and is given as an injection into the eye. It has been shown to stabilise eyesight in most patients and 30–40% of patients experience an improvement in their visual acuity.

P1.52   C: Surgery is indicated in patients who do not wish to take long-term medication

Indications for surgery include severe oesophagitis, long-term complications, and inability or unwillingness to take long-term medication. Surgical options include laparoscopic fundoplication, laparoscopic placement of a Silastic prosthesis or use of the falciform ligament to reduce the hernia and maintain it, and open fundoplication. Long-term follow-up studies suggest that about a third of patients need proton pump inhibitors after surgery, compared with two-thirds of patients managed medically. Surgery is useful in sliding and rolling hernias; rolling hernias are more likely to obstruct. Patients should be able to eat normally after surgery.

P1.53   A: Ankylosing spondylitis

The presence of morning stiffness, age of onset <40 years, limited spinal flexion and improvement with exercise rather than rest is suggestive of ankylosing spondylitis. This can be confirmed with an X-ray of the lumbosacral spine showing sacroiliitis and HLA-B27 testing. Patients should be referred early for consideration of anti-TNF therapy. Fifty per cent of patients have associated non-spinal pathology such as iritis.

P1.54   D: Methotrexate frequently causes menstrual disturbances

Full blood count and LFTs should be done pre-treatment, after the initial dose and dose changes. Once stable, they can be done every 2–3 months. Falls in WCC and platelets, or increase in LFTs by a threefold factor or more, should prompt cessation. A mild increase in LFTs is common but a fall in albumin of >5 g/l is an early sign of liver toxicity. Folic acid is given on the 6 days a week when methotrexate is not taken. Methotrexate is teratogenic.

P1.55   A: Asperger syndrome

This child has typical features of Asperger syndrome. Children with this condition have a specific impairment in social functioning but have a normal IQ and often excel in certain areas. Patients can have a normal vocabulary but struggle with abstract language and metaphors, and have significant difficulties interpreting and using non-verbal communication.

Sleep disturbance

P1.56   A: Bed-time restriction

P1.57   E: Melatonin

P1.58   C: Intermittent short-term hypnotics

P1.59   D: Light therapy

Once other causes of sleep disturbance have been excluded, such as restless legs syndrome or chronic pain, insomnia should be classified as primary insomnia or delayed sleep phase syndrome (cannot get to sleep at night, cannot get up in morning). Delayed sleep phase syndrome is thought to be a disturbance of circadian rhythm and may respond to melatonin. Failing this, use of light boxes or exposure to natural light may help. Primary insomnia responds to a trial of at least 2 weeks of sleep restriction. Failing this, short-term intermittent use of hypnotics may be justified, with appropriate counselling.

P1.60   E: Ulipristal acetate

In this patient who has already tried anti-inflammatories and contraceptive pills and is awaiting surgery, the next step would be to try ulipristal acetate orally for 3 months. This is a progesterone receptor modulator and has been shown to be superior to placebo and GnRH analogues in both side effects and efficacy, reducing bleeding by 80%. It is licensed for use for up to 3 months before surgery. Danazol is not recommended for routine use by NICE due to side effects, whereas GnRH analogues are licensed to be used before planned surgery, but are associated with significant side effects. Mefenamic acid is unlikely to help if other NSAIDs have failed and HRT is unlikely to be effective in a premenopausal women.

P1.61   A: Cinnarazine is an effective treatment

Hyoscine is the most effective treatment, especially when used as a patch. Cinnarazine and promethazine are helpful but promethazine causes sedation and for most patients this limits its use, although it may be useful in children. Patients should be advised to stay on deck where possible, with a view of the horizon, and to try to stay in the middle of the boat where motion is minimal. Alcohol, heavy meals and pungent odours can exacerbate symptoms. Homeopathic treatments might be effective but trials have not shown any benefit from acupressure bands.

P1.62   D: Quantiferon testing is the investigation of choice in screening contacts

Quantiferon is a highly sensitive and specific test for TB-sensitised T cells, and patients with a positive test should be given chemoprophylaxis. Heaf testing is suitable for mass screening of populations whereas Mantoux testing is more specific and is a better choice for screening healthcare workers where Quantiferon is not available, although false positives can occur. Chest X-rays will pick up only pulmonary TB. Heaf testing might be positive in patients who have had avian TB or previous BCG vaccination.

P1.63   B: Oral doxycycline 100 mg once daily for 6 weeks

Blepharitis is a chronic condition and is managed in most cases with regular lid cleaning and compresses, with short courses of topical antibiotics for flare-ups. Where this is not helping and the diagnosis is not in question a 6-week course of a tetracycline is often helpful. Prednisolone drops should not be used in a red eye without ophthalmological review in case of underlying herpes simplex keratitis. Prolonged use of topical antibiotics is unlikely to help and will promote resistance.

P1.64   E: Refer immediately to the emergency department for an X-ray

This patient has symptoms of a fractured fibula, commonly seen after a fall wearing ski boots or inline skates. The common peroneal nerve might be damaged, causing numbness over the lateral border of the foot and weak dorsiflexion. Surgery might be necessary to keep the fibula reduced. Undisplaced fractures of the mid-shaft might not need a cast, but where there are signs of damage to the common peroneal nerve this should be treated actively to avoid lasting disability.

Abdominal pain

P1.65   G: Diverticulitis

This pattern of recurring attacks of left iliac fossa pain is usually due to diverticulitis. Colonic cancer would be the main differential in this age group and can be differentiated on barium enema or colonoscopy. In younger patients, irritable bowel syndrome can cause similar symptoms.

P1.66   K: Renal colic

Renal colic tends to radiate to the scrotum or labia and typically comes in waves. Dipstick testing usually shows haematuria.

P1.67   E: Crohn's disease

Crohn's disease usually starts in the terminal ileum or proximal colon and a mass can form in this part of the bowel. Diarrhoea, weight loss and fever are common. Diagnosis is usually made on endoscopy.

P1.68   C: Acute cholecystitis

Referred pain to the shoulder is usually a sign of diaphragmatic irritation, in this case due to inflammation of the gallbladder. Ectopic pregnancy or chlamydial perihepatitis should also be considered as possible causes in women. In cholecystitis there is right upper quadrant tenderness that is worse on inspiration.

P1.69   H: Gastric carcinoma

Progressive dysphagia with weight loss suggests a diagnosis of gastric or oesophageal cancer. An epigastric mass might be palpable and hepatomegaly is common.

P1.70   A: Ezetimibe has been reported to be associated with an increased risk of cancer

The SEAS (Simvastatin and Ezetimibe in Aortic Stenosis) trial looked at use of ezetimibe in combination with simvastatin in patients with mild aortic stenosis. It found no significant reduction in cardiovascular endpoints but did find increased incidence of all cancers. Ezetimibe is a cholesterol absorption inhibitor that has been shown in trial data to reduce low-density lipoproteins (LDLs), but it did not reduce clinical endpoints. Patients with a mixed hyperlipidaemia should be treated with a statin initially. Macrolides, amlodipine and antifungals interact with simvastatin and atorvastatin and should be used with caution in all patients on statins. Sleep problems are common, and there are increasing reports of impotence with statins. Patients with familial hyperlipidaemias should be treated to target.

P1.71 E: No treatment needed

Dead eggs (nits) often persist for many months after an episode of hair lice infestation and are not themselves an indication for treatment. If live lice are seen, wet combing with conditioner or simeticone is efficacious and not associated with resistance. Nits close to the scalp suggest recent infection, whereas those some distance from the scalp are likely to be old.

P1.72 C: Clinically asymptomatic cancers are being diagnosed earlier

The most likely explanation for the increase in cancer diagnoses over a short period is improved case finding. The time course is too short for a change in true prevalence and prostate cancer has a long lead time before symptoms appear. The lack of change in the death rate suggests that these cancers are not associated with reduced life expectancy, ie they are being diagnosed earlier but treatment and individual life expectancy are the same. Changes in life expectancy with new treatments can be compared only on a case–control basis. Advances in treatment might have led to improved life expectancy for individual patients, but many patients are treated with watchful waiting and die of other causes.

P1.73 A: The trial demonstrated significant benefits in treating hypertensive patients with calcium antagonists and ACE inhibitors compared with β blockers and thiazides

The ALLHAT study showed that thiazides were as effective as calcium antagonists and ACE inhibitors in preventing coronary heart disease. The ASCOT study showed that aggressive treatment with calcium antagonist followed by ACE inhibitor was significantly superior to β blockade followed by thiazide for overall mortality, stroke and diabetes. The study was a primary prevention study involving hypertensive patients with at least one other risk factor.

P1.74 A: Glossopharyngeal neuralgia

Glossopharyngeal neuralgia is less common than trigeminal neuralgia but causes similar symptoms in the distribution of the glossopharyngeal nerve. Initial assessment should aim to exclude facial nerve involvement, tonsillar tumour and herpes zoster. Treatment usually aims to provide reassurance and avoidance of trigger factors where possible. Anticonvulsants can be helpful in some cases.

P1.75 D: Sedation is usually transient

Constipation is near universal with patients on strong opioids, regardless of preparation. It usually persists and patients should start a laxative when they start the opioids. In chronic kidney disease (CKD) stages 4 or 5, fentanyl or oxycodone is a better choice due to the risk of toxicity with morphine and diamorphine. Pain should be rated on an out-of-10 scale; visual analogue scales are better for children. Although sedation and nausea are usually seen at the onset of treatment only, constipation is persistent.

P1.76   C: Retrospective studies are quicker to conduct than prospective studies

Retrospective studies are more prone to bias but are cheaper and quicker to conduct. They have the advantage that the two groups are known to have different rates of a disease, whereas prospective studies do not have this advantage. It is not uncommon for an intervention group and a control group to have a statistically insignificant difference in event rates at the end of a long and expensive trial.

Skin lesions

P1.77   C: Keratoacanthoma

P1.78   E: Pyogenic granuloma

P1.79   B: Basal cell carcinoma

P1.80   A: Actinic keratosis

P1.81   C: Dermovate

Dermovate is a high-potency steroid that is suitable for short-term treatment of psoriasis and eczema that is not responding to treatment with milder steroids. It should be applied for a maximum of 4 weeks and a maximum of 50 g should be applied per week.

P1.82   E: Refer directly to the antenatal unit for biophysical profile

Reduced fetal movements are a common concern in the third trimester. Mothers should be asked to choose a set time every day and record how long it takes to feel 10 movements. If these are not felt by that time she should be referred to the antenatal unit for a biophysical profile, comprising cardiotocography (CTG), ultrasound examination of liquor volume, fetal tone, movements and breathing movements, giving a numerical score with 10 the maximum. If the score is between 0 and 2, immediate delivery is indicated, whereas a score of 8 or more is normal.

P1.83   E: Systematic desensitisation therapy

Antidepressants may help if there is associated depression or anxiety but anxiety is often secondary to the agoraphobia. Benzodiazepines should be avoided due to a risk of addiction. Systematic desensitisation consists of graded exposure and agreement of goals and homework where the patient continues to practice in real life. Up to 70% of patients report improvement although complete recovery of all symptoms is less common. The aim should be for a patient to be able to function normally. Hypnosis is sometimes used as part of this process but the graded exposure to the stimulus is key.

P1.84   B: Avoidance of nail rubbing

This condition is seen in people under stress who rub their thumbnails, causing typical central nail damage. Where this condition is unilateral, trauma to the nail bed should be considered. In fungal nail infections the infection normally starts distally, with discoloration of the nail, whereas a low calcium level causes brittle nails. Reassurance alone will not improve the condition and sometimes CBT might be appropriate to break up the stress response.

P1.85   D: Lymphoedema

Lymphoedema is a common incurable complication of breast cancer surgery, particularly where this involves axillary clearance. The arm is typically oedematous with no erythema and with non-pitting oedema. Infection can develop and fibrosis is common. Management involves elevation and massage, and four-layer bandaging, followed by compression hosiery, can be effective. Lymphoma would not normally affect a whole arm, although cellulitis and DVT are usually associated with erythema and tenderness.

P1.86   D: Start a smoking cessation programme and repeat the blood tests in 4 weeks

This pattern of blood results usually reflects secondary polycythaemia due to chronic hypoxia from COPD and smoking. Smoking cessation might be sufficient to bring his haemoglobin back to normal limits. If this fails to occur he should be investigated to confirm whether this is primary or secondary polycythaemia. Primary polycythaemia is associated with the *JAK2* mutation and can be tested in most laboratories. The mainstay of management is venesection once secondary causes have been addressed.

P1.87   C: Suggest that she sees another doctor at the practice

GMC guidelines state that you should avoid treating people to whom you are close. Obviously, in life-or-death situations this can be waived, but convenience is not a reason to enter into a clinical situation where one's judgement might be impaired. If one has serious concerns about patient safety, it would be appropriate to raise these but clash of personalities is not an appropriate reason to instigate a complaint. GMC guidance further recommends that you should provide treatment only where you have adequate knowledge of the patient's health, and in the scenario described here there could be issues in your mother's medical history of which you are unaware.

Upper gastrointestinal disorders

P1.88   E: MALToma

Non-Hodgkin's lymphoma affecting the mucosa-associated lymphoid tissue (MALT) of the stomach is the most common non-epithelial malignancy of the stomach and accounts for 3% of stomach tumours. These tumours are associated with *Helicobacter pylori* infection and in low-grade tumours regression can occur after eradication of the infection.

P1.89   A: Achalasia

Achalasia is due to failure of relaxation of the gastro-oesophageal junction, resulting in progressive dilatation of the oesophagus. Regurgitation is common and many patients develop aspiration pneumonia. The symptoms progress more slowly than oesophageal cancer but often cause chronic malnourishment. In South America this condition is often seen in association with cardiomegaly in Chagas' disease, a trypanosomal infection.

P1.90   B: Barrett's oesophagus

Barrett's oesophagus is associated with a small risk of developing cancer and many authorities advocate routine endoscopic surveillance. The presence of dysplasia in biopsies is suspicious but at repeat endoscopy 75% of these will have resolved on treatment with a proton pump inhibitor (PPI). Where this has not occurred surgery should be considered.

P1.91   H: Oesophageal stricture

Oesophageal stricture is usually caused by acid reflux and often presents as bolus obstruction, but upper gastrointestinal endoscopy and biopsy are mandatory to exclude an underlying malignancy. Dilatation can be carried out at the time of endoscopy.

P1.92   I: Plummer–Vinson syndrome

Plummer–Vinson syndrome (also know as Patterson–Brown–Kelly syndrome) causes an oesophageal web and therefore dysphagia, together with iron-deficiency anaemia. It is associated with a significant increase in risk of oesophageal cancer.

P1.93   A: PSA screening has been shown to increase diagnosis of early prostate cancer

Large-scale studies of prostate cancer screening using PSA blood tests show that it increases the diagnosis of early prostate cancer but this does not translate into improved overall mortality or improved quality of life. Radical surgery for early screen-detected prostate cancer was shown in the PIVOT trial to have significant adverse effects, with no improvement in total or prostate cancer-related mortality.

P1.94   C: Each child has a 0% chance of being affected

Huntington's disease is an autosomal dominant trait that presents in middle age. Children of affected parents therefore have a 50% risk of inheriting the gene (assuming that the named parent is indeed the biological parent) and, in time, of becoming affected. If they are affected they will therefore have a 50% chance of passing the disease to each of their children, but if they are unaffected they will not have any risk of being a carrier or of developing the disease.

P1.95   E: Ultraviolet light used at the onset of symptoms may abort the attack

Cold sores are caused by reactivation of latent herpes simplex in the trigeminal ganglion, rather than primary infection. There is no evidence that topical aciclovir is effective but there is some evidence of efficacy for oral aciclovir. However, oral aciclovir is expensive and is not considered cost-effective. Where attacks are triggered by UV light, sunscreens might be effective. Small hand-held UV light emitters are available on FP10, to be used at the onset of tingling, and have been shown to abort or shorten the duration of an attack.

P1.96   B: De Quervain's tenosynovitis

De Quervain's tenosynovitis is inflammation of the extensor pollicis brevis and abductor pollicis longus tendons. Finkelstein's test is positive if resisted abduction is painful. Treatment is usually steroid injection and a splint, but surgical decompression might be required in chronic cases. Carpal tunnel syndrome causes pain on pressure over the carpal tunnel (Tinel's test) or through forced flexion of the wrist (Phalen's test). Medial and lateral epicondylitis cause tenderness over the medial and lateral epicondyles respectively.

P1.97   B: Pelviureteric junction obstruction is more common in patients with duplex ureters

A Duplex ureter is seen in 0.2% of live births, and is more common in patients with a positive family history. It is usually picked up on antenatal ultrasound but in older patients might be discovered on routine ultrasound scanning. PUJ obstruction and urinary tract infection are more common in patients with this condition and this might require active management. Surgery is seldom necessary.

P1.98   E: Refer under the 2-week rule

This child has symptoms of retinoblastoma and should be referred under the 2-week rule. Early treatment carries a good prognosis because these tumours tend to metastasise late. Any child with new-onset squint, leukocoria or uveitis needs urgent assessment. The condition is familial and often there will be an affected first-degree relative.

P1.99   A: Bimanual examination

This woman has symptoms of an ovarian tumour and abdominal examination alone will miss pelvic tumours. Vaginal examination is mandatory in these cases, and where a mass is found referral under the 2-week rule is indicated. Ovarian tumours are often clinically silent in their early stages, becoming apparent only when they reach sufficient size to cause pressure effects or ascites, and a high index of suspicion should be maintained in patients with new symptoms, particularly those affecting the bladder or bowel, or those who have clinical evidence of ascites.

P1.100   B: IgA nephropathy

IgA nephropathy is the underlying pathology in 50% of cases of recurrent frank haematuria. It is usually seen in children and young adults and is more common in boys. Episodes are usually triggered by viral infections and usually resolve over days or weeks. Oral steroids are often used. Most patients have a good prognosis, but 15–20% of patients go on to develop chronic renal failure. Poor prognosis is associated with heavy proteinuria and hypertension. Bladder cancer would be very unusual in this age group. Wilms' tumours usually present in infancy and are palpable on examination as a flank mass, with microscopic haematuria. Polycystic kidneys are usually evident from birth in children, or develop in adulthood in the case of adult polycystic kidney disease.

P1.101   D: Traumatic depigmentation

Long-term eczema can result in lichenification (thickening of the skin), thinning due to long-term steroid use or loss of pigment due to scratching. Vitiligo can produce a similar appearance but is usually evident elsewhere. Tinea causes colour changes but there is usually scaling. Drug reactions usually cause darker macules.

P1.102   E: Presence of cataracts

The Guthrie test is done shortly after birth and involves taking a heel-prick test for congenital hypothyroidism. Coordination and patch testing are done at a later date when these skills have started to develop, usually by health visitors at the 8- and 18-month checks, and by an orthoptist around the age of 3 years. Newborn babies all have otoacoustic emission testing shortly after birth. Congenital cataracts must be picked up early to avoid amblyopia.

P1.103   D: Optic neuritis

This patient is suffering from retrobulbar neuritis, usually caused by multiple sclerosis. Papilloedema typically causes a peripheral visual field loss with normal acuity. CRVO usually causes engorgement of the retinal veins and a sunset appearance of the retina. Acute glaucoma causes severe pain in the eye, whereas amaurosis fugax causes retinal pallor and loss of vision in the whole eye and lasts for seconds or minutes.

P1.104   E: His TSH should be <0.01 μU/l

Patients with a previous history of thyroid cancer should be treated until they have a TSH <0.01 μU/l to prevent stimulation of any residual thyroid tissue. Often this requires higher doses of levothyroxine than are normally used, but there is no set dose and the dose should be given at the lowest level that suppresses TSH, to avoid excess symptoms of hyperthyroidism. T_4 and T_3 levels do not need to be measured because the goal of treatment is suppression of TSH rather than biochemical euthyroidism.

Statistical terms

P1.105   I: Standard deviation

P1.106   D: Odds ratio

The odds ratio is the ratio of the risk for a condition in one group compared with another.

P1.107   E: The *p* value

A *p* value of <0.05 is generally accepted as the threshold of statistical significance, ie the risk of the finding occurring by chance is 1:20.

P1.108   C: Incidence

The incidence is the rate of new diagnoses; the prevalence is the number of people with a condition at a given time.

P1.109 H: Specificity

Specificity is the number of true negatives; sensitivity is the number of true positives.

P1.110 D: There is a 1% annual risk of developing malignancy in patients with Barrett's oesophagus

Barrett's oesophagus is metaplastic change in the distal oesophagus caused by longstanding acid reflux. There is a 1% annual risk of malignant transformation and many centres carry out routine surveillance. Treatment is of the underlying reflux, with proton pump inhibitors for life. Photodynamic therapy is available in some centres. There is no association between *H. pylori* and Barrett's oesophagus.

P1.111 E: Tiotropium should be considered at step 2 in COPD management

The POET-COPD trial (*N Engl J Med* 2011) compared long-acting β agonists and tiotropium in stage 2 of COPD management and found evidence of reduced exacerbations in the tiotropium group. There is mounting evidence that β blockers are safe and effective in patients with COPD, because these patients often have coexistent ischaemic heart disease, and there is some evidence that exacerbations of COPD are reduced with β blockers. Indacaterol is a new long-acting β agonist that can be given once a day, and studies suggest a beneficial impact on FEV_1 compared with salmeterol. Patients with a resting SpO_2 of >95% can usually fly without oxygen, whereas those with a resting SpO_2 of <92% will need supplemental oxygen. A hypoxic challenge test can be carried out in these patients.

P1.112 A: Acute angle-closure glaucoma

This is a typical history of acute angle-closure glaucoma. On examination the pupil is often fixed in a semi-dilated position and is oval. The eye feels stony-hard and the pain is extreme. Cluster headache can cause pain localised around the eye, but is not usually associated with fixation of the pupil. Anyone with a temporal headache should be examined to exclude temporal arteritis. Migraine would not normally cause pupillary changes and subarachnoid haemorrhage causes a more generalised headache with no loss of vision, although cranial nerve lesions can be seen.

P1.113 B: Each patient has a 70% chance of improving after the intervention

Cates's plots are designed to assist patients in understanding the likely pros and cons of a treatment. They are usually expressed as a table of 100 people, with patients improving being represented as a smiling face and patients being worse off as a sad face. Patients harmed by treatment may also be shown, eg for antibiotics in otitis media, patients with resultant diarrhoea are represented by a face with a cross through, and patients who are prevented from having an adverse outcome (ie saved) by a different colour smiling face. If the number of sad and smiling faces is equal, there is a 50% chance of improving and 50%

chance of deteriorating with a treatment, ie no net effect. If there are >50% of the faces smiling, the chance of an individual being better off is >50%. This relates to individual chance of improvement, not level of improvement in an individual. No conclusions regarding cost-effectiveness can be drawn without data on cost.

P1.114   B: Achilles tendinopathy

Quinolone antibiotics are associated with tendinopathy. This usually settles with cessation of the drug, rest and ice, together with non-steroidal anti-inflammatories. Rupture would usually be suggested by a palpable step in the tendon and reduced plantarflexion. Overuse injury may cause tendonitis but is usually seen when there has been a change in training or footwear. Polymyalgia rheumatica tends to cause a pelvic girdle rather than an ankle pain.

P1.115   D: Extrinsic allergic alveolitis

This patient has symptoms of farmers' lung, an acute extrinsic allergic alveolitis. Symptoms typically come on 4–8 hours after exposure to fungal spores and in time the condition can progress to pulmonary fibrosis. Similar symptoms are seen with bird fanciers, maltworkers and mushroom farmers. An occupational history is vital in diagnosing these patients. Management is with avoidance and steroids if severe. Bronchiectasis would tend to present with recurrent chest infections from childhood, whereas pulmonary fibrosis would usually be associated with chronic rather than relapsing and remitting symptoms, and clubbing.

P1.116   B: The combined oral contraceptive has a number needed to treat of 5 for management of primary dysmenorrhoea

A Bandolier review found that, in general, NSAIDs are the most effective treatment, with ibuprofen having the best risk:benefit ratio. Aspirin was the least effective. COX-2 inhibitors are effective, with good tolerability. There is no evidence to support the use of spinal manipulation and paracetamol has very weak efficacy in pain relief in this condition.

P1.117   E: Where a partnership agreement does not exist, the partnership can be terminated at any time by one of the partners

Where no formal partnership agreement exists, the partnership is considered a 'partnership at will' and can be terminated at any time without prior discussion. A partnership agreement should include all names and profit shares and therefore should be updated with all partnership changes. All decisions are by a majority, unless specified in the partnership agreement. Non-GP partners are legal, but might require complex calculations regarding remuneration.

Learning and teaching methods

P1.118   F: Socratic

P1.119   B: Counselling

P1.120   D: Heuristic

P1.121   C: Didactic

Didactic teaching is the traditional form of medical school teaching typified by lectures. The Socratic approach encourages the learner to become more self-aware and the role of the teacher is to raise this self-awareness, whereas the heuristic approach aims to empower the learner to practise lifelong, self-directed learning. The counselling style is particularly useful for mentoring roles. A detailed discussion on this subject can be found in Roger Neighbour's book, *The Inner Apprentice*.

P1.122   Trephining

Subungal haematoma is caused by trauma to the nailbed. Untreated the nail will be lost, and the haematoma causes acute pain. This can be relieved with a red-hot paperclip or a bevelled needle used as a drill. The nail is often lost over the next few weeks and can take some months to re-grow. This appearance in the absence of trauma may be a sign of subungal melanoma.

P1.123   C: The earliest possible fertile ovulation is around 28 days postpartum

Ovulation precedes the onset of a period so patients should be advised not to have unprotected sex before their first period after childbirth. The pill should not be used in the early postpartum phase due to the risk of thromboembolism. In the absence of breastfeeding, the earliest the pill should be considered is 21 days, but patients who have suffered from HELLP syndrome or pregnancy-induced hypertension are at increased risk of thrombosis and should not start the COCP until biochemically normal and normotensive. The COCP interferes with breastfeeding, so the mini-pill is a better choice in lactating mothers. Mothers should be warned that breastfeeding has poor efficacy as a contraceptive.

Management of back pain

P1.124   E: Red flag symptoms
P1.125   B: GP management
P1.126   H: Review in 2 weeks
P1.127   D: Physiotherapy
P1.128   G: Refer to secondary care
P1.129   C: He should have an MMR booster immediately

A single dose of MMR confers immunity in 70–85% of patients. In the case of an outbreak, a booster dose is recommended which will boost coverage to 95%, and can be given from 4 weeks after the previous dose. Single measles vaccines are not licensed or available in the UK. Failure to vaccinate with the booster at this time makes him prone to infection and carriage of the vaccine. Where children have received a booster before the age of 18 months, the usual pre-school booster should also be given because response below the age of 18 months can be suboptimal.

P1.130 **D:** **It can be associated with palpitations**

The typical patient with mitral valve prolapse is a young slim woman. It is frequently asymptomatic and is often picked up on routine examination as a diastolic murmur or systolic click. It is associated with atypical chest pain and palpitations, and rarely causes congestive cardiac failure or embolic phenomena. β Blockers or antiplatelet therapy might be indicated. Patients with no other abnormalities on echocardiography and no other cardiac risk factors have a long-term survival rate similar to that of the general population.

P1.131 **D:** **Nasal polyps**

Nasal polyps are by far the most common cause of reduced smell and taste. Tumours of the frontal lobe, meningiomas or ethmoid tumours are all very rare and usually associated with other symptoms. Overuse of decongestants causes rhinitis rather than loss of smell. Nasal polyps can cause reduced sense of smell without complete nasal obstruction and are often not visible without Thudichum's speculum. A trial of steroids, either nose drops or orally, will produce a dramatic improvement if nasal polyps are the cause. They can be removed surgically, but 50% recur within 2 years.

Causes of pneumonia

P1.132 **G:** *Mycoplasma pneumoniae*

Mycoplasma pneumoniae causes a flu-like respiratory illness that affects children. It can be associated with erythema multiforme, myalgia and diarrhoea. Treatment is with a macrolide or tetracycline for 10–14 days.

P1.133 **F:** **Measles**

Measles starts with a prodromal illness with respiratory symptoms and can go on to develop into pneumonia in around one in six patients, with bronchiectasis as a late complication.

P1.134 **A:** **Aspergillosis**

Aspergillosis tends to affect people with HIV or on immunosuppressants, or chronically ill individuals. It is usually diagnosed in patients who fail to respond to antibiotic therapy. It has been noted *post mortem* in 4% of patients dying in hospital.

P1.135 **L:** **Varicella**

Varicella frequently causes a primary viral pneumonia in adults but less commonly in children. X-rays show multiple small pulmonary lesions. Treatment is with aciclovir.

P1.136 **E:** **Legionnaires' disease**

Legionella sp. has an incubation period up to 10 days and is often associated with altered mental status. Respiratory symptoms and signs are often mild initially, and renal failure can develop. Treatment is with a macrolide and supportive care.

P1.137   C: This condition often has an infectious cause

There are many causes of erythema multiforme. Mycoplasma and herpesvirus infections are common causes and should be excluded, particularly if oral steroids are contemplated. Itch often responds to antihistamine or topical steroids. This condition can be associated with mouth and genital ulcers in Stevens–Johnson syndrome or with toxic epidermal necrolysis. Erythema nodosum causes tender nodules on the legs that fade to look like bruises.

P1.138   D: She should be referred for an ultrasound examination

Multinodular goitres are common but where there is a dominant nodule the patient should be referred for excision in order to prevent malignant change. This occurs in about 5% of multinodular goitres. Indications of malignancy that should prompt 2-week referral include rapid growth, tracheal compression, laryngeal nerve involvement, irregular nodules, lymphadenopathy and a history of neck irradiation.

P1.139   C: Ventricular bigeminy

This ECG shows ventricular bigeminy, where a normal sinus beat is followed by a premature ventricular contraction. There is often a compensatory pause after the ectopic beat. In the absence of other cardiovascular disease it is seldom of consequence. A history should be taken, aimed at identifying any factors that might increase ectopic activity, such as thyroid disease, caffeine or alcohol, but usually no treatment is needed. Paroxysmal atrial fibrillation consists of runs of atrial fibrillation interspersed with normal sinus rhythm whereas Wenckebach's phenomenon is characterised by an increasing PR interval until a ventricular beat is missed. AV dissociation shows atrial activity and ventricular activity that are not coordinated, whereas 2:1 heart block shows two P waves for each QRS complex.

P1.140   B: Basal cell carcinoma

The appearance of an ulcerated lesion on the ear suggests either an SCC or a BCC. In this case there is a pearly rolled edge with telangiectasia, suggestive of a BCC. Keratoacanthomas usually develop over a fairly rapid time course, but are similar histologically and clinically, often making excision necessary for diagnosis. Chondrodermatitis is usually seen higher up on the pinna and is a painful nodule. Actinic keratosis does not usually ulcerate.

Difficult patients

P1.141   B: Entitled demanders

Entitled demanders seek medical attention and try to control the direction through intimidation and induction of guilt. They might also attempt to use litigation or the threat of this to get their own way.

P1.142   D: Heartsink patient

'Heartsinks' are a function of the doctor–patient relationship rather than purely a character trait of the patient. Female GPs identify fewer heartsinks than their male colleagues, and doctors who are stressed and showing signs of burnout typically report higher numbers of heartsinks.

P1.143   F: Self-destructive denier

The possibility of underlying depression should be considered in these patients, but often these patients seem to derive satisfaction from their plight, in an extension of the sick role. An example would be the patient with poorly controlled diabetes who is rapidly going blind but continues to ignore advice on diet and medication.

P1.144   E: Manipulative help rejector

Manipulative help rejectors are usually pleasant in a consultation but believe that they are beyond help and seem to enjoy the physician's inability to cure them of their symptoms, which are usually mild and not life threatening. Where a symptom is cured they will often present with a new, equally difficult symptom.

P1.145   C: Frequent attenders

One should always avoid subjective terms that imply a character judgement such as 'dependent clinger' or 'heartsink' when writing in medical notes.

P1.146   A: Check thyroid autoantibodies

The most likely cause in this patient is thyroid eye disease, usually seen in Graves' disease, but it can precede the development of hyperthyroidism. Myasthenia gravis causes ptosis rather than proptosis and can be tested for with anti-acetylcholine receptor antibodies. A brain tumour would not usually cause proptosis and tumours in the orbit would usually cause visual signs and pain. Orbital cellulitis can cause proptosis but is usually clinically obvious, with erythema, pain and fever, together with ophthalmoplegia and, later, loss of colour vision. Following blood tests for Graves' disease, she should be referred to ophthalmology.

P1.147   B: Cryptosporidia can be resistant to chlorination of water

Some strains are resistant to chlorination, although all strains of these organisms should be killed by chlorine dioxide ozone if used correctly. Transmission is faeco-oral, with humans or animals passing spores in the faeces. Affected children should remain off school until 48 hours after symptoms have settled. Most cases are mild but children and immunocompromised individuals can develop a chronic illness. Transmission is usually through drinking, but can also be through swimming in lakes and rivers, drinking from streams (eg when hiking) or sexual intercourse.

Hypertension trials

P1.148   B: ALLHAT

The ALLHAT (Antihypertensive and Lipid Lowering Treatment to Prevent Heart Attack trial) study showed benefits for treatment with thiazides, but not for doxazosin, which was shown to increase risk of CVD and heart failure.

P1.149   D: DASH

The DASH (Dietary approaches to stop hypertension) study used a low-sodium, low-fat, high-fruit-and-vegetable diet. The effects were independent of weight reduction.

P1.150   H: HYVET

The HYVET (Hypertension in the very elderly trial) showed that treating patients with a systolic blood pressure >160 reduced morbidity and mortality and was well tolerated.

P1.151   I: STOP

The STOP (Swedish Trial in Old Patients with Hypertension-2 Study) randomised primary care hypertensive patients to conventional treatment (β blockers or thiazides), ACE inhibitors or calcium antagonists. It found no difference between the three groups.

P1.152   C: CAMBO

The CAMBO (Conventional versus Automated Measurement of Blood pressure in the Office) trial found that leaving a patient in a room with an automated blood pressure machine, set to take six readings over 12 min, eliminated the white coat effect and were close to the ambulatory reading.

P1.153   B: It is a cause of sudden death in young athletes

HOCM is the most common genetic cardiac disease and is inherited as an autosomal dominant trait, although many cases are the result of spontaneous mutation. It frequently presents with sudden death in young athletes, and in some countries high-school athletes are required to have echocardiography as a screening test. Less frequently it can present with chronic heart failure or arrhythmia, but treatment usually controls symptoms only without affecting outcome. It can also be detected as an asymptomatic finding in older patients.

P1.154   E: Transdermal opioid patches do not reach steady-state analgesic levels for 24 hours

Transdermal patches require 24 hours to reach a steady state and additional breakthrough analgesia might be required during this time. Co-proxamol is toxic in overdose but is available on a named-patient basis. Buprenorphine is a partial agonist but can be taken with other opioids.

P1.155   B: Change to a triphasic pill

Breakthrough bleeding is common in the first 6 months on the combined pill. If it persists and no other cause can be found, the patient should be changed to a higher oestrogen dose pill or a triphasic pill. There is little justification for taking two combined pills a day because the dose of oestrogen would pose a significant risk of side effects. The mini-pill is a common cause of spotting and would not be an appropriate alternative in this instance. A Mirena IUS would be technically difficult to fit in a nulliparous woman, but might be appropriate if symptoms could not be controlled with medication or if estrogen was contraindicated.

P1.156   A: Acamprosate reduces the desire to drink

Acamprosate works on CNS GABA receptors to reduce the desire for alcohol and is licensed for use in prevention of relapse. Antabuse produces an unpredictable reaction and can cause severe illness. It should only be used under consultant supervision for new patients, although it might be an effective longer-term treatment once abstinence has been established. Brief interventions, with assessment, education and advice on drinking, have been shown to reduce alcohol consumption by 20%. Many patients with no long-term damage can safely reduce their drinking to normal levels without the need for abstinence, which in many cases is socially difficult, eg in remote communities. Long-term follow-up of survivors shows that, at 4 years, 28% of patients have been abstinent for 6 months and 18% are drinking asymptomatically (Rand report).

Treatment of prostate cancer

P1.157   E: External-beam radiotherapy

Approximately 12% of patients receiving external-beam radiotherapy suffer proctitis and haemorrhage. This is significantly less common with brachytherapy.

P1.158   I: Watchful waiting

Radical prostatectomy was shown to reduce deaths from prostate cancer but not overall mortality when compared with watchful waiting.

P1.159   D: Docetaxel

Docetaxel chemotherapy can be effective in non-hormone-responsive recurrences. Bisphosphonates might be useful in managing bone pain as an adjunct to radiotherapy or NSAIDs.

P1.160   G: Orchidectomy

NICE recommend offering bilateral orchidectomy to all patients with hormone-sensitive tumours as an alternative to LHRH agonists.

P1.161   F: LHRH analogue

LHRH analogues cause an initial flare in testosterone production followed by suppression to the equivalent of castration. Initial treatment should be covered with an anti-androgen to prevent tumour flare, especially where there are spinal metastases. Cord compression has been reported in some patients in whom LHRH analogues are used alone.

P1.162   E: Patients who are intolerant of colchicine or NSAIDs should be treated with prednisolone

Most cases of gout are due to an inherited metabolic defect or are iatrogenic, common triggers including thiazides, furosemide and low-dose salicylates. The traditional purine-rich duet is rarely seen as a cause. Uric acid often drops during an acute attack. Joint aspiration reveals clear fluid, with crystals seen on microscopy. Colchicine should be given as 500 µg three times a day. Prophylaxis should be considered if patients are having more than two attacks a year, but should not be started during an acute attack, and patients should be warned that prophylaxis can trigger an acute attack.

P1.163   D: Seborrhoeic keratosis

Seborrhoeic keratoses are common lesions usually seen on the torso from the age of 40 onwards. No evidence of viral infection has been found, and although unsightly no treatment is needed, other than on cosmetic grounds.

P1.164   C: Candidal infection is more common in pregnancy

A fishy smell suggests bacterial vaginosis or infection with *Trichomonas* sp. These are both treated with metronidazole orally or clindamycin pessaries. There is no need for condoms or partner treatment with bacterial vaginosis. Bacterial vaginosis is often discovered incidentally on swabs or smears. Thrush is more common in sexually active people, pregnant women and immunocompromised individuals. Trichomoniasis is a sexually transmitted infection that causes a urethritis in men and a foul-smelling mucopurulent discharge in women. Diagnosis is on microscopy.

P1.165   B: The data show a statistically significant weight loss at 3 months

The data show an 80% drop-out rate by 12 months. The data are not presented on an intention-to-treat basis. Assuming that the patients who drop out regain their weight loss, the average weight loss is likely to be <1 kg. The high drop-out rates imply poor concordance with treatment. Weight loss is maintained in the 20% of patients who are still in the programme at 12 months.

Viral infections

P1.166   E: Human papillomavirus

P1.167   H: Norovirus

P1.168   I: Parvovirus B19

P1.169   B: Coxsackievirus

P1.170   C: Epstein–Barr virus

HPV is responsible for increasing numbers of cases of oral cancer, often in patients without the traditional risk factors of alcohol and smoking. Norovirus is the leading cause of infectious gastroenteritis in developed countries and is highly infectious, causing particular problems in hospitals, hotels and cruise ships. Slapped cheek is a common viral condition affecting preschool children. It is rarely dangerous in children but unexposed pregnant women have a small risk of fetal hydrops. Hand, foot and mouth disease affects toddlers and causes characteristic vesicles on the buccal mucosa, hands and feet. It is self-limiting and usually caused by Coxsackie A virus or enteroviruses. Both the sporadic and the endemic (usually equatorial Africa) forms of Burkitt's lymphoma are associated with EBV infection.

P1.171   C: Perthes' disease

Perthes' disease, avascular necrosis of the femoral head, is usually seen in children between the ages of 5 and 10 years, and 80% of cases are seen in boys. Initially it presents as an irritable hip but later the joint becomes fixed and movements improve, albeit with a positive Trendelenburg gait. Congenital dislocation of the hip usually presents earlier as asymmetrical creases, or is picked up at child health surveillance. Slipped upper femoral epiphysis is typically seen in boys between the ages of 10 and 15 years, and presents with a shortened and rotated leg. Septic arthritis is usually associated with a raised CRP and WCC. The main differential is irritable hip but this does not usually persist as long and can be excluded on X-ray.

P1.172   C: Patients diagnosed with osteoporosis should be investigated for coeliac disease

Bisphosphonates are available in oral and intravenous formulations. They have been shown to increase bone density and reduce fractures. In patients who are intolerant, strontium can be used as a second-line treatment. A T score <2.5 is diagnostic, and all patients should be assessed to exclude secondary osteoporosis, eg due to coeliac disease or hypogonadism. Bisphosphonates should usually be prescribed for 5 years. Where patients have refractory osteoporosis, PTH or teriparatide can be used under specialist supervision.

P1.173   A: All patients should be advised to exercise regularly

All patients with clinical symptoms and signs of osteoarthritis should be advised to exercise regularly, although they should be advised to avoid high impact or twisting/loading movements (eg basketball). X-rays seldom add to clinical findings and correlate poorly with symptoms. Patients should be screened for associated depression or anxiety, which may impede progress. All patients who are overweight or obese should try to lose weight, aiming for $>5\%$ of initial body weight. Patients who fail to respond to oral or topical analgesia, lifestyle changes and physiotherapy, or who have severe symptoms should be referred for consideration of joint replacement. Arthroscopy is indicated only for mechanical symptoms such as locking.

P1.174   B: Benign intracranial hypertension

Benign intracranial pressure causes headache in the mornings and evenings, relieved by standing. It is associated with papilloedema and in time visual field may be lost and a nerve VI palsy may develop. It usually affects young obese women and is due to impaired absorption of cerebrospinal fluid. It is usually idiopathic or may be seen in endocrine abnormalities, pregnancy or as a reaction to medication such some drugs. Treatment with lumbar puncture provides rapid relief at presentation, and recurrence may be prevented with acetazolamide or shunt insertion in refractory cases. Acute glaucoma affects the pupils early and is constant, whereas pre-eclampsia would not normally be seen at this stage of pregnancy, and would be associated with hypertension and proteinuria. The main differential diagnosis is a space-occupying lesion.

Management of abnormal smears

P1.175   A: Refer for colposcopy

Patients with 'borderline change with endocervical changes' should be referred for colposcopy after one abnormal smear. Patients with 'borderline smear with squamous changes' should be referred after three abnormal smears.

P1.176   D: Repeat in 6 months

Three inadequate smears should prompt referral for colposcopy.

P1.177   H: Smear no longer necessary

Local protocols vary but most areas invite women for their first smear at 25, then 3-yearly to 49 and 5-yearly to 64. Patients aged over 65 need have a smear only if they have had a previous abnormal result.

P1.178   D: Repeat in 6 months

Again, local protocols vary but it is considered acceptable after one smear showing mild dyskariosis to repeat this and refer for colposcopy if the follow-up smear is abnormal.

P1.179   B: Refer under 2-week rule

Smears that are suspicious of cancer should be referred under the 2-week rule. Note that cervical smears are a screening test rather than a diagnostic test and cannot rule out cancer. Where a cervix looks abnormal or there is a suspicious history, a clinical diagnosis should prompt a 2-week referral.

P1.180   C: Prescribe vitamin D analogues

This patient has psoriasis. The use of emollients will often improve the dry scaly appearance, leaving red papules. The improvement in symptoms with ultraviolet light is characteristic. Steroids will often produce a dramatic improvement, which relapses, however, on cessation of the steroid. Vitamin D analogues are the first-line treatment for most patients. Patients with new-onset psoriasis should have a thorough drug history to exclude causative agents such as β blockers.

P1.181   A: She should be offered incision and curettage

Chalazions are cysts that develop in the meibomian glands. They often enlarge slowly but a third resolve within 3 months and almost all resolve within 2 years. If they become infected they should be treated with a short course of antibiotic ointment. Definitive treatment is incision and curettage, which can be done in general practice if the right equipment is available. If large they can compress the eyeball, causing astigmatism. Lesions around the eye should always be examined for evidence of malignancy (eg basal cell carcinoma, squamous cell carcinoma), although this would be unusual in this age group. Cryotherapy is not appropriate in this area due to the risk of cicatrising scars.

P1.182   A: All pregnant women should take vitamin D supplements

Patients with pre-existing hypertension are at increased risk of pre-eclampsia and should be monitored for this. Consideration should be given to using aspirin and changing antihypertensives to nifedipine, labetalol or methyldopa. ACE inhibitors and angiotensin receptor blockers are teratogenic. All patients should take folic acid 400 µg and vitamin D. Doses of these should be higher in high-risk patients, eg patients with diabetes, those with a personal or family history of neural tube defects and those on anticonvulsants should take 5 mg folic acid a day. Alcohol should be limited to 1–2 units once or twice a week and every effort should be made to stop smoking. Nicotine replacement therapy is safe in pregnancy. Overweight patients should be advised and supported to lose weight pre-conception, because obesity increases risk of diabetes and hypertension. Attention should also be paid to patients with a history of substance abuse.

P1.183   C: *Salmonella* sp.

Salmonellosis has an incubation period of 12–48 hours and typically causes vomiting followed by diarrhoea, which usually settles over 72 hours. In some cases it can cause a reactive arthritis and approximately 1% of patients go on to become carriers. Treatment is supportive, and antibiotics are not recommended for most patients. *Campylobacter* sp. causes diarrhoea and malaise but vomiting is rare; prolonged excretion can occur and this might be relevant for care-home or nursing staff. *Shigella* sp. is unusual in the UK but should be suspected in travellers who return with bloody diarrhoea. *Cryptosporidium* sp. usually affects children, whereas typhoid has a much longer incubation period and a more protracted clinical course.

P1.184   B: Cupping of the disc indicates damage to the eye despite normal intraocular pressure

Normal pressure glaucoma is a condition where there are signs of damage to the optic nerve with normal pressure. These patients should be started on treatment and have regular visual field monitoring. Laser iridotomy is useful for acute angle-closure glaucoma. Relying on patient symptoms is a poor indicator of disease progression because most patients are unaware of their peripheral visual field loss.

P1.185   C: Multiple myeloma

This pattern of symptoms and blood results is suggestive of myeloma. Urine should be sent for Bence Jones protein and he should be referred under the 2-week rule. CLL would usually cause a raised white cell count and symptoms are unusual, whereas lung cancer would usually cause respiratory symptoms. Metastatic prostate cancer can cause bony pain but would be unusual in patients without urinary symptoms. Persistent backache in young patients with systemic signs should prompt investigation to exclude sarcoma or infection.

P1.186   C: Patients should be monitored with regular βhCG levels for 2 years

Around 10% of molar pregnancies go on to develop neoplastic disease, but if treated early there is a very good prognosis. Recurrence risk for molar pregnancy is approximately 1 in 80 and most women go on to have a normal pregnancy afterwards. The COCP should not be used until βhCG levels are undetectable because it can delay tumour regression. All patients should be referred to specialist centres for follow-up.

The Mental Health Act

P1.187   I: None of the above

Detention is specifically excluded in patients without mental illness who are sexually deviant, suffer from drug and alcohol addiction, or commit disorderly acts, or on the grounds of religious or cultural beliefs.

P1.188   H: Section 136

Section 136 allows the police to take a patient to a place of safety for up to 72 hours. They cannot enter a private residence without consent to do so, however.

P1.189   C: Section 4

Section 4 of the Mental Health Act allows admission for 72 hours for assessment and allows for emergency detention and assessment. It requires one doctor and the application can be made by the nearest relative or an Approved Mental Health Professional. It should be used only where delay would pose a significant risk of harm to the patient or others.

P1.190   I: None of the above

Severe learning disabilities in the absence of other mental health problems are specifically excluded under the 2007 amendments to the Mental Health Act. This situation would best be resolved through the courts of protection.

P1.191   F: Section 17

Section 17 is an amendment introduced in 2007 to allow supervised community treatment orders and includes provision for failure to comply and the conditions under which re-admission would be needed.

Management of heavy menstrual bleeding

P1.192   C: **Fibroids present on ultrasound**

P1.193   H: **Refer under 2-week rule**

P1.194   A: **Contraceptive pill**

P1.195   I: **Tranexamic acid**

P1.196   E: **Mirena**

P1.197   B: **Check thyroid function**

Simple snoring can have a significant impact on quality of life of spouses and many snorers present only because of spousal pressure. Sleep apnoea should be excluded on the history and significant causes of obstruction such as large tonsils, a large tongue base or nasal obstruction identified. Simple measures that can help include weight loss, avoidance of sedatives and alcohol, and positional measures if the snoring is postural. Thyroid function should always be checked. Where simple measures fail, UVPP might be considered but it is very painful and is associated with a significant risk of nasal escape.

P1.198   B: **A 23-year-old man who has recently returned from a year travelling in south-east Asia with a new tattoo**

At-risk groups include those who have had blood transfusions before 1987, those who have had dental treatment, invasive medical procedures or body piercing in the developing world, those with a history of intravenous drug use, people with a raised ALT level and people who have had contact with these groups. Singapore is a developed country and not high risk; patients who live abroad as expats, but who do not use local facilities for health care, are not at high risk.

P1.199   E: **Women with Down syndrome should be screened for premature menopause**

Patients with Down syndrome suffer a number of health problems. Hearing difficulties are common, both sensorineural and conductive, as are cataracts. Women with Down syndrome enter the menopause on average 6 years early and dementia is increasingly prevalent beyond the age of 40. A third of patients with Down syndrome will develop hypothyroidism so screening is recommended as part of the Quality and Outcomes Framework. Atlantoaxial instability is seen in 20% of patients and often presents with cervical myelopathy. Altered gait and continence issues are signs of this condition.

P1.200   C: Moderate depression

PHQ-9 is an assessment tool for classifying the severity of depression based on the nine criteria listed in DSM-IV, looking at symptoms in the 2 weeks before the test. It is not a diagnostic test. The classification of depression severity according to PHQ-9 score is as follows:

0−4:	Normal
5−9:	Mild
10−14:	Moderate
15−19:	Moderately severe
20−27:	Severe

Paper 2
Questions

Total time allowed is three hours.

P2.1 **Minor injuries**
While working in the local minor injury unit a young man comes in
with the injury shown below.

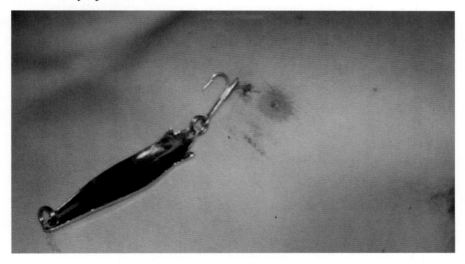

**Which one of the following would be the most appropriate strategy to
remove the hook?**

○   A   Cut the hook where it enters the skin and push the distal end
through the skin

○   B   Making an incision along the skin overlying the barb and removing
the hook

○   C   Pull the hook back out through the entry wound

○   D   Push the hook through and out of the skin before cutting off the
barb

○   E   Refer to on-call plastic surgery team to remove under general
anaesthetic

P2.2 **Joint pain**
A 7-year-old boy is seen with his mother complaining of a 6-week history of joint pain, lethargy and headache. He has been getting recurrent episodes of sore throat and has persistently enlarged lymph nodes. On examination he is pale and has some petechiae on his back. Which of the following is the most appropriate next step in this patient? Select one option only.

○ A Prescribe a 10-day course of phenoxymethylpenicillin (penicillin V)

○ B Reassure the mother that he probably has post-viral fatigue and review in 6 weeks if no better

○ C Check his full blood count (FBC)

○ D Prescribe a non-steroidal drug for his arthralgia

○ E Reassure the mother that the probable diagnosis is Henoch–Schönlein purpura, which should resolve without any complications

Lower urinary tract symptoms in men

P2.3–2.7

Options

A 5α-Reductase inhibitor
B α Blocker
C α Blocker plus 5α-reductase inhibitor
D Anticholinergic
E Bladder training
F Desmopressin
G GnRH analogue
H None of the above

Complete the table below describing the management of lower urinary tract symptoms. Each option may be used once, more than once or not at all.

Symptoms	Moderate-to-severe LUTS	Detrusor instability	LUTS with enlarged prostate	LUTS with enlarged prostate despite treatment with 3	Nocturnal polyuria
Treatment	P2.3	P2.4	P2.5	P2.6	P2.7

P2.8 **Psoriasis**
A 14-year-old girl with psoriasis comes to see you begging for something to be done for the lesions on her face. These respond to short courses of potent topical steroids but quickly return on stopping. Which one of the following would be the single most appropriate management option for her?

○ A Betamethasone cream for 8 weeks

○ B Coal tar

○ C Emollients

○ D Topical tacrolimus

○ E Vitamin D

P2.9 Hip dislocation
Which of the following statements about screening for congenital dislocation of the hip is true? Select one option only.

○ A The Ortolani test is used to detect a dislocatable hip

○ B The Barlow test is used to detect a dislocated hip

○ C Ultrasonography is much more sensitive and specific than clinical testing

○ D Most children who are discovered to have the condition will require surgery

○ E Breech presentation is a risk factor

P2.10 Rectal bleeding
A 37-year-old man complains of severe pain every time that he passes a stool, with fresh blood on the toilet paper. This has not improved with Anusol. Examination reveals a small skin tag and exquisite tenderness just inside the anal margin, but no mass. Which of the following is the most appropriate management in this case? Select one option only.

○ A Topical glyceryl trinitrate

○ B Anal stretch

○ C Instillagel

○ D Ciprofloxacin

○ E Haemorrhoidectomy

P2.11 Pain relief
A 67-year-old man has been suffering from metastatic lung cancer for the last 18 months. He has been using fentanyl patches at home for the last few weeks but is now getting very distressed. You decide to start a syringe driver. Which of the following statements is correct about the use of syringe drivers in palliative care? Select one option only.

○ A Morphine may suppress respiration and therefore should not be used in patients with lung pathology

○ B When converting a patient to a morphine syringe driver from fentanyl, it is best to start at a low dose and titrate upwards to achieve pain control

○ C Levomepromazine (Nozinan) will help with agitation and nausea

○ D Morphine is effective only for visceral pain

○ E Midazolam and morphine cannot be mixed in the same syringe driver because of precipitation

P2.12 **Shortness of breath**
A 74-year-old former boilermaker complains of progressive dyspnoea and weight loss over the last 18 months. He is an ex-smoker but has no other previous medical history of note. On examination he has bilateral inspiratory crackles and is clubbed. You arrange a chest X-ray, which shows diffuse shadowing and pleural plaques. What is the most likely diagnosis? Select one option only.

○   A   Asbestosis

○   B   Bronchogenic carcinoma

○   C   Extrinsic allergic alveolitis

○   D   Left ventricular failure

○   E   Chronic obstructive pulmonary disease

P2.13 **Hypoglycaemia**
You visit a 24-year-old man with type 1 diabetes who is drowsy, slurred and confused. He has had gastroenteritis and his mother thinks that he has not been eating. You measure his blood sugar level at 1.6 mmol/l. You decide to give him intramuscular glucagon. Write the appropriate dose in milligrams in the box below.

Common infections

Options

A   1 day
B   4 days
C   1 week
D $2\frac{1}{2}$ weeks
E   3 weeks
F   6 weeks
G   3 months

For each of the common self-limiting infections seen in primary care, select the usual duration of symptoms from the list of options above. Each option may be used once, more than once or not at all.

P2.14   **Acute tonsillitis**
P2.15   **Acute bronchitis**
P2.16   **Acute sinusitis**
P2.17   **Acute otitis media**

P2.18 **Heel pain**

A 37-year-old recreational marathon runner complains of recurrent pain in his right heel. He has tried anti-inflammatories and several different insoles and different shoes with no benefit. He has seen a sports therapist who has taped his foot to no avail. Examining him he has marked local tenderness. You give him a steroid injection into the point of maximal tenderness but when he fails to improve arrange an X-ray, which shows a heel spur. Which one of the following would be appropriate in his management at this stage?

○   A   Bed rest

○   B   Botox injections

○   C   Refer for excision of his heel spur

○   D   Refer for lithotripsy

○   E   Repeat cortisone injection

P2.19 **Fatigue**

A 67-year-old woman presents with dizziness and fatigue. Her electrocardiogram (ECG) is shown below.

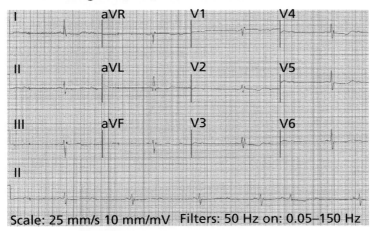

Scale: 25 mm/s 10 mm/mV   Filters: 50 Hz on: 0.05–150 Hz

Heart rate: 32 bpm
QT interval: 604 ms

Which one of the following statements is true with regard to this case?

○   A   The diagnosis is Möbitz type 2 heart block

○   B   She should be treated with a cardioselective β blocker

○   C   This condition is usually iatrogenic

○   D   If the patient is well in herself she can be referred to the outpatient department

○   E   She should be treated with a permanent pacemaker

P2.20 **Vasectomy**
One of your patients comes to see you to request a vasectomy. He has four children already and feels that he cannot afford to have any more. You counsel him about the pros and cons of vasectomy. Which of the following statements about vasectomy is true? Select one option only.

○ A It is usually carried out under general anaesthetic

○ B Sterility is immediate after the procedure

○ C Bruising is uncommon and should be investigated

○ D The lifetime failure rate is approximately 1%

○ E Vasectomy is reversible in only 50% of cases

P2.21 **Nose bleeds**
With regard to the management of epistaxis in a 76-year-old man, which of the following statements is correct? Select one option only.

○ A Most bleeds are posterior

○ B Bleeding comes from branches of the internal jugular vein

○ C The majority of cases are caused by high blood pressure

○ D Anterior bleeds are never fatal

○ E Silver nitrate cautery may cause septal perforation

P2.22 **Eye symptoms**
A 56-year-old office worker with no previous history of note presents with a painful red eye of 3 days' duration. There is no history of trauma or foreign body, and he does not wear contact lenses. He has tried over the counter chloramphenicol with no benefit. Examination reveals reduced corneal sensation and fluorescein staining reveals the appearance below.

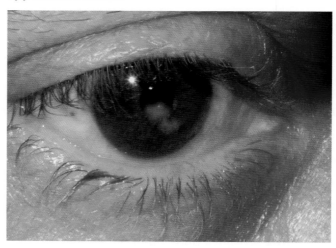

Which of the following is the most likely diagnosis?

○   A   Dendritic ulcer

○   B   Iritis

○   C   Acute conjunctivitis

○   D   Corneal foreign body

○   E   Recurrent corneal erosion

P2.23   Assisted suicide
Which one of the following statements about assisted suicide is true?

○   A   Assisted suicide is legal in the UK as long as certain legal criteria are met

○   B   Rates of physician-assisted suicide have risen consistently since legalisation in the Netherlands

○   C   Physician-assisted suicide accounts for 17% of deaths in the Netherlands

○   D   Neuromuscular relaxants are the drug of choice in the Netherlands

○   E   The 'doctrine of double effect' refers to the use of a drug primarily to bring about death in assisted suicide

P2.24   Memory problems
A 76-year-old man is brought into the surgery by his wife. He claims not to know why he is there but she tells you that she is worried that he may be starting to develop dementia. Which of the following statements is NOT true about dementia? Select one option only.

○   A   Dementia is usually associated with altered cognition and consciousness

○   B   It is usually seen in many spheres of intellectual function

○   C   All patients should have baseline biochemical and haematological investigations before referral

○   D   *Gingko biloba* is of some benefit in slowing memory impairment

○   E   HIV testing is appropriate in young patients

Liver function tests

Options

A Gallstones
B Gilbert syndrome
C Haemochromatosis
D Haemolysis
E Hepatitis
F Iatrogenic
G Malnutrition
H Physiological

For each of the descriptions below, select the most appropriate diagnosis from the list of options. Each option may be used once, more than once or not at all.

P2.25 A 34-year-old man has recently suffered flu-like symptoms. His bloods show a raised bilirubin only and a normal FBC.

P2.26 A 56-year-old man with epilepsy attends for liver function tests (LFTs) as part of an insurance medical. He has a raised γ-glutamyltransferase (GGT), normal bilirubin, ALT (alanine transaminase) and alkaline phosphatase (ALP).

P2.27 A 12-year-old girl has blood tests as part of investigations for recurrent urinary tract infections. Her ALP level is raised, although bilirubin and ALT are normal.

P2.28 A 34-year-old man has recently returned from a holiday where he had a brief romance. He has now developed jaundice. His blood tests show an ALT five times normal levels, bilirubin elevated and a normal ALP.

P2.29 A 47-year-old woman presents with acute abdominal pain. Her urine has darkened and her stools are pale. Bloods show raised ALT, raised bilirubin and raised ALP. GGT is normal.

P2.30 **Wound management**
A 76-year-old woman who has been treated for a recurrence of breast cancer has a fungating wound. She is particularly concerned about the odour. She has been told that she is incurable. Which of the following palliative treatments may help? Select one option only.

○ **A** An absorbent dressing will remove exudates and minimise odour

○ **B** Admission for a short course of intravenous antibiotics will reduce bacterial load and thus the odour

○ **C** Topical metronidazole is effective

○ **D** Skin grafting will close the wound and reduce the odour

○ **E** Treatment should be directed at helping her cope psychologically

P2.31 **Abdominal pain**

A 45-year-old man presents with acute onset of severe pain in his loin that is radiating to the flank and groin. On examination he is slightly tender in the renal angle but has no fever. His urine is positive to blood on dipstick testing. Which one of the following statements about this situation is true?

○   A   He should be given fluids and a broad-spectrum antibiotic

○   B   This condition is usually the result of raised urate levels

○   C   A non-steroidal anti-inflammatory drug (NSAID) is contraindicated due to the risk of renal failure

○   D   Plain radiographs will usually show a stone if one is present

○   E   This could be a presentation of a renal tumour

Erectile dysfunction

Options

A   All of them
B   Caverject
C   MUSE (medicated urethral system for erection)
D   None of them
E   Sildenafil
F   Tadalafil
G   Vacuum pump

For each statement relating to treatments for erectile dysfunction, select the most appropriate treatment from the list of options. Each option may be used once, more than once or not at all.

P2.32   **The treatment may cause disturbance of colour vision.**
P2.33   **It is contraindicated in sickle cell disease.**
P2.34   **It is contraindicated in urethral stricture.**
P2.35   **Its efficacy may persist for 36 hours after use.**
P2.36   **It may be prescribed on the NHS to men with Parkinson's disease.**

P2.37 **Data interpretation**
A local reflexologist writes to your practice asking if you would like to set up a reflexology service under practice-based commissioning. She cites a recent paper that showed significant benefits for patients with depression. You look the paper up on the internet and find the following abstract:

Qualitative study of the efficacy of reflexology in patients with mild depression
A retrospective postal survey was sent to 18 patients who had received reflexology for mild depression in the 6 months before the survey. The survey dealt with efficacy and satisfaction measures using a 10-point scale. The results showed that 16/18 (89%) of patients reported improvement in their depression after treatment, while no patients reported adverse effects; 13/18 described themselves as very satisfied with the service and 5/18 were quite satisfied. The mean number of sessions was 11, with each session lasting 45 minutes. These data suggest that reflexology is a cost-effective and efficacious alternative to drugs in the management of depression.

Which one of the following statements is true with regard to this research?

○   A   The data support the suggestion that reflexology is a cost-effective alternative to drug therapy

○   B   The study follows a valid protocol

○   C   Qualitative studies are less prone to bias than quantitative studies

○   D   The results should be treated with caution because of inclusion bias

○   E   The improvement rates are significantly better than those seen with antidepressants

P2.38 **Abdominal pain**
A 53-year-old woman presents with mild right iliac fossa pain of 2 months' duration. Examination shows no abnormality but blood tests show a mild iron-deficiency anaemia. Which of the following statements regarding investigation is correct? Select one option only.

○   A   Refer for colonoscopy

○   B   Refer for sigmoidoscopy

○   C   If a barium enema is normal she may be reassured

○   D   Refer for ultrasonography

○   E   A raised ESR suggests that infection is a probable cause

P2.39 Suicide
Which one of the following statements about suicide is true?

○   A   Approximately 4000 people a year commit suicide in England and Wales

○   B   Young women are a high-risk group

○   C   It is more likely in those living in rural communities

○   D   Cutting the wrists is the most common mode of attempted suicide

○   E   There is a 20% risk of a patient who has had an episode of deliberate self-harm committing suicide within the next 12 months

Paediatric syndromes

Options

A   Charcot–Marie–Tooth syndrome
B   Down syndrome
C   Edwards' syndrome
D   Fragile X syndrome
E   Klinefelter syndrome
F   Noonan syndrome
G   Patau syndrome
H   Turner syndrome
I   Williams' syndrome

For each description below, select the most appropriate diagnosis from the list of options. Each option may be used once, more than once or not at all.

P2.40   A chromosome 18 trisomy with a ventricular septal defect and pulmonary stenosis.

P2.41   A child with upslanting eyes, prominent epicanthic folds, reduced muscle tone and spots on the iris.

P2.42   It accounts for 5–10% of severe learning difficulties in boys; often skips a generation.

P2.43   It affects boys only, with delayed puberty, cryptorchidism and learning difficulties.

P2.44   It is characterised by elfin facies, aortic stenosis and hypercalcaemia.

P2.45 Private fees
Your practice manager has been reviewing the private fees charged in your practice and has suggested that these be increased. Which one of the following statements is true with regard to private services?

○ A Private fees can be set at whatever level the practice wishes

○ B The British Medical Association publishes recommended levels for each service annually

○ C Private fees cannot increase by more than the level of inflation

○ D Private fees are covered by the GMS Contract

○ E Private fees can be charged only if the practice is registered for VAT

P2.46 Hip surgery
A 61-year-old woman comes to see you for advice about whether she should have her hip replaced (as recommended by her orthopaedic surgeon). Which one of the following statements about hip replacements is true?

○ A Ninety per cent of hip replacements last for more than 10 years

○ B There is a 10% infection risk for hip replacement surgery

○ C Once pain free, there are no restrictions on movement

○ D The incidence of DVT is 10% after total hip replacement

○ E Hip resurfacing is superior to conventional arthroplasty in advanced osteoarthritis

Headache

P2.47–2.51

Options

A Cluster headache
B Cervicogenic headache
C Medication overuse headache
D Migraine
E Tension headache
F None of the above

Complete the diagnosis row in the table below designed to aid in the classification of headache, using the list of options above. Each option may be used once, more than once or not at all.

Frequency	1 to several per month	Variable	Alternate days to 8/day	Daily for weeks	>15 days a month
Severity	Moderate – severe	Mild– moderate	Severe	Moderate– severe	Mild–severe
Site of headache	Unilateral or bilateral	Bilateral	Unilateral	Posterior unilateral	Bilateral
Pain type	Throbbing/ pulsing	Pressure/ tightening	Severe unilateral pain	Ache from occipital region	Diffuse ache/ pressure
Aura?	In 33%	None	In some patients	None	None
Duration	4–72 h	Variable	15–180 min	Hours/ constant	Hours/ constant
Photophobia	Severe	Mild	Mild, may be ipsilateral	None	None
Nausea/ vomiting	Moderate– severe	Mild	Mild– moderate	Mild	None
Patient activity	Lie still	Normal	Agitated	Worse with head movement	Normal
Examination findings	Normal	Trigger points in scalp	Epiphora	Pain on neck movement	Normal
Diagnosis	P2.47	P2.48	P2.49	P2.50	P2.51

P2.52 Febrile illness in childhood
A 3-year-old boy is brought in by his mother with a 6-day history of fever, conjunctivitis, cracked lips and a red tongue, with red swollen hands and feet. She reports that in the first few days of the illness he had a rash on his abdomen, but this has now faded. On examination of his heart sounds he has a gallop rhythm and the heart sounds appear muffled. Which of the following is the likely diagnosis? Select one option only.

○   A   Kawasaki's disease

○   B   Takayasu's disease

○   C   Measles

○   D   Rubella

○   E   Scarlet fever

P2.53 **Oedema**

A 73-year-old man with a history of hypertension and diabetes presents with 4 weeks of increasing breathlessness on exertion. Over the last 10 days he has had trouble sleeping and cannot get his shoes on as a result of swollen legs. On examination he is afebrile with bilateral basal crepitations and a regular pulse, which you measure as 100 at rest. Which of the following diagnoses is probable in this case? Select one option only.

○   A   New-onset atrial fibrillation (AF)

○   B   Pulmonary fibrosis

○   C   Right ventricular failure

○   D   Cor pulmonale

○   E   Biventricular failure

P2.54 **Sore penis**

A 5-year-old boy is brought in by his father because he says that it hurts to pass urine. On examination he has balanitis. Which of the following statements is true with regard to management of this condition? Select one option only.

○   A   *Staphylococcus aureus* is the most common organism

○   B   Topical treatment is rarely helpful

○   C   All patients should be referred for circumcision

○   D   It may cause phimosis

○   E   Ninety per cent of 6-year-olds should be able to retract the foreskin

P2.55 **Emergency contraception**

A 21-year-old woman asks for the morning-after pill. She suffered condom failure the night before. She is taking phenytoin for epilepsy but is otherwise fit and well. You discuss her options and she is not happy to have a coil. What dose of oral levonorgestrel would be appropriate in this case? Write the answer in the box below.

P2.56 **Visual problems**

A 24-year-old man comes to see you for advice. He has been told by his optician that he has keratoconus and has been referred to see an ophthalmologist. He is understandably concerned and would like to know more about the condition. Which one of the following is correct regarding this condition?

- A The condition is always bilateral
- B The condition is caused by nutritional deficiency
- C The condition is non-progressive
- D The condition may be associated with corneal thinning
- E The only treatment for this condition is corneal grafting

P2.57 **Back problems**

A 13-year-old girl attends with her mother. She is becoming increasingly concerned about the appearance of her back and has stopped going swimming because of this. On examination she has a prominent scoliosis. Which of the following statements about scoliosis is true? Select one option only.

- A Spontaneous resolution never occurs
- B Scoliosis is always evident from infancy
- C Scoliosis in adolescence is more common in boys
- D Scoliosis usually affects the lumbar spine
- E Scoliosis may be associated with deformity of the skull and ribcage

Bleeding in early pregnancy

Options

A Blighted ovum
B Cervical incompetence
C Complete abortion
D Ectopic pregnancy
E Missed abortion
F Septic abortion
G Threatened abortion

For each of the descriptions below, select the most appropriate diagnosis from the list of options. Each option may be used once, more than once or not at all.

P2.58 A woman with heavy bleeding in week 7 of pregnancy, which initially settled. She now feels unwell and has an offensive vaginal discharge.

P2.59 A woman with a positive pregnancy test has bleeding and abdominal pain in the sixth week of her pregnancy. Ultrasonography shows an empty uterus. Her quantitative βhCG (β-human chorionic gonadotrophin) level is maintained over 72 hours.

P2.60 A woman with a previous history of dilatation and curettage presents with bleeding and mild cramps in week 14 of pregnancy.

P2.61 A woman with painless bleeding in week 7 of pregnancy. On examination her external os is closed.

P2.62 This is usually accompanied by light bleeding only and severe abdominal pain.

P2.63 Respiratory problems in babies

A 3-month-old baby is brought to the out-of-hours treatment centre by his parents with a cough and failure to feed. He had previously been well and was born after an uneventful pregnancy. He has had coryzal symptoms for the last 3 days. On examination he is tachypnoeic, cyanosed and has a temperature of 40°C. Examination of his chest reveals widespread wheeze and crepitations. What is the most likely diagnosis? Select one option only.

○   A   Pneumonia

○   B   Inhaled foreign body

○   C   Asthma

○   D   Bronchiolitis

○   E   Pertussis

P2.64 **Discrimination**
One of your receptionists decides to retire and you advertise for a replacement. Several of the applicants are aged over 60 years. The practice retirement age is set at 60. Which one of the following statements is true about this situation?

○   A   Age discrimination laws are designed specifically to protect elderly people

○   B   Mandatory retirement is 60 years for women and 65 years for men

○   C   Employers must write to employees in advance of their retirement date and advise them of their rights to apply to work beyond this date

○   D   Employment benefits with length of service are legal as long as the length of service to qualify is no more than 10 years

○   E   Dismissal on the basis of age is unlawful regardless of age

P2.65 **Hirschsprung's disease**
The parents of a boy newly diagnosed with Hirschsprung's disease come to see you for advice. She is 4 months into her second pregnancy and is concerned that her unborn child may also be affected. Which one of the following statements regarding this situation is correct?

○   A   Hirschsprung's disease affects females more than males

○   B   Hirschsprung's disease is associated with Down syndrome

○   C   Prenatal testing is routinely available for affected families

○   D   The condition is sporadic, hence the unborn child is not at increased risk

○   E   The risk of a second affected sibling is <10%

P2.66 **Treatment of chest infections**
A 76-year-old man with controlled hypertension is diagnosed with pneumonia. Which of the following statements about management is correct? Select one option only.

○   A   He should receive a broad-spectrum cephalosporin

○   B   He should be treated with a macrolide

○   C   First-line treatment should be amoxicillin 250 mg three times daily

○   D   If he fails to respond to a first-line antibiotic the dose should be increased

○   E   If *Staphylococcus* sp. is suspected flucloxacillin should be added

P2.67 **Premature ejaculation**

A 28-year-old man and his partner are seen together. Since being together he has been plagued by premature ejaculation and this is starting to cause problems in their relationship. Which of the following statements about management of this condition is true? Select one option only.

○ A The problem affects 5% of men questioned in surveys

○ B Clomipramine taken before intercourse is no more effective than placebo

○ C Paroxetine can increase the period before ejaculation up to eight times longer than placebo

○ D Fluoxetine is very effective when taken once a day

○ E Chlorpromazine is the treatment of choice for resistant patients

Management of epididymitis

P2.68–2.70

Options

A Amoxicillin
B Benzylpenicillin
C Ciprofloxacin
D Contact tracing
E Doxycyline
F Screen for *Chlamydia* sp.
G Trimethoprim

Complete the algorithm below for the management of acute epididymo-orchitis, from the list above. Each option may be used once, more than once or not at all.

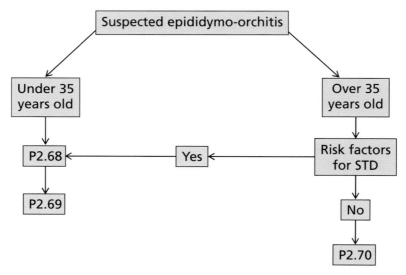

P2.71 Lithium
Your practice decides to do an audit of lithium prescribing as a result of a significant event. Which one of the following statements is correct regarding the use of lithium in general practice?

○ A   Lithium has a wide therapeutic range

○ B   Lithium has few side effects

○ C   Lithium is associated with an increase in risk of hypothyroidism

○ D   Lithium is safe to use in renal impairment

○ E   Lithium toxicity is rare

P2.72 Whiplash
A 67-year-old man has been involved in a car crash earlier in the day. He tells you that he was shunted from behind and his airbag deployed. He was assessed by a first responder at the scene and told that he had whiplash, but was advised to attend the surgery for a prescription for analgesia. He reports pins and needles in his right hand and, on examination, has limited rotation in his neck. There is some tenderness in the lower cervical spine and numbness over the lateral aspect of his right arm. Which one of the following would be appropriate management in this situation?

○ A   Gentle manipulation

○ B   Immobilisation with a soft collar

○ C   Muscle relaxants and anti-inflammatories, with gastric protection

○ D   Refer to physiotherapy

○ E   Stabilise cervical spine, refer to local accident and emergency department for imaging

P2.73 Infertility
A 31-year-old woman presents with her 32-year-old husband about their inability to have children. They are concerned that it might be a result of her age and would like referral. You take a full history and examine them both. Which one of the following is NOT a cause of infertility?

○ A   Endometriosis

○ B   Alcohol consumption

○ C   Smoking

○ D   High body mass index (BMI)

○ E   Tight underwear

P2.74 Use of ACE inhibitors

A 67-year-old hypertensive woman is started on aspirin and ramipril after suffering a transient ischaemic attack. One week after starting the ramipril she attends for renal function testing and her creatinine has increased from 83 μmol/l to 133 μmol/l. Which of the following statements about her management is true? Select one option only.

   ○   A   The dose of ramipril should not be increased further and she should have a repeat blood test in 1 week

   ○   B   As long as she is not hypotensive and her creatinine <150 μmol/l she can be reassured

   ○   C   The ramipril should be stopped and specialist advice sought

   ○   D   The ramipril should be changed to an angiotensin II receptor blocker

   ○   E   She should have her aspirin stopped

P2.75 Working with colleagues

After morning surgery one of the practice nurses comes to see you with concerns about the competence of one of your colleagues. She reports that she has noticed several occasions recently where he has given inappropriate medical treatment and feels duty bound to report her concerns. When you attempt to bring this up with the doctor concerned, he becomes aggressive and irritable. Which one of the following would be the appropriate step to take at this stage?

   ○   A   Report him to the General Medical Council

   ○   B   Discuss his performance with other members of the practice team to see if there are other concerns

   ○   C   Contact his appraiser to express your concerns

   ○   D   Refer him to the National Clinical Assessment Authority (NCAA)

   ○   E   Refer him to the local medical committee

P2.76 Vertigo

A 54-year-old woman presents with vertigo. Which of the following symptoms would be consistent with a diagnosis of benign paroxysmal positional vertigo? Select one option only.

   ○   A   Hallpike testing provokes instantaneous onset of symptoms

   ○   B   It worsens with repeat Hallpike testing

   ○   C   It is typically triggered by particular head movements

   ○   D   It is associated with unilateral tinnitus

   ○   E   It may be treated with Stemetil

P2.77 Moles

A 32-year-old woman attends for a mole check after reading a newspaper article about skin cancer. The lesion shown below is particularly worrying her, because it has recently grown significantly.

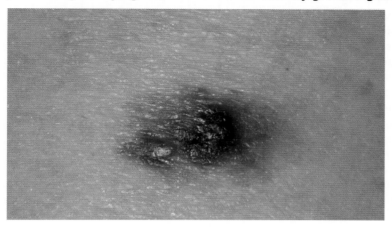

What is the likely diagnosis? Select one option only.

○ A Seborrhoeic keratosis

○ B Intradermal naevus

○ C Histiocytoma

○ D Malignant melanoma

○ E Squamous cell carcinoma (SCC)

P2.78 Eating disorders

Which one of the following statements is true with regard to anorexia nervosa?

○ A Patients can be screened for this condition using the SCOFF questionnaire

○ B The prevalence in the UK is estimated to be 10%

○ C It is seen exclusively in females

○ D It is characterised by obsession with exercise

○ E It can be diagnosed in those with a BMI <20 kg/m^2 and food avoidance

Cardiovascular drugs

Options

A   Amiodarone
B   Atorvastatin
C   Clopidogrel
D   Dipyridamole
E   Flecainide
F   Furosemide
G   Indapamide
H   Isosorbide mononitrate
I   Metoprolol
J   Ramipril
K   Simvastatin
L   Sotalol
M   Spironolactone
N   Valsartan
O   Verapamil
P   Warfarin

For each clinical scenario above, select the most appropriate therapy from the list of options. Each option may be used once, more than once or not at all.

P2.79   It reduces triglycerides as well as total cholesterol.
P2.80   It is used for prophylaxis of atrial fibrillation.
P2.81   It may be used in left ventricular dysfunction where ACE (angiotensin-converting enzyme) inhibitors are not tolerated.
P2.82   It is contraindicated in patients on β blockers.
P2.83   It often causes headache, flushing and postural hypotension.
P2.84   It should be considered in patients with heart failure already on an ACE inhibitor and thiazide.
P2.85   It may cause corneal microdeposits and phototoxicity.
P2.86   It may be safely used in young patients with hypertension and renal artery stenosis.

P2.87   **Aspirin**
A 52-year-old businessman comes to see you for a well man check. He is normotensive and his cholesterol and glucose levels are normal. He asks you about the merits of taking daily aspirin. Which one of the following statements is correct regarding the pros and cons of aspirin in primary prevention?

○   A   Aspirin may increase the risk of cancer

○   B   Aspirin use in primary prevention reduces risk of non-fatal myocardial infarction

○   C   Clopidogrel should be used for primary prevention due to an improved safety profile

○   D   The risk of gastrointestinal bleeding remains constant regardless of duration of aspirin use

○   E   There are no significant side effects from taking aspirin

P2.88   **Treatment of skin lesions**
A 12-year-old girl has had the skin lesion below for 18 months. She has tried topical salicylic acid and topical glutaraldehyde without benefit.

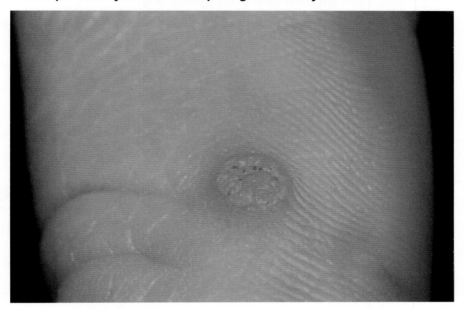

Which one of the following would be the single most appropriate next step in her treatment?

○   A   Bleomycin

○   B   Cryotherapy

○   C   Excision

○   D   Podophyllin

○   E   No treatment

P2.89 Palpitations
A 33-year-old marketing executive complains of palpitations at night. These come and go and, although he does not feel unwell with them, he gets a fluttering sensation in his chest for 30–60 seconds. He is otherwise well and takes no regular medication. His bloods and ECG are normal; however, a 24-hour ECG reveals short runs of atrial fibrillation. Which of the following statements about paroxysmal atrial fibrillation are true? Select one option only.

A   It affects approximately 10% of the population at some time in their lives

B   All patients should be anticoagulated because of the risk of stroke

C   Digoxin is effective in this patient group

D   Lifestyle has little effect on symptoms

E   Patients with recurrent symptoms can use flecainide as a 'pill-in-the-pocket' treatment

P2.90 Abdominal pain
A 37-year-old woman complains of recurrent severe pain in the right upper quadrant after meals. On examination she is tender in the right upper quadrant on deep inspiration. Which one of the following statements is true?

A   If caused by gallstones the pain usually settles within a few minutes

B   When associated with jaundice the cause is usually malignant

C   Symptoms usually settle spontaneously with a change in diet

D   She should be referred for endoscopic retrograde cholecystopancreatography

E   A raised alkaline phosphatase (ALP) suggests that the diagnosis is gallstones

P2.91 Sore throat
A 21-year-old who was started on antibiotics for tonsillitis 2 days ago presents with signs of a quinsy. Which of the following statements about this condition is true? Select one option only.

A   It is usually caused by infection with *Haemophilus influenzae* type B

B   It is an abscess within the tonsillar crypts

C   Earache, trismus and dysphagia are typical symptoms

D   It should be treated by adding in metronidazole tablets

E   It does not recur

P2.92 **Rash**

A 19-year-old girl complains of an itchy weeping rash on her abdomen. She thinks this may have started a few days after having her navel pierced. The appearance is shown below.

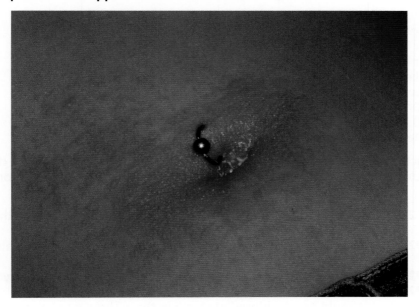

Which one of the following is the most likely cause of this rash?

○   A   Infection

○   B   Irritant dermatitis to the surgical spirit she has used to clean the piercing

○   C   Nickel dermatitis

○   D   Psoriasis

○   E   None of the above

Management of chronic stable asthma

Options

A	Check inhaler technique
B	Infliximab
C	Inhaled β_2 agonist as needed
D	Inhaled high-dose steroids
E	Inhaled regular-dose steroids
F	Leukotriene receptor antagonist
G	Long-acting bronchodilator
H	Omalizumab
I	Oral theophylline
J	Regular oral steroids

For each clinical scenario below, select the most appropriate therapeutic choice from the list of options. Each option may be used once, more than once or not at all.

P2.93 **It is licensed for use in severe persistent allergic asthma with proven IgE-mediated sensitivity to inhaled allergens.**

P2.94 **This is add-on therapy in a patient using an inhaled β_2 agonist 5 days a week on average.**

P2.95 **It may be associated with increased morbidity and mortality.**

P2.96 **It has an additive effect with inhaled steroids.**

P2.97 **It should be considered at step 5 in the asthma management protocol.**

P2.98 **Deafness**
A 35-year-old woman presents with steadily increasing deafness that is causing her to struggle to hear on the telephone. Which of the following statements about otosclerosis is true? Select one option only.

○ A It causes a sensorineural deafness, worse in low frequencies

○ B It typically presents in the fifth decade

○ C Its incidence is rising

○ D It often gets worse during pregnancy

○ E Hearing aids are the only treatment

P2.99 **Boils**
A 25-year-old woman presents complaining of recurrent boils in her axillae. These come on for no obvious reason and she has had numerous courses of antibiotics over the last 5 years. She says that she is fed up and has had to stop shaving her armpits, which she finds very distressing. Which of the following statements about treatment of this condition is true? Select one option only.

○ A Botox injections may reduce the frequency of attacks

○ B Anhydrol Forte may be helpful in place of antiperspirant

○ C A low-dose combined oral contraceptive may be helpful

○ D Long-term oral tetracycline is effective in reducing frequency of attacks

○ E She should be referred at this point for surgical excision and skin grafting

P2.100 Arm pain
A 73-year-old woman noticed a sudden popping sensation in her left arm. On examination her arm has the following appearance.

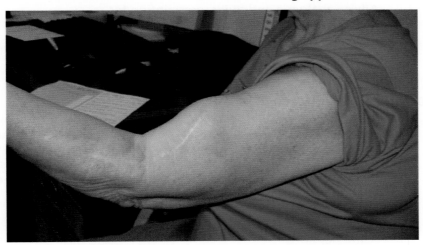

What treatment is required?

○ A Referral to physiotherapy for ultrasound therapy

○ B Referral to orthopaedics for repair

○ C Collar-and-cuff sling

○ D Steroid injection into the rotator cuff

○ E None

P2.101 Epiglottitis
Which of the following are NOT features of epiglottitis? Select one option only.

○ A The patient is unwell and looks septic

○ B The voice is muffled

○ C There is increasing dysphagia

○ D There is drooling

○ E It is exclusively seen in children

P2.102 Sore throat
A 54-year-old woman complains of a sore throat for the last 2 days and a fever. Examining her she has bilaterally enlarged tonsils with exudate. Her previous medical history includes hypertension, depression and thyrotoxicosis. She is taking ramipril, fluoxetine, levothyroxine and carbimazole. Which one of the following would be the most appropriate management in this situation?

A   Admit under on-call ear, nose and throat team

B   Advice analgesia and fluids, issue a deferred prescription for antibiotics to use if there is no improvement after 48 hours

C   Advice analgesia and fluids, prescription for phenoxymethylpenicillin to use immediately

D   Advise analgesia and fluids, together with advice on review criteria

E   Check full blood count immediately

P2.103 Abdominal pain
A 68-year-old man with no previous medical history of note complains that over the last few days he has gone yellow. He has no pruritus but for some weeks has had epigastric pain and intermittent nausea with some diarrhoea. He has lost 5 kg in weight. On examination he is tender in his right upper quadrant and his liver is palpable on deep inspiration. What is the single most likely diagnosis?

A   Acute cholecystitis

B   Acute hepatitis

C   Cholangiocarcinoma

D   Chronic cholecysitis

E   Primary biliary cirrhosis

P2.104 Hand injuries
You see a 23-year-old man at the walk-in centre who has cut his knuckles on someone else's teeth during a pub fight the night before. On examination he has several puncture wounds over the knuckles and the hand is swollen. Which of the following statements about his management is NOT true? Select one option only.

A   He should be given co-amoxiclav 625 mg three times daily and advised to return for review the following day

B   The wounds should be cleaned with saline, and closed

C   An X-ray should be taken of the hand to exclude underlying fracture or broken teeth

D   Consideration should be given to HIV testing

E   He should receive a tetanus booster

P2.105 Tennis elbow

An audit of minor surgery carried out in the surgery reveals that a significant number of patients treated with cortisone injections for tennis elbow return for further treatment. You review the evidence with a view to creating a practice protocol. Which one of the following statements is correct regarding current evidence-based management of this condition?

A All patients not improving after 4 weeks of physiotherapy should be referred for consideration of Botox therapy

B Graduated loading with eccentric exercises should be used as first-line treatment

C Most cases are seen in racket sport players, and they should be advised to modify their technique

D Steroid injections provide long-term benefit, although they may cause side effects

E Topical non-steroidal anti-inflammatory drugs do not have any effect in this condition

Drug management of Parkinson's disease

Options

A Amitriptyline
B Chlorpromazine
C Citalopram
D Clozapine
E Domperidone
F Levodopa and dopa decarboxylase inhibitor
G Pramipexole
H Rivastigmine
I Selegiline
J None of the above

For each of the statements regarding drug management of Parkinson's disease below, select the most appropriate option from the list above. Each option may be used once, more than once or not at all.

P2.106 Associated with impulse control symptoms, particularly in young men

P2.107 Useful for depressive symptoms in patients with Parkinson's disease

P2.108 Co-prescription with levodopa agents allows a lower dose of dopamine

P2.109 Indicated for psychotic symptoms

P2.110 Dizziness

You visit an 82-year-old man with a history of ischaemic heart disease who complains of dizziness. He reports that he has developed vertigo and double vision, and has dysarthria when you speak to him. Neurological examination also shows some loss of sensation and loss of power in both arms. He has no signs of middle-ear disease and his cardiovascular observations are normal. Which one of the following is the most likely diagnosis?

 ○ A Labyrinthitis

 ○ B Ménière's disease

 ○ C Migraine

 ○ D Vestibular neuronitis

 ○ E Vertebrobasilar stroke

P2.111 Rash

A 3-year-old girl presents with a vesicular rash on her face and body. She was previously well until she developed a flu-like illness 3 days ago. She has no eye or chest symptoms. Her face has the following appearance.

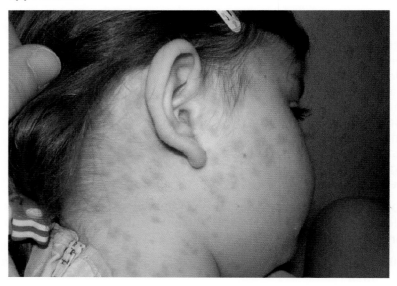

What is the diagnosis?

 ○ A Measles

 ○ B Rubella

 ○ C Shingles

 ○ D Parvovirus B19

 ○ E Chickenpox

Prescription charges

Options

A   Apply under low-income scheme
B   Automatically entitled to free prescriptions
C   Entitled to free NHS dental treatment
D   Entitled to free NHS sight tests
E   Entitled to free prescriptions on applying for an exemption certificate
F   Not entitled to free dental treatment
G   Not entitled to free NHS sight test
H   Not entitled to free prescriptions
I   Prescription pre-payment certificate

For each of the patients described below, select the most appropriate rule about health charges. Each option may be used once, more than once or not at all.

P2.112   **A 56-year-old businessman with diet-controlled diabetes who needs antibiotics.**

P2.113   **A 33-year-old woman who gave birth 9 months ago needs a dental crown.**

P2.114   **A 57-year-old accountant who takes thyroxine needs an eye test.**

P2.115   **An 18-year-old student who needs antibiotics.**

P2.116   **A 35-year-old person with newly diagnosed epilepsy taking phenytoin.**

P2.117 Skin problems

A 76-year-old man presents with a rash on both legs for 2 years. It is itchy and he has been using E45. He has no previous history of note and is otherwise well. The rash is shown below.

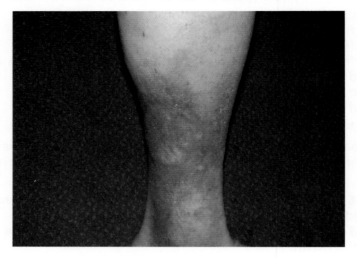

What is the diagnosis?

○ A Asteatotic eczema

○ B Varicose eczema

○ C Pompholyx

○ D Psoriasis

○ E Contact dermatitis

Examination of the eye

Options

A Acute angle-closure glaucoma
B Cataract
C Chronic glaucoma
D Corneal abrasion
E Keratoconus
F Optic atrophy
G Recurrent uveitis
H Retinoblastoma

For each of the scenarios described below, select the most appropriate diagnosis from the list of options. Each option may be used once, more than once or not at all.

P2.118 The red reflex appears white.

P2.119 On fundoscopy the disc appears pale compared with the other eye.

P2.120 The pupil is fixed but round.

P2.121 The pupil is fixed but irregular.

P2.122 The disc has a cupped appearance.

P2.123 **Birthmarks**

A 5-year-old girl is noted to have the lesion below by her grandmother, who is looking after her while her parents are on holiday. She is concerned as to the significance. The child has no previous history of note and there is no family history of note. Examination reveals a total of two such lesions on her body both <1 cm in diameter.

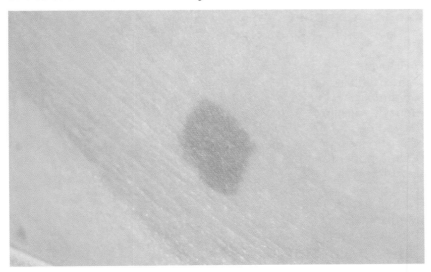

What is the single most likely diagnosis?

○   A   Albright syndrome

○   B   Bloom syndrome

○   C   Neurofibromatosis

○   D   Tuberous sclerosis

○   E   None of the above

P2.124 Eyelid problems

A 21-year-old man presents with a painless swelling in his left lower eyelid for 3 months. On examination there is no erythema or discharge. Which of the following is the most likely diagnosis? Select one option only.

○ A Basal cell carcinoma

○ B Stye

○ C Xanthelasma

○ D Chalazion

○ E Conjunctivitis

Antibiotic prescribing

Options

A Aciclovir
B Amoxicillin
C Co-amoxiclav
D Benzylpenicillin
E Cefradine
F Ciprofloxacin
G Chloramphenicol
H Erythromycin
I Flucloxacillin
J Fusidic acid
K Metronidazole
L Nitrofurantoin
M Phenoxymethylpenicillin
N Trimethoprim

For each infection described below, select the most appropriate antibiotic from the list of options. Each option may be used once, more than once or not at all.

P2.125 A 67-year-old woman who requires prophylaxis against recurrent urinary tract infections and has had a severe allergic reaction to Septrin (co-trimoxazole).

P2.126 A 21-year-old student who has been in close contact with a patient with meningococcal meningitis.

P2.127 A 4-year-old child with tonsillitis.

P2.128 A 35-year-old man with a chest infection who is allergic to penicillin.

P2.129 A 34-year-old veterinary nurse who has received a dog bite to the hand.

P2.130 Diabetic ketoacidosis
Which of the following statements about the management of diabetic ketoacidosis (DKA) is true? Select one option only.

○   A   Emergency treatment involves an immediate insulin injection and fluid rehydration

○   B   DKA usually has no prodromal phase

○   C   The respiratory rate is often reduced

○   D   Polydipsia often causes fluid overload and hyponatraemia

○   E   Initial treatment should include stat injection of intramuscular glucagons

P2.131 Shin lesions
A 21-year-old student presents with a 1-week history of tender lumps on her shins. She is otherwise fit and well and takes no regular medication. A photograph of her shins is shown below.

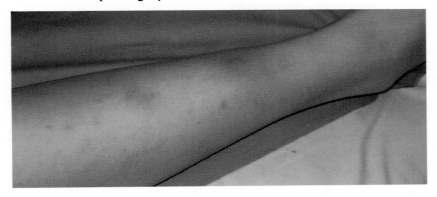

Which of the following statements about this condition is NOT true? Select one option only.

○   A   It may be caused by cat scratch disease

○   B   Patients should have a throat swab and chest X-ray as routine investigations

○   C   It may be caused by the oral contraceptive pill

○   D   Non-steroidal anti-inflammatory drugs (NSAIDs) may provide symptomatic relief

○   E   It is usually a sign of underlying malignancy

Child development

Options

A   3 months
B   5 months
C   5 years
D   8 weeks
E   10 months
F   18 months
G   30 months

For each of the developmental milestones below, select the most appropriate age from the list of options. Each option may be used once, more than once or not at all.

> **P2.132 Walks unsupported.**
> **P2.133 Uses single words appropriately.**
> **P2.134 Smiles responsively.**
> **P2.135 Able to sit unsupported.**
> **P2.136 Uses phrases.**
> **P2.137 Reaches for objects presented.**
> **P2.138 Maintains eye contact.**

P2.139 Rheumatological treatments
    With regard to drug treatments for rheumatological conditions, which of the following statements is true? Select one option only.

○   A   Infliximab is licensed for the prevention of recurrence in rheumatoid arthritis

○   B   Hydroxychloroquine will reduce pain, swelling and stiffness in systemic lupus erythematosus (SLE)

○   C   Penicillamine is given by intramuscular injection

○   D   Methotrexate produces immediate benefit in rheumatoid arthritis

○   E   Sulfasalazine has no effect on fertility, so it can be safely used in younger patients

P2.140 Hand pain

A 53-year-old woman presents with 6 weeks of malaise and fatigue associated with swelling and erythema affecting her metacarpophalangeal joints in both hands. These are particularly stiff first thing in the morning. Which of the following is a likely diagnosis? Select one option only.

○ A Primary nodal osteoarthritis

○ B Rheumatoid arthritis

○ C Reiter syndrome

○ D Gout

○ E Rheumatic fever

P2.141 Audit

Which one of the following statements is true with regard to audit in primary care?

○ A Audit involves researching the effects of new treatment protocols

○ B Standards must be defined and agreed before an audit is carried out

○ C The 'audit cycle' refers to the continual need to refine our audit criteria

○ D The implementation of change is implicit in the audit cycle

○ E Audits should be doctor led

P2.142 Glue ear

Which of the following statements about the management of glue ear in a 27-month-old child is correct? Select one option only.

○ A All children with glue ear that persists for more than 3 months should have grommets fitted

○ B Oral amoxicillin will treat most cases of glue ear if used early

○ C Adenoidectomy at the time of grommet insertion significantly reduces the risk of recurrence

○ D Grommets are the only long-term solution to glue ear

○ E Glue ear causes sensorineural hearing loss

Shoulder problems

Options

A   Cervical spondylosis
B   Frozen shoulder
C   Osteoarthritis
D   Referred pain
E   Ruptured supraspinatus
F   Shoulder dystocia
G   Shoulder–hand syndrome
H   Subluxation of the glenohumeral joint
I   Supraspinatus tendonitis

For each of the cases described below select the most appropriate choice from the list of options. Each option may be used once, more than once or not at all.

P2.143 **A 19-year-old girl who is 5 weeks pregnant presents with vaginal bleeding and pain in the tip of her left shoulder. On examination she has a full range of movement in the shoulder.**

P2.144 **A 56-year-old man presents with several years of pain and reduced range of movement in his right shoulder. On examination there is limited range of movement and extensive crepitus.**

P2.145 **A 67-year-old woman with a history of chronic neck pain complains of pain in her right shoulder with weakness in abduction. She also reports paraesthesiae in her arm at times.**

P2.146 **A 45-year-old man is seen with a 12-week history of reduced range of movement in his left shoulder. This started without obvious cause and on examination you note that external rotation is particularly affected.**

P2.147 **A 23-year-old man presents with pain and reduced range of movement in his left shoulder. He thinks that he may have fallen on to his shoulder the previous night after drinking, but cannot remember. On examination his shoulder looks flattened and, in addition to inability to abduct his shoulder, he has a numb patch on the side of his humerus.**

P2.148 Hand lesions

A 73-year-old woman attends the surgery complaining about a lesion on her hand that appeared 2 months ago and has rapidly grown in size. The lesion is shown below.

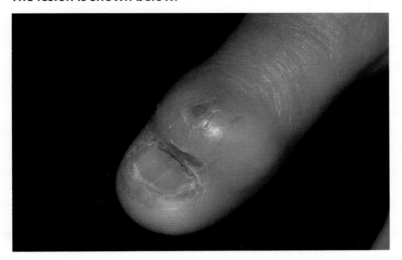

Which of the following statements about this lesion is true? Select one option only.

○   A   This lesion is likely to be a squamous cell carcinoma

○   B   This lesion is a ganglion and may be treated with needle aspiration

○   C   Biopsy is necessary to differentiate between a keratoacanthoma and an SCC

○   D   These lesions should always be treated because resolution is rare

○   E   Small lesions may be treated successfully with liquid nitrogen

○   F   These lesions are more common in men

Medical records legislation

Options

A   Access to Health Records Act
B   Access to Medical Reports Act
C   Children's Act
D   Community Care Act
E   Data Protection Act
F   Freedom of Information Act
G   Mental Health Act 1983
H   Public Records Act

For each of the scenarios below, select one of the most appropriate Acts from the list of options.

> **P2.149** It allows patients to see entries in their medical records made since 1991.
> **P2.150** It allows patients to access and request alterations to be made to computer records.
> **P2.151** It allows a charge of up to £10 to be made for access to records, plus copying expenses.
> **P2.152** It assumes that a mother automatically has responsibility for a child.
> **P2.153** It allows patients to attach a codicil to the record in question if he or she disagrees with it.
> **P2.154.** It allows doctors to withhold information from a patient's record that would be damaging to his or her mental health.

Red eye

P2.155–2.160

Options

A   Acute glaucoma
B   Anterior uveitis
C   Conjunctivitis
D   Episcleritis
E   Keratitis
F   Scleritis

Complete the table opposite from the list of options above. Each option may be used once, more than once, or not at all.

Suspected condition	P2.155	P2.156	P2.157	P2.158	P2.159	P2.160
Common symptoms	Severe pain, photophobia, haloes, no discharge	Photophobia, foreign body sensation, purulent discharge	Photophobia, pain, blurred vision	Severe pain without discharge, insidious onset, history of connective tissue disease	Minimal pain, no discharge, no photophobia. Foreign body sensation	Foreign body sensation, discharge
Common signs	Hazy cornea, fixed pupil, reduced acuity	Corneal defect visible with fluorescein, pus in anterior chamber	Circumcorneal erythema, irregular pupil, reduced acuity	Acuity maybe normal	Localised erythema, normal acuity	Conjunctival injection and mucopurulent discharge, normal visual acuity

P2.161 Colic

A new mum comes to see you at the end of her tether. Her 4-week-old son has had awful colic every night for the last 2 weeks. He is otherwise well but she demands that something be done. On examination no abnormalities are found. Which of the following statements about colic is true? Select one option only.

   ○   A   It is usually associated with vomiting at the end of an attack

   ○   B   It occurs in 1% of infants

   ○   C   It usually resolves over 1–2 weeks

   ○   D   It may be helped with dicyclomine

   ○   E   It may be helped with lactase added to feeds

Gynaecological malignancies

Options

A   Cervical carcinoma
B   Cervical intraepithelial neoplasia
C   Choriocarcinoma
D   Endometrial carcinoma
E   Ovarian carcinoma
F   Vulval carcinoma
G   Vulval intraepithelial neoplasia

For each of the descriptions below, select the most appropriate diagnosis from the list of options. Each option may be used once, more than once or not at all.

    P2.162 It tends to be multifocal.
    P2.163 It causes post-coital bleeding.
    P2.164 It is associated with raised βhCG.
    P2.165 It has a 30% 5-year survival rate.
    P2.166 It is associated with diabetes.

P2.167 Haemoptysis

A 67-year-old man who has been a lifelong smoker presents with haemoptysis, progressive shortness of breath and weight loss. His hands have the appearance shown below.

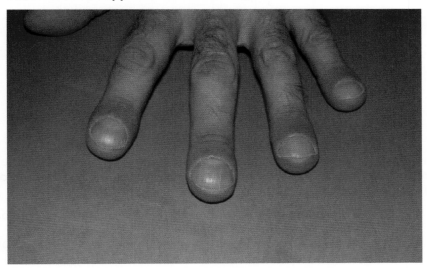

What is the probable underlying diagnosis? Select one option only.

○ A Inflammatory bowel disease

○ B Congenital heart disease

○ C Pneumonia

○ D Cystic fibrosis

○ E Lung cancer

P2.168 Urinary problems in babies

You are referred a 3-month-old baby boy by the health visitor after his mother noticed that he is leaking urine from the middle of his penis. On examination there seems to be a small pit on the underside of the penis. Which of the following statements about this condition is true? Select one option only.

○ A The condition is rare, with an incidence of 1:5000

○ B It always presents in infancy

○ C Surgery is always indicated

○ D It is usually associated with other abnormalities of the urogenital tract

○ E It may be a sign of female virilisation

Hirsutism

Options

A   Combined oral contraceptive
B   Cyproterone acetate
C   Dianette
D   Electrolysis
E   Finasteride
F   Metformin
G   Minoxidil
H   Referral
I   Spironolactone
J   Weight loss

For each of the patients described below, select the most appropriate therapy from the list of options. Each option may be used once, more than once or not at all.

P2.169 A 22-year-old woman with excessive facial hair and irregular periods. Blood tests are normal.

P2.170 A 47-year-old woman with hirsutism who has a history of DVT on the contraceptive pill and who has not found electrolysis or camouflage effective.

P2.171 A 27-year-old woman of Mediterranean origin with normal periods who has a prominent hair on her upper lip only and is unable to take the pill.

P2.172 An 18-year-old girl with hirsutism and acne, not responding to the combined oral contraceptive pill (COCP).

P2.173 A 23-year-old woman who is hirsute with irregular periods and primary infertility.

Dizziness and vertigo

Options

A   Acoustic neuroma
B   Benign paroxysmal positional vertigo
C   Cardiogenic syncope
D   Cervical vertigo
E   Hyperventilation
F   Ménière's disease
G   Ramsay Hunt syndrome
H   Round window rupture
I   Migraine
J   Vestibular neuronitis

For each scenario described below, select the single most likely diagnosis from the list of options. Each option may be used once, more than once or not at all.

P2.174 Recurrent attacks of pressure in the ear are associated with tinnitus, deafness and vertigo.

P2.175 There is an acute onset of severe vertigo with vomiting, which usually settles over several days.

P2.176 It is associated with a sensation of light-headedness and palpitations before fainting.

P2.177 It is associated with vertigo only on moving the head in certain planes.

P2.178 Vertigo is accompanied by facial palsy and deafness.

P2.179 Prostate tests
A 63-year-old man requests a PSA (prostate-specific antigen) test to see if he has prostate cancer. Before testing you spend some time counselling him about the test and its use. Which of the following statements about PSA testing is true? Select one option only.

○   A   The test is highly sensitive

○   B   The test is highly specific

○   C   A raised PSA may be caused by urinary infection

○   D   PSA testing is a proven diagnostic test

○   E   Anyone with a PSA >4.0 mmol/l should be referred

P2.180 Drug abuse
A 29-year-old man registers at the practice, having just moved to the area. At his first consultation he admits that he has been injecting heroin for the last 8 months and would like help in stopping. Which one of the following statements about this area of practice is NOT true?

○   A   He should be converted to a twice-daily maintenance dose of methadone and this should be gradually reduced

○   B   He should be advised about the importance of safe sex

○   C   GPs are not obliged under the terms of the GMS contract to provide substitution treatment for opiate dependency

○   D   A treatment contract should be agreed with the patient that covers the responsibilities of each party

○   E   A hierarchy of goals is recommended that will initially minimise harm and aim for eventual abstinence

P2.181 Breathlessness
A 19-year-old man presents complaining of an acute onset of breathlessness and pain in his left chest. He has no previous history of note. On examination he is tall and lean, and seems to be in good health. He has reduced air entry on the left side of his chest and is tachypnoeic. Which of the following is the most likely diagnosis? Select one option only

○ A Pleurisy

○ B Pulmonary embolus

○ C Panic attack

○ D Pneumothorax

○ E Bronchopneumonia

P2.182 Travel advice
A 24-year-old girl who is about to go travelling for a year consults you for advice on antimalarials. Which of the following statements about prevention of malaria is true? Select one option only.

○ A Malarone is taken weekly starting 1 week before travel until 4 weeks after return from a malaria region

○ B Patients who are entitled to free prescriptions can get antimalarials on an FP10

○ C As long as patients take antimalarials as prescribed they are at very low risk of catching malaria

○ D Mefloquine is associated with neuropsychiatric side effects in up to 10% of patients

○ E Doxycycline is associated with photosensitivity

P2.183 Patient complaints
You receive a letter of complaint from a patient. Which one of the following is a requirement relating to the practice response?

○ A A written response must be received by the patient within 10 working days

○ B The complaint must be acknowledged within 5 working days

○ C The complaint needs to be considered only if it is received on paper

○ D If the patient's concerns are not satisfied by the practice response, the patient can take the complaint to the Healthcare Commission

○ E There is a time limit of 12 months for practice complaints

P2.184 Mumps

You are telephoned by the mother of a 15-year-old boy who is away on school camp. One of his classmates has just been diagnosed with mumps and his mother is concerned that he is at risk. Which of the following statements about mumps is true? Select one option only.

○   A   The incubation period is 7–10 days

○   B   Salivary gland swelling is pathognomonic and seen in all cases

○   C   Ten per cent of patients with mumps develop symptomatic meningeal involvement

○   D   Of postpubertal males 80% develop bilateral orchitis

○   E   Of those with orchitis 70% become infertile

P2.185 Data interpretation

A trial comparing a new intervention for acute stroke with standard care is carried out, with disability score at 12 months as the primary outcome. The disability score was ranked from 1 to 3, with 1 being the least disabled and 3 the most disabled. The results of the trial are shown below.

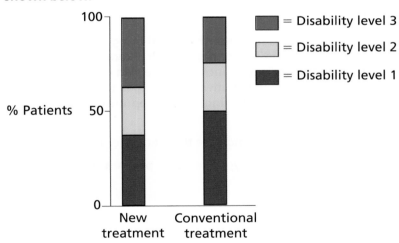

Which one of the following statements is correct regarding these data? Select one option only.

○   A   The new treatment increases severe disability compared with standard treatment

○   B   The new treatment reduces disability at all levels compared with standard treatment

○   C   The new treatment reduces severe disability but has no effect on minor disability, compared with conventional treatment

○   D   The results are not statistically significant

○   E   The results are prone to bias

P2.186 Cholesterol

A 42-year-old man attends having read an article in a newspaper suggesting that people with arcus cornea are at high risk of heart disease and should have statins. He is concerned because he has this condition. His blood pressure is 124/70 mmHg and he does not smoke, is of normal weight and has recently been tested for diabetes as part of a private insurance well man check. Which of the following statements is true regarding this condition?

○ A Arcus cornea is a sign of high triglycerides rather than high cholesterol and he should be prescribed a fibrate

○ B He is at high risk of cardiovascular disease and should be prescribed aspirin and a statin regardless of his cholesterol level

○ C He should be referred to an endocrine clinic due to the association of this condition with the metabolic syndrome

○ D He should have his cholesterol measured and be treated according to his calculated cardiovascular risk score, using QRISK or a similar method

○ E He should start simvastatin 40 mg once daily

P2.187 Nappy rash

Parents of a formula-fed 4-month-old girl bring her in to see you for a second opinion regarding her nappy rash. Examining her you note a florid rash on the perineum, including the skin creases. They have tried zinc oxide barrier cream and medicated wipes to no avail. Which one of the following would be the single most appropriate next step in her management?

○ A Advise the parents to increase the frequency of nappy changes

○ B Change her milk to a hypoallergenic preparation

○ C Clotimazole

○ D Hydrocortisone

○ E Tacrolimus

P2.188 Breast cancer

You see a 62-year-old woman after she has been diagnosed with ductal carcinoma *in situ* (DCIS) on routine mammography. She asks you to tell her what the diagnosis means for her. Which one of the following statements is true regarding DCIS?

○ A It is associated with Paget's disease of the nipple

○ B It is not usually sensitive to tamoxifen

○ C It is not associated with invasive disease

○ D It is rare

○ E Patients with confirmed DCIS can be treated with watchful waiting

P2.189. Earache

A 9-month-old boy has had earache for the last 2 days. In spite of regular analgesia he is inconsolable and febrile. Examining him his right tympanic membrane is bulging. You decide to prescribe amoxicillin. Write the correct dose in milligrams based on his age in the box below.

Management of autism

Options

A   Amitriptyline
B   Aripiprazole
C   Fluoxetine
D   Methylphenidate
E   Quetiapine
F   Paroxetine
G   Risperidone
H   None of the above

For each of the statements below regarding drug management of autism, select the most appropriate option from the list above. Each option may be used once, more than once or not at all.

P2.190 Helpful where sleep problems predominate.
P2.191 Used where inattention occurs.
P2.192 Limits the impact of maladaptive behaviour.
P2.193 May be useful for restricted repetitive behaviours where methylphenidate is not tolerated.

P2.194 Spasticity

A 9-year-old boy comes to see you with his parents. He has cerebral palsy and attends a specialist school where he has regular physical therapy. In spite of this he gets frequent episodes of pain throughout the day due to muscle spasm. He asks if there is anything that can be done to help. Which one of the following would be the most appropriate management option at this stage?

- A Baclofen
- B Botox
- C Clonazepam
- D Diazepam
- E Dorsal rhizotomy

P2.195 Haematuria

A 34-year-old man with no previous medical history of note attends for a new patient check. He brings in a urine sample as instructed, but on dipstick testing is strongly positive for blood. He is asymptomatic and there are no nitrites or leukocytes detected on urinalysis. Which one of the following would be the most appropriate action at this point in his management?

    A Check blood pressure

    B Digital rectal examination

    C Refer for renal ultrasound

    D Refer to 2-week wait clinic

    E Send urine for microscopy to confirm haematuria

P2.196 Shortness of breath

A 73-year-old man who is an ex-smoker complains of several months of increasing shortness of breath. On examination he has a few fine crepitations in both lung bases. ECG and blood tests including BNP are normal. You arrange for spirometry at your local hospital, the results of which are shown below.

	FEV_1	FVC	FEV_1/FVC	Transfer factor
Patient reading	2.48	3.26		2.91
Percentage predicted	77	78	76	35

What is the most likely diagnosis? Write your answer in the box below.

P2.197. Dementia

Mr Smith has just been diagnosed with vascular dementia. He comes to see you with his wife to discuss the diagnosis and treatments that may help. Which one of the following interventions has been shown to have a significant impact on the rate of decline in cognitive function in patients with vascular dementia?

    A Acetylcholinesterase inhibitors

    B Aggressive control of blood pressure

    C Antiplatelet treatment

    D Memantine

    E Statins

P2.198 Hearing problems

A 76-year-old woman complains of difficulty hearing and bilateral tinnitus. Her audiogram is shown below. What is the most likely diagnosis? Select one option only.

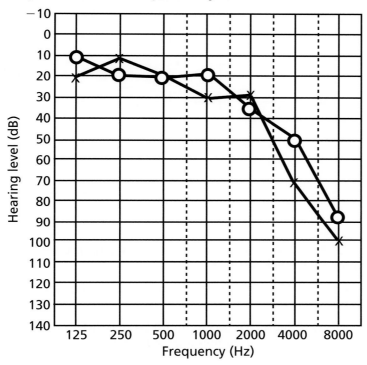

○ A Sudden-onset sensorineural hearing loss

○ B Presbyacusis

○ C Acoustic neuroma

○ D Noise-induced hearing loss

○ E Otosclerosis

P2.199 Data interpretation
Your local commissioning group is looking at the variation in emergency admission rates across the area in an attempt to reduce referrals. They present the following data:

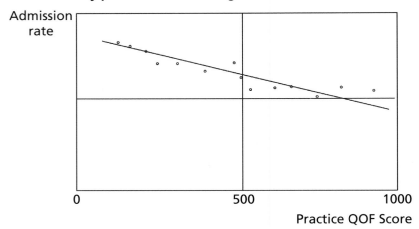

Which one of the following statements is true with regard to possible explanations for these results?

○ A Practices with high QOF scores are more likely to be located in areas with high deprivation scores

○ B Practices with high QOF scores might be making more earlier diagnoses, resulting in higher admission rates for elective treatment

○ C Practices with high QOF scores might be exception reporting the most sick patients to inflate their QOF scores artificially

○ D It is easier to obtain high QOF scores in areas of high morbidity where there are naturally high admission rates

○ E Practices with high QOF scores have devolved much of their routine work to non-medical staff, who are better able to manage complex medical problems

P2.200 Fainting

A 74-year-old woman complains of recurrent episodes where she feels dizzy and has fallen on two occasions. She is being treated for hypertension but is otherwise well. On examination her pulse is 84 and regular, and her heart sounds are normal. Her blood pressure is 124/62 mmHg. What would be the most appropriate examination to carry out at this stage? Select one option only.

○ A 24-hour blood pressure

○ B 24-hour tape

○ C Electrocardiogram

○ D Full blood count

○ E Standing blood pressure

Paper 2 Answers

P2.1   **D:**   **Push the hook through and out of the skin before cutting off the barb**

The best technique to remove barbed fishing hooks is to inject local anaesthetic around the likely exit point of the barb (or use a ring block for digits) before pushing the hook out through the skin. Once the barb is clear of the skin it can be cut off and the hook then pulled back out through the entry wound. This gives two small scars rather than a much larger scar with incision along the hook or pulling it back out of the wound without removing the barb first. Tetanus status should be checked and wound toilet carried out afterwards.

P2.2   **C:**   **Check his FBC**

This child has symptoms of leukaemia, which is the most common malignant disease in children and often presents with muscle and joint pain. Signs of marrow failure include anaemia, frequent infections and thrombocytopenia, although blast activity may also cause headache, fits and gum hypertrophy.

Lower urinary tract symptoms in men

P2.3   **B:**   **α Blocker**
P2.4   **D:**   **Anticholinergic**
P2.5   **A:**   **5α-Reductase inhibitor**
P2.6   **C:**   **α Blocker plus 5α-reductase inhibitor**
P2.7   **F:**   **Desmopressin**

NICE recommend the following as drug treatment for patients bothered by LUTS. An alternative to desmopressin for nocturnal polyuria is a loop diuretic in the late afternoon.

Symptoms	Moderate-to-severe LUTS	Detrusor instability	LUTS with enlarged prostate	LUTS with enlarged prostate despite treatment with 3	Nocturnal polyuria
Treatment	α Blocker	Anticholinergic	5α-Reductase inhibitor	α Blocker + 5α-reductase inhibitor	Desmopressin

P2.8   D: Topical tacrolimus

Vitamin D analogues and coal tar are not suitable for facial psoriasis. If lesions fail to respond to short courses of topical steroids or continuous treatment is needed, topical tacrolimus is more suitable due to a lower risk of side effects. Emollients are unlikely to be effective in this situation.

P2.9   E: Breech presentation is a risk factor

Breech presentation and positive family history are risk factors. Ortolani testing involves attempting to relocate a dislocated hip whereas Barlow testing attempts to dislocate a hip. Ultrasound screening has a high pickup rate but is associated with a high false-positive rate. Most children require splinting only.

P2.10   A: Topical glyceryl trinitrate (GTN)

This patient has symptoms suggestive of an anal fissure; where this is not settling with dietary changes or topical treatment, GTN or diltiazem application may be of benefit.

P2.11   C: Levomepromazine will help with agitation and nausea

Fentanyl or MST dose should be converted to 24-hour subcutaneous morphine dose according to the conversion chart in the BNF. Morphine is an excellent painkiller for all types of pain, but in less severe cases NSAIDs may be useful for bone pain. Morphine is the drug of choice for respiratory symptoms because it also reduces dyspnoea.

P2.12   A: Asbestosis

Asbestosis is a progressive lung fibrosis caused by inhalation of blue asbestos. It increases the risk of lung cancer 5-fold and in smokers by 55-fold. Industrial compensation is available. The prognosis is poor. Spirometry shows a restrictive defect; however, a chest X-ray may miss fibrosis and CT (computed tomography) may be more appropriate.

P2.13   1 mg

Hypoglycaemia should be treated if possible with oral glucose. If they are unconscious they should be given glucagon. The dose for glucagon is 1 mg for patients over 8 years and 500 µg for those under 8 kg (or <25 kg). Both oral glucose and glucagon produce a short-lived rise in blood glucose levels and close monitoring is necessary to spot relapse. If not responding 50 ml of 20% intravenous glucose may be given.

Common infections

P2.14   C: 1 week
P2.15   E: 3 weeks
P2.16   D: $2\frac{1}{2}$ weeks
P2.17   B: 4 days

Explaining to patients the natural history of self-limiting infections encourages appropriate use of antibiotics and may potentially improve the utilisation of health resources, through reduced use of appointments for self-limiting illness.

P2.18   D: Refer for lithotripsy

Plantar fasciitis usually responds to orthotics and taping. Where there is no response a steroid injection may provide short-term relief. Where a heel spur is shown on X-ray, lithotripsy is often helpful. Botox is indicated for patients with pes cavus, but is not suitable for athletes. Further injection is unlikely to help.

P2.19   E: She should be treated with a permanent pacemaker

The diagnosis is complete heart block. She should be referred immediately for a pacemaker. The most common cause is ischaemic heart disease. If compromised, atropine 1 mg can be used.

P2.20   E: Vasectomy is reversible in only 50% of cases

The lifetime failure rate is <1:1000. Bruising is very common and the most common long-term complication is pain. It is usually performed under local anaesthetic and sterility should not be assumed until 3 months and two negative sperm counts have passed.

P2.21   E: Silver nitrate cautery may cause septal perforation

Most bleeds are anterior and unilateral with bleeding from Little's area, the plexus of capillaries derived ultimately from the internal and external carotid. The most common cause is idiopathic followed by iatrogenic, with aspirin and warfarin therapy being particular culprits. Bleeding points may be cauterised with silver nitrate but over-zealous or too frequent use of this may result in perforation of the nasal septum. Where pressure fails to settle the bleeding, Merocel packs are easily inserted by nurses or doctors and are extremely effective. BIPP packing is seldom used.

P2.22   A: Dendritic ulcer

This is a typical history of a dendritic ulcer. The appearance could also be seen in corneal abrasion or corneal ulcer in a contact lens wearer, but not with this history. Treatment is with aciclovir five times a day.

P2.23   D: Neuromuscular relaxants are the drug of choice in the Netherlands

Rates of physician-assisted suicide have fallen slightly since legalisation in the Netherlands. Physician-assisted suicide accounts for 1.7% of deaths in the Netherlands. The 'doctrine of double effect' refers to the use of a drug for its analgesic properties, which also accelerates death as a side effect, eg diamorphine syringe drivers. It is legal to give the drug in this circumstance.

P2.24   A: Dementia is usually associated with altered cognition and consciousness

Dementia does not affect consciousness. Where consciousness is affected, consider causes of delirium. Young patients may have metabolic defects, eg Wilson's disease or HIV.

Liver function tests

P2.25   B: Gilbert syndrome

Isolated hyperbilirubinaemia is almost never of pathological significance. This can be demonstrated by taking a fasting bilirubin after an overnight fast.

P2.26   F: Iatrogenic

Enzyme-inducing drugs and alcohol can elevate GGT levels.

P2.27   H: Physiological

ALP may be elevated in adolescence, bone tumours and Paget's disease.

P2.28   E: Hepatitis

Acute hepatitis usually presents with a greatly elevated ALT.

P2.29   A: Gallstones

LFTs usually return to normal after the obstruction has been removed.

P2.30   C: Topical metronidazole is effective

Topical or oral metronidazole is often effective if regular cleaning with povidone–iodine is ineffective.

P2.31   E: This could be a presentation of a renal tumour

Renal colic can be due to direct obstruction by tumour or bleeding from the tumour. Calcium levels can be raised and should be measured. Signs of infection should prompt admission. Stones are not usually visible on a plain film. An NSAID should be used unless contraindicated.

Erectile dysfunction

P2.32   E: Sildenafil

Sildenafil may cause chromatopsia, usually green.

P2.33   A: All of them

Patients who are predisposed to priapism should not take treatments for erectile dysfunction.

P2.34   C: MUSE

MUSE is a transurethral system and should not be used in urethral stricture.

P2.35   F: Tadalafil

Tadalafil should be taken at least 30 minutes before sexual activity and the effect may persist for up to 36 hours.

P2.36   A: All of them

Patients with neurological disease, renal failure, diabetes or prostate cancer, or who have had radical pelvic surgery qualify for impotence drugs on the NHS.

P2.37   D: The results should be treated with caution because of inclusion bias

Qualitative studies are notoriously prone to bias. This study has no standardised measure of depression scores at either the outset or the end, consists of self-reporting by patients who self-refer and pay for a treatment in which they presumably have faith, has no control group and relies on the use of only one therapist. It is therefore prone to inclusion bias, reporting bias and a strong placebo effect. The economic analysis is not valid because most patients with mild depression would not need drug treatment. The number needed to treat (NNT) cannot be calculated because there is no comparison group.

P2.38   A: Refer for colonoscopy

This patient has symptoms of a right-sided colonic cancer. Sigmoidoscopy will not visualise the area and barium enema, although the first-line investigation, can miss up to 20% of lesions. Raised ESR is consistent with cancer.

P2.39   A: Approximately 4000 people a year commit suicide in England and Wales

There is a bimodal social-class distribution, with middle classes being at lowest risk. Older divorced men who have just lost their jobs and live in towns are most likely to commit suicide. Overdose is the most common method, and violent attempts, such as hanging, are the most likely to succeed. There is a 1–2% risk of deliberate self-harmers committing suicide within 12 months.

Paediatric syndromes

P2.40   C: Edwards' syndrome

Edwards' syndrome is associated with heart abnormalities.

P2.41   B: Down syndrome

Patients with Down syndrome also frequently have congenital heart disease.

P2.42   D: Fragile X syndrome

Fragile X syndrome is associated with abnormalities of DNA structure and prenatal testing may be possible in females with affected relatives.

P2.43   E: Klinefelter syndrome

Klinefelter syndrome has the karyotype 47XXY and occurs in 1:1000 liveborn babies.

P2.44   I: Williams' syndrome

Williams' syndrome is inherited on chromosome 7 and is often associated with learning difficulties.

P2.45   A: Private fees can be set at whatever level the practice wishes

Private fees can be set on a free-market basis but practices should beware exploiting patients where they have no option to go elsewhere, eg for occupational medicals where their registered GP is required to complete a report. The Monopolies Commission banned the BMA from setting recommended fees some years ago. Private work is not covered by the GMS Contract. Private fees should be displayed prominently and patients made aware of these before services are provided.

P2.46   A: Ninety per cent of hip replacements last for more than 10 years

The infection rate is approximately 1%. Crossing the surgical leg over the non-surgical leg is associated with dislocation. The incidence of deep vein thrombosis (DVT) is 1.5% and of pulmonary embolus (PE) 1.1%. Hip resurfacing is superior to conventional arthroplasty for survival of the prosthesis and preservation of bone mineral density, but is usually indicated only in early disease.

Headache

P2.47   D: Migraine

P2.48   E: Tension headache

P2.49   A: Cluster headache

P2.50   B: Cervicogenic headache

P2.51   C: Medication overuse headache

P2.52   A: Kawasaki's disease

This child has Kawasaki's disease, a febrile vasculitis affecting children. It may cause coronary artery aneurysms in a third of patients and has a mortality rate of around 3%. ECG changes are seen including arrhythmias and long QT interval. Treatment is with aspirin or intravenous immunoglobulin.

P2.53   E: Biventricular failure

This patient has signs of right- and left-sided heart failure. Cor pulmonale is right-sided heart failure secondary to pulmonary disease. The presence of a regular pulse precludes new-onset AF as a diagnosis.

P2.54   D: It may cause phimosis

Balanitis is usually caused by *Candida* sp. or coliforms. Topical antifungals and sometimes fusidic acid are often helpful. Recurrent attacks may cause phimosis and need circumcision. Fifty per cent of 6-year-olds cannot fully retract their foreskin.

P2.55   3 mg

Patients taking anticonvulsants that are potent enzyme inducers should ideally have the IUD as first choice of emergency contraception. Where this is not possible, a double dose of levonorgestrel should be taken as soon as possible after unprotected sexual intercourse.

P2.56   D: The condition may be associated with corneal thinning

Keratoconus may be unilateral or bilateral and is characterised by progressive irregularity of the cornea, resulting in astigmatism. In some patients it progresses to corneal thinning and eventually corneal transplantation is required. It can be inherited as either an autosomal recessive or dominant trait, and may be associated with syndromes such as Down, Marfan or Ehlers–Danlos. Milder cases can be treated with contact lenses or glasses, or corneal implants to modify the corneal distortion.

P2.57   E: Scoliosis may be associated with deformity of the skull and ribcage

Of infants with scoliosis 50% will resolve spontaneously. Primary scoliosis often presents in adolescence where it is more common in girls. It is usually mid-thoracic and the curve is usually concave to the right. It may be associated with plagiocephaly in infants and prominence of the posterior rib cage in teenagers. Treatment where indicated usually involves insertion of rods.

Bleeding in early pregnancy

P2.58   F: Septic abortion

She should be admitted for intravenous antibiotics and ERPC (evacuation of retained products of conception).

P2.59   D: Ectopic pregnancy

An empty uterus and a climbing or static quantitative βhCG suggests a non-uterine pregnancy.

P2.60   B: Cervical incompetence

Cervical incompetence typically causes mid-trimester loss with few contractions.

P2.61   G: Threatened abortion

Of threatened abortions 75% settle spontaneously.

P2.62   D: Ectopic pregnancy

All women with abdominal pain should have a pregnancy test because there may be few gynaecological signs.

P2.63   D: Bronchiolitis

Bronchiolitis occurs in epidemics in winter, caused by respiratory syncytial virus. It is particularly severe in those under 6 months old and can be fatal. High-risk patients (eg congenital heart disease), those with apnoeas or tachypnoeas, and those with failure to feed should be admitted to hospital. Well children can often be managed at home.

P2.64   C: Employers must write to employees in advance of their retirement date and advise them of their rights to apply to work beyond this date

Age discrimination protects elderly and young people. Mandatory retirement cannot be lower than 65 years for men *and* women. The maximum qualifying length of service for benefits is 5 years. Dismissal on the basis of age is legal from 65 onwards, as long as it can be justified.

P2.65   B: Hirschsprung's disease is associated with Down syndrome

The incidence of Hirschsprung's disease is 1:5000, and it is more common in babies with Down syndrome (1.5% prevalence) and affected siblings (risk in future pregnancies 12–33%). Genetic markers have been identified and carrier testing is available in some areas, although there is currently no prenatal test available. The male:female ratio is 4:1, although where the whole bowel is affected it is 1:1.

P2.66   E: If *Staphylococcus* sp. is suspected flucloxacillin should be added.

The first-line treatment for community-acquired pneumonia is amoxicillin at a dose of 500–1000 mg three times daily (BTS guidelines), which should cover intermediate resistant strains of *Streptococcus pneumoniae*. In allergic individuals or where atypical pneumonia is suspected, a macrolide is appropriate. During flu outbreaks staphylococcal pneumonia has a high mortality and should be treated with flucloxacillin.

P2.67   C: Paroxetine can increase the period before ejaculation up to eight times longer than placebo

Up to 31% of male respondents to surveys reported premature ejaculation. Clomipramine is useful when taken before intercourse or as a once-daily treatment, but has an adverse side-effect profile in many patients. Paroxetine once daily is the most effective treatment.

Management of epididymitis

P2.68   E: Doxycyline
P2.69   D: Contact tracing
P2.70   C: Ciprofloxacin

Epididymo-orchitis in men <35 is usually caused by sexually transmitted infection such as chlamydial infection, although, in men >35 without risk factors for STIs, it is usually caused by enteric Gram-negative organisms. All patients presenting with symptoms of epidymo-orchitis should have a sexual history taken and antibiotic choice should be guided by this history.

P2.71 C: Lithium is associated with an increase in risk of hypothyroidism

Lithium toxicity is still seen frequently, particularly in the elderly, despite the QOF targets on monitoring and frequent safety advice. Patients should have renal and thyroid function monitored before and regularly after starting treatment, and patients should be warned of common side effects such as tremor, dry mouth, thirst and urinary frequency. Lithium has a narrow therapeutic window and toxicity may develop rapidly with dehydration, pregnancy or renal impairment. There is also a reported association with hyperparathyroidism so calcium levels should also be monitored

P2.72 E: Stabilise cervical spine, refer to local accident and emergency department for imaging

This patient has symptoms of significant cervical spine injury, with limited rotation, paraesthesia in the hands and focal neurological signs, with age >65 years. Urgent X-ray is indicated and he should be transferred by ambulance with spinal immobilisation.

P2.73 E: Tight underwear

The NICE guidelines advise that, although there is evidence that scrotal temperature can reduce sperm quality, there is no evidence that wearing looser-fitting underwear makes any difference. Caffeine consumption has not been shown to be harmful either.

P2.74 C: The ramipril should be stopped and specialist advice sought

NICE guidance suggests that an increase of 50% in creatinine or a rise to >200 μg/ml should prompt referral. Most cases are caused by occult renal artery stenosis which may cause secondary hypertension. Angiotensin receptor antagonists (ARBs) have the same effect and NICE recommend that both be started under specialist supervision if baseline creatinine >150 μg/ml.

P2.75 B: Discuss his performance with other members of the practice team to see if there are other concerns

This situation might have arisen for a number of reasons and it would be inappropriate to invoke disciplinary procedures at this stage. The behaviour may be a sign of burn-out or stress, and this should be addressed sensitively by someone whom he trusts. If these concerns are found to be genuine, referral might be appropriate if in-house procedures fail to bring about resolution. The local medical committee provides invaluable support in this situation and should be considered before going outside the practice.

P2.76 C: It is typically triggered by particular head movements

BPPV is rotatory vertigo brought on by head movements in a certain plane, eg lying back in a dentist's chair. It is not associated with any other neuro-otological symptoms and can be demonstrated with Hallpike testing, whereby torsional nystagmus is provoked after a latent period of 15–30 seconds. This fatigues with repeat testing. The presence of other neuro-otological symptoms should prompt further investigations to exclude alternative diagnoses, eg Ménière's disease or cholesteatoma. Acoustic neuromas rarely cause vertigo without other otoneurological symptoms.

P2.77   D: Malignant melanoma

This lesion has the following features of melanoma: asymmetry, size >6 mm, irregular edges or surface and non-uniform pigmentation.

P2.78   A: Patients can be screened for this condition using the SCOFF questionnaire

Anorexia requires a BMI <17.5 kg/m^2 and an inability to eat. Prevalence is 1–2% in women, much lower in men. Over a 4- to 8-year follow-up 2% of patients died and 65% achieved normal weight. The SCOFF questionnaire includes the following questions:

Do you make yourself **S**ick because you feel uncomfortably full?
Do you worry that you have lost **C**ontrol over how much you eat?
Have you recently lost more than **O**ne stone in a 3-month period?
Do you believe yourself to be **F**at when others say that you are too thin?
Would you say that **F**ood dominates your life?

A score of ≥2 indicates a likely case of anorexia nervosa or bulimia.

Cardiovascular drugs

P2.79   B: Atorvastatin

P2.80   L: Sotalol

Sotalol is effective in prophylaxis of AF and may be used while awaiting DC cardioversion to try to cardiovert patients chemically.

P2.81   N: Valsartan

Angiotensin II receptor antagonists are licensed in heart failure and after myocardial infarction.

P2.82   O: Verapamil

Verapamil should not be used in patients with bradycardias or heart block, or those who take β blockers.

P2.83   H: Isosorbide mononitrate

P2.84   M: Spironolactone

P2.85   A: Amiodarone

Amiodarone has a long half-life and is associated with ophthalmic, dermatological and thyroid dysfunction.

P2.86   G: Indapamide

ACE inhibitors and angiotensin II receptor antagonists are first-line treatment in young hypertensive patients, but where renal artery stenosis is present a thiazide is a better choice.

P2.87   B: Aspirin use in primary prevention reduces risk of non-fatal myocardial infarction

Aspirin in primary prevention studies has been shown to reduce the risk of myocardial infarction, but the gains are offset by an increase in risk of gastrointestinal bleeding. The risk of bleeding seems highest in the first 1–2 years and falls off with duration of use. There is a large body of evidence that aspirin will reduce the risk of cancer, particularly colorectal, and also reduce the risk of metastases. There is also a transient increase in risk of MI on stopping aspirin. At present, the consensus is that there is insufficient evidence to recommend aspirin or other antiplatelets for primary prevention in patients who are otherwise well.

P2.88   B: Cryotherapy

Cryotherapy given at 3-weekly intervals will cure 75% of warts after four treatments. Side effects such as pain and blistering are common, and patients should be warned of the risk of hypopigmentation and tendon damage. Excision should be avoided due to risk of scarring, and all patients should be advised that two-thirds of cases of warts spontaneously resolve within 2 years, and a third within 6 months. Podophyllin and bleomycin are not usually used for simple warts due to their side-effect profile.

P2.89   E: Patients with recurrent symptoms can use flecainide as a 'pill-in-the-pocket' treatment

AF affects 0.4% of the general population, but incidence increases sharply with age. Patients should be anticoagulated if they have persistent prolonged attacks and are at high risk, eg coexisting hypertension, smoking. Reductions in alcohol, caffeine, stress and smoking help to reduce the incidence of the condition. In patients with a structurally normal heart flecainide is effective as treatment.

P2.90   E: A raised ALP suggests that the diagnosis is gallstones

Gallstones cause either a flatulent dyspepsia or biliary colic. Colic tends to be severe and can require treatment with pethidine injection. Pain usually comes 60–120 minutes after fatty meals and can last several hours. It is usually associated with raised ALP and stones can cause pancreatitis or obstructive jaundice. Where associated with weight loss, cancer should be considered in the differential diagnosis.

P2.91   C: Earache, trismus and dysphagia are typical symptoms

Most cases are caused by streptococcal infections, and the abscess is outside the tonsillar capsule close to the upper pole of the tonsil. The patient is usually unwell and unable to swallow fluids or solids. Intravenous fluids and intravenous broad-spectrum antibiotics, with interval tonsillectomy, are the usual management options.

P2.92   C: Nickel dermatitis

Allergic contact dermatitis is a type IV hypersensitivity reaction and affects 1–2% of the population, with nickel being a common precipitant. These are commonly seen with jewellery such as piercings and watch bracelets. Treatment is by avoidance, with topical steroids if necessary for short periods.

Management of chronic stable asthma

P2.93   H: Omalizumab

Omalizumab (Xolair) is given by subcutaneous injection.

P2.94   E: Inhaled regular dose steroids

P2.95   G: Long-acting bronchodilator

Salmeterol and formoterol have been shown, in some studies, to be associated with increased admissions to hospital and increased mortality.

P2.96   F: Leukotriene receptor antagonist

Leukotriene receptor antagonists seem to be synergistic with inhaled steroids and these may be of particular benefit in patients with exercise-induced asthma or allergic rhinitis.

P2.97   J: Regular oral steroids

In regular oral steroid use, always consider the need for bisphosphonates.

P2.98   D: It often gets worse during pregnancy

Otosclerosis is an autosomal dominant disease with incomplete penetrance that affects 0.5–2% of the population, sex ratio 2 females:1 male, more common in white people. It tends to worsen during pregnancy, menstruation and the menopause. Most patients present before the age of 30. It causes a conductive hearing loss, slightly worse at lower frequencies, often with a dip in the bone-conduction thresholds at 2 kHz. Stapedectomy is an effective treatment but there is a risk of hearing loss, so many patients choose to wear hearing aids instead. There is some evidence that the incidence is falling, thought to be a result of the use of fluoride in drinking water.

P2.99   D: Long-term oral tetracycline is effective in reducing frequency of attacks

Hidradenitis suppurativa is not a disease of apocrine glands, but rather an acne-like condition. Treatment options include short courses of antibiotics and oral steroids or local steroid injections. Long-term antibiotics may be useful and as a last resort some patients may require surgery. Dianette may be helpful in women because of the cyproterone acetate component.

P2.100   E: None

This patient has ruptured the long head of biceps, which produces a characteristic Popeye appearance. No treatment is needed.

P2.101   E: It is exclusively seen in children

Epiglottitis is usually seen in young children, but may be seen in adults, where the principal complaint is of severe pain on swallowing. The most common differential is croup, but children with epiglottitis are much sicker and should be admitted as an emergency before attempting to examine the child.

P2.102   E: Check full blood count immediately

Carbimazole is associated with a risk of agranulocytosis and patients should be advised to report any signs of infection, eg sore throat, immediately. Patients with signs of infection should have a full blood count checked as a matter of urgency, and should be treated with antibiotics. If there are signs of sepsis or quinsy admission should be considered.

P2.103   C: Cholangiocarcinoma

Cholangiocarcinoma usually affects patients in the age range 5–70. It may be misdiagnosed in the early stages as gallstones but tends to cause jaundice followed by pruritus, with weight loss, anorexia and diarrhoea. Abdominal examination may reveal a palpable gallbladder or hepatomegaly. Survival rates are poor, with a 5% 5-year survival rate. Acute cholecystitis tends to cause a febrile illness with severe right upper quadrant pain, whereas chronic cholecystitis would not usually cause weight loss. In primary biliary cirrhosis, pruritus usually precedes jaundice.

P2.104   B: The wounds should be cleaned with saline, and closed

The human mouth is full of anaerobes and aerobes that can rapidly cause severe illness. All patients in whom the skin is punctured should receive antibiotics and a tetanus booster, and those with any signs of spread should be admitted to either orthopaedics or plastic surgery according to the site of the bite. Always consider a foreign body as a cause of infection in traumatic wounds.

P2.105   B: Graduated loading with eccentric exercises should be used as first-line treatment

Steroid injections provide good short-term relief of symptoms, but there is evidence that they increase the risk of recurrence and may delay healing. Avoidance of the irritating action together with eccentric muscle loading is the first-line treatment. There is some evidence for the short-term use of topical NSAIDs and GTN patches in resistant cases. Where these treatments fail, referral for surgery or Botox should be considered.

Drug management of Parkinson's disease

P2.106   G: Pramipexole

Pramipexole and ropinirole are associated with impulse control disorders, with a 14% lifetime risk. Common symptoms are hypersexuality and pathological gambling.

P2.107   C: Citalopram

SSRIs are the first-line choice for depression, which affects up to 50% of patients. Tricyclics should be avoided due to sedation and risk of falls.

P2.108   I: Selegiline

MAO-B inhibitors such as selegiline are useful on their own or in combination with dopamine.

P2.109   D: Clozapine

Psychotic symptoms such as hallucinations are very common in Parkinson's disease in advanced stages. Clozapine is an effective treatment.

P2.110   E: Vertebrobasilar stroke

The presence of brain-stem symptoms with dizziness is suggestive of a brain-stem ischaemic event, rather than a labyrinthine process. Labyrinthitis would normally cause rotatory vertigo, with nystagmus but not dysarthria or upper limb symptoms. Ménière's disease causes vertigo, fluctuating hearing and tinnitus, which recur, with asymptomatic periods in between. Vestibular neuronitis causes acute severe rotatory vertigo with unilateral tinnitus and nausea, without associated neurological symptoms. Migraine may cause labyrinthine or isolated neurological symptoms but this pattern is much more suggestive of a brain-stem event.

P2.111   E: Chickenpox

Chickenpox typically presents with a non-specific febrile illness followed by the development of a vesicular rash. Measles usually starts on the back of the neck and is also associated with conjunctival symptoms. Parvovirus B19 causes a slapped cheek appearance.

Prescription charges

P2.112   H: Not entitled to free prescriptions

Patients with diabetes treated with drugs are entitled to free prescriptions.

P2.113   C: Entitled to free NHS dental treatment

Women who are pregnant and up to 12 months postpartum are entitled to free dental treatment and NHS prescriptions.

P2.114   G: Not entitled to free NHS sight test

Myxoedema gives exemption from prescription charges not eye tests.

P2.115   B: Automatically entitled to free prescriptions

People aged 16, 17 or 18 and in full-time education are exempt from charges.

P2.116   E: Entitled to free prescriptions on applying for an exemption certificate

Those patients who need replacement therapy, or have medically treated diabetes, epilepsy or a fistula, are entitled to free prescriptions on applying and receiving an exemption certificate.

P2.117   B: Varicose eczema

Asteatotic eczema results from loss of lubricating fluid from the skin; it presents as a crazy paving pattern on the lower legs. Psoriasis causes thickened plaques of skin over flexor aspects, eg elbows. Pompholyx affects the soles of the feet and the palms of the hands.

Examination of the eye

P2.118   H: Retinoblastoma

Retinoblastoma is often diagnosed by loss of red reflex and has been picked up from family photos when one person has no red eye.

P2.119   F: Optic atrophy

Optic neuritis causes disc pallor; in the acute phase the disc may also be swollen.

P2.120   A: Acute angle-closure glaucoma

Unlike uveitis, the pupil is fixed but round.

P2.121   G: Recurrent uveitis

Recurrent uveitis causes adhesions around the periphery of the iris.

P2.122   C: Chronic glaucoma

The cup:disc ratio is used to monitor the progression of glaucoma.

P2.123   E: None of the above

Café-au-lait patches are brown macules, usually present from birth. They affect up to 10% of people and, when there are fewer than four patches <0.5 cm and no patches >1.5 cm, they are of no significance. Multiple patches are suggestive of neurofibromatosis or Albright syndrome, characterised by cystic bone lesions and precocious puberty. Tuberous sclerosis is characterised by shagreen patches that fluoresce under UV light. Patients with Bloom syndrome have short stature, telangiectasia and facial erythema.

P2.124   D: Chalazion

Chalazions are retention cysts in meibomian glands. They are similar in appearance to styes but lack signs of acute inflammation. Often settling spontaneously, ones that do not may be treated surgically. Infected chalazions are treated in the same way as styes.

Antibiotic prescribing

P2.125   L: Nitrofurantoin

Nitrofurantoin is the most appropriate choice in this case. Co-trimoxazole (Septrin) is a combination of trimethoprim and sulfamethoxazole.

P2.126   F: Ciprofloxacin

Ciprofloxacin is a useful alternative to rifampicin as prophylaxis.

P2.127   M: Phenoxymethylpenicillin

Phenoxymethylpenicillin is the first-line treatment for tonsillitis in patients who do not have penicillin allergy.

P2.128   H: Erythromycin

Erythromycin has a similar spectrum of activity to amoxicillin and also covers atypical pneumonia.

P2.129   C: Co-amoxiclav

All dog and cat bites or scratches should be treated with co-amoxiclav or doxycycline and metronidazole if penicillin allergic.

P2.130   A: Emergency treatment involves an immediate insulin injection and fluid rehydration

DKA may follow a prodromal illness or present acutely as a consequence of an intercurrent illness. There is often abdominal pain and vomiting, and polydipsia with polyuria. Patients are often significantly dehydrated, although frequently they have an apparent hyperkalaemia on blood testing. Examination findings include tachypnoea and ketotic breath.

P2.131   E: It is usually a sign of underlying malignancy

Common causes of erythema nodosum include streptococcal infections, sarcoidosis, infections and drugs. Treatment is conservative and aimed at the underlying cause.

Child development

Ninety per cent of children achieve the developmental stage by the ages below. Failure to achieve one or more of these milestones by the age suggests that further assessment may be indicated.

P2.132   F: 18 months

P2.133   F: 18 months

P2.134   D: 8 weeks

P2.135   E: 10 months

P2.136   G: 30 months

P2.137   B: 5 months

P2.138   A: 3 months

P2.139   B: Hydroxychloroquine will reduce pain, swelling and stiffness in SLE

Hydroxychloroquine is effective in SLE and RA. Infliximab is for use in active RA only. Sulfasalazine causes reversible effects on fertility. Methotrexate may take some weeks to become effective.

P2.140   B: Rheumatoid arthritis

Primary nodal osteoarthritis affects the distal interphalangeal joints of the fingers. Reiter syndrome usually involves iritis or conjunctivitis. Gout would be unlikely to affect both sides simultaneously.

P2.141   D: The implementation of change is implicit in the audit cycle

The audit cycle is the process of setting standards, measuring performance, diagnosing the problem, implementing change and then re-measuring. Standards can be 'soft', such as the number of complaints, or 'hard', such as the number of patients treated to a blood pressure target.

P2.142   C: Adenoidectomy at the time of grommet insertion significantly reduces the risk of recurrence

Long-term studies suggest that adenoidectomy at the time of grommet insertion greatly reduces the risk of recurrence. Glue ear is not caused by bacterial infection; however, grommets are sometimes used to try to prevent recurrent otitis media. The major clinical significance of glue ear is that it can cause conductive hearing loss at critical stages in a child's development; most children have glue ear at some time in their lives, although very few go on to develop hearing impairment as a result. Treatment is reserved for those with demonstrable hearing loss that fails to resolve naturally. Alternatives to surgery include temporary hearing aids, but there is no evidence at the present time that dietary modification or osteopathy helps, although the natural tendency to resolution may be responsible for a powerful placebo effect.

Shoulder problems

P2.143   D: Referred pain

Pain in the shoulder may be a sign of diaphragmatic irritation, eg cholecystitis or ruptured ectopic.

P2.144   C: Osteoarthritis

Long-standing pain and reduced range of movement suggest osteoarthritis rather than rotator cuff and the history is too long for frozen shoulder. There is often prominent lipping of the joint.

P2.145   A: Cervical spondylosis

Cervical spondylosis may be present with or without neurological symptoms.

P2.146   B: Frozen shoulder

Frozen shoulder affects all movements but external rotation is particularly affected.

P2.147   H: Subluxation of the glenohumeral joint

This is a typical description of a dislocated shoulder.

P2.148   E: Small lesions may be treated successfully with liquid nitrogen

This is a myxoid cyst. These soft rubbery nodules are usually seen on the distal interphalangeal joints of fingers or toes. They usually arise after trauma and are 1.0–1.5 cm in diameter. They are not derived from the joint or tendon sheath, and are not ganglia or synovial cysts. They may cause a groove to develop in the nail. More common in women >40, they often burst and treatment is indicated only for cosmetic reasons or discomfort. They may be treated with liquid nitrogen, intralesional steroid or excision, but often recur.

Medical records legislation

P2.149   A: Access to Health Records Act

P2.150   E: Data Protection Act

P2.151   A: Access to Health Records Act

P2.152   C: Children's Act

P2.153   B: Access to Medical Reports Act

P2.154   A: Access to Health Records Act

Red eye

P2.155   A: Acute glaucoma

P2.156   E: Keratitis

P2.157   B: Anterior uveitis

P2.158   F: Scleritis

P2.159   D: Episcleritis

P2.160   C: Conjunctivitis

P2.161   E: It may be helped with lactase added to feeds

Colic is a disease of unknown origin but some evidence suggests that it may be caused by temporary lactose intolerance. It occurs in 20% of infants and usually lasts up to 3 months of age. Dicyclomine is contraindicated in those aged under 6 months. Vomiting suggests alternative diagnoses, eg constipation, Hirschsprung's disease.

Gynaecological malignancies

P2.162   G: Vulval intraepithelial neoplasia (VIN)

Unlike CIN, VIN tends to be multifocal and regular follow-up is needed even if the primary lesion is removed completely.

P2.163   A: Cervical carcinoma

Cervical cancer tends to present with bleeding, usually postcoital but also intermenstrual or postmenopausal. A high index of suspicion is needed in these situations.

P2.164   C: Choriocarcinoma

Women who have a molar pregnancy are monitored for 2 years to detect choriocarcinoma. Rising βhCG levels suggest that this has occurred, hence after a molar pregnancy patients are advised not to get pregnant for 2 years.

P2.165   E: Ovarian carcinoma

Ovarian cancer tends to be diagnosed late because of the non-specific nature of the symptoms.

P2.166   D: Endometrial carcinoma

Endometrial carcinoma is associated with diabetes and usually presents with postmenopausal bleeding.

P2.167   E: Lung cancer

With a smoking history, clubbing and weight loss, cancer is the most likely diagnosis. Cystic fibrosis and congenital heart disease cause shortness of breath and clubbing but present earlier. Pneumonia would not normally cause clubbing; however, bronchiectasis may cause shortness of breath and clubbing.

P2.168   E: It may be a sign of female virilisation

Crypto-orchidism and hypospadias raise the possibility of female virilisation. The condition is seen in 1:300 male births. Epispadias, where the opening is on the upper, dorsal side of the penis, may be associated with bladder abnormalities. Mild cases of hypospadias may present in adulthood.

Hirsutism

P2.169   A: Combined oral contraceptive

In women with no biochemical evidence of hormonal imbalance a combined oral contraceptive is the best initial treatment.

P2.170   E: Finasteride

In women who are unable to take the COCP, or in whom it is not effective, finasteride may be effective. Adequate contraception is essential.

P2.171   D: Electrolysis

Cosmetic techniques should be considered for all women, particularly where hair is localised.

P2.172   C: Dianette

Dianette is licensed for the treatment of hirsutism and acne. It is preferable to cyproterone alone because adequate contraception is needed to prevent feminisation of a male fetus.

P2.173   H: Referral

This woman probably has polycystic ovary syndrome. Referral is indicated to optimise chances of conception and control symptoms.

Dizziness and vertigo

P2.174   F: Ménière's disease

This is a classic description of Ménière's disease.

P2.175   J: Vestibular neuronitis

Vestibular neuronitis tends to produce severe vertigo, which often causes people to take to their beds for several days. It is thought to be viral.

P2.176   C: Cardiogenic syncope

Vestibular disease causes rotatory vertigo. Light-headedness without vertigo is seldom caused by otological disease.

P2.177   B: Benign paroxysmal positional vertigo

A benign paroxysmal positional vertigo causes maximal symptoms when the affected semicircular canal is stimulated more than the others.

P2.178   G: Ramsay Hunt syndrome

Herpes zoster affecting the geniculate ganglion may cause facial nerve paralysis, vertigo and sensorineural deafness. It should be treated with aciclovir and steroids.

P2.179   C: A raised PSA may be caused by urinary infection

PSA is neither highly specific nor sensitive. A significant number of people with prostate cancer are missed by PSA testing and many undergo prostate biopsy without having cancer confirmed. Old age, prostatic hyperplasia, infection and instrumentation can all elevate the PSA. There are age-specific cut-offs for elevated PSA.

P2.180   A: He should be converted to a twice-daily maintenance dose of methadone and this should be gradually reduced

Methadone is given once daily and has a long half-life. Buprenorphine is safer in overdose and less addictive than methadone. Management of opiate abuse includes a holistic approach to lifestyle risk factors.

P2.181   D: Pneumothorax

Spontaneous pneumothorax is often idiopathic but, where recurrent, CT may demonstrate bullae. In this instance surgical pleurodesis may be indicated. In spontaneous pneumothorax cyanosis is rare and can often be treated with needle aspiration.

P2.182   E: Doxycycline is associated with photosensitivity

Malarone needs to be taken only from 2 days before entering a malaria zone until 1 week after leaving. It is taken daily. Antimalarials are available only on private prescription. Mefloquine causes neuropsychiatric side effects in less than 1% of patients. All patients should use insect repellents, long trousers and sleeves, and consider insect nets.

P2.183   A: A written response must be received by the patient within 10 working days

There is a time limit of 6 months for practice complaints. The complaint must be acknowledged within 2 working days. Complaints may be verbal, written or emailed to the practice. The Healthcare Commission deals with the *process* of the complaint, not the substance. There is a time limit of 6 months from the incident, but this can be extended, eg if a patient was too ill to complain. Out-of-hours complaints should be made to the relevant PCO (primary care organisation).

P2.184   C: Ten per cent of patients with mumps develop symptomatic meningeal involvement

The incubation period is usually around 18 days. Of patients 70% develop salivary gland involvement, and infection is by droplets or fomites. Although 25% of postpubertal males develop orchitis, it is unilateral in 80% and hence the risk of infertility is low.

P2.185   A: The new treatment increases severe disability compared with standard treatment

The graph suggests that more patients in the new treatment group will experience severe disability than in the usual treatment group. This type of study is prone to recording and inclusion bias but without information on study design and confidence intervals it is not possible to comment on statistical significance or possible bias.

P2.186.   D: He should have his cholesterol measured and be treated according to his calculated cardiovascular risk score, using QRISK or a similar method

The Copenhagen Heart Study found that xanthelasmas are a predictor of ischaemic heart disease, myocardial infarction, atherosclerosis and death independent of other risk factors, including lipid levels. Arcus cornea, on the other hand, was not associated with increased risk. This patient is not therefore at increased risk due to his arcus but he should have his cholesterol measured so that he can be reassured about his 10-year risk scores. It is unlikely, however, that he would reach the threshold for intervention given his normal blood pressure, lack of smoking and diabetes.

P2.187   C: Hydrocortisone

Nappy rash that affects the skin creases is usually caused by *Candida* sp. Less commonly it can be caused by bacterial infection or dermatitis. Treatment with clotrimazole and more regular nappy changes/leaving the nappy off help. Where nappy rash spares creases, it is usually caused by irritant dermatitis. Barrier creams, regular nappy changes and use of baby wipes all help in this situation.

P2.188   A: It is associated with Paget's disease of the nipple

Eczematous lesions on the nipple, often associated with discharge, are frequently associated with DCIS. The rate of progression to invasive cancer is 30–50% and the tumours are usually estrogen receptor positive. DCIS is frequently picked up at an early stage on mammography due to the presence of microcalcification.

P2.189   62.5 mg three times daily

The dose for amoxicillin based on age is 62.5 mg three times daily up to 1 year, from 1 year to 8 years 125 mg three times daily, and >8 years 250 mg three times daily.

Management of autism

P2.190   G: Risperidone

Risperidone is recommended as an adjunct treatment where there is hyperactivity, irritability or sleep problems.

P2.191   D: Methylphenidate

Methylphenidate is helpful for inattention but often less so than in children with ADHD.

P2.192   B: Aripiprazole

Aripiprazole is effective for maladaptive behaviour. Risperidone may also be used in this context but frequently causes weight gain.

P2.193   C: Fluoxetine or ecitalopram

Fluoxetine or ecitalopram has been used with some benefit in restricted repetitive behaviour, but there is limited evidence for their use. Methylphenidate is also used for this problem.

P2.194   A: Baclofen

NICE guidance for management of spasticity in patients with cerebral palsy advises that all patients should have physical therapy as part of a multidisciplinary team approach, with consideration of orthoses. Where these fail to control symptoms, oral baclofen is the most appropriate medication for day-time use. Benzodiazepines are helpful at night where sedation is less of a problem. Focal spasticity affecting motor function, eg in the hand, can be treated with Botox, whereas intrathecal baclofen or dorsal rhizotomy may help if medication fails.

P2.195   A: Check blood pressure

Persistent microscopic haematuria is common, and usually benign, but may be a sign of renal disease. The most common cause is infection, so this should be excluded with urinary culture. A blood pressure check as part of the initial assessment is mandatory to pick up renal disease and, if elevated, should prompt a routine referral. All patients with persistent haematuria should have baseline renal function and urine protein assessment. Urine microscopy, unless on very fresh urine, has low sensitivity and prostate cancer is an unlikely cause for microscopic haematuria in asymptomatic men. Renal ultrasound is indicated if there are symptoms suggestive of renal colic.

P2.196   Pulmonary fibrosis

Pulmonary fibrosis causes a restrictive lung defect so the FEV_1 and FVC will both be reduced, hence the normal FEV_1/FVC. The transfer factor is markedly reduced, however, confirming the probable diagnosis of pulmonary fibrosis.

P2.197   B: Aggressive control of blood pressure

Unlike Alzheimer's disease, vascular dementia is usually unresponsive to acetylcholinesterase inhibitors or memantine. Slight benefits in cognition have been reported in some trials, but these are thought to be due to presumed coexistent Alzheimer's disease-type neuropathology. Aggressive treatment of blood pressure has been shown to reduce the risk of the disease and also slow its rate of decline if used early in the disease. This has not been shown to be true for antiplatelet or statin use.

P2.198   B: Presbyacusis

A symmetrical, high-frequency, sensorineural loss is characteristic of presbyacusis. Bilateral tinnitus is not a sign of acoustic neuroma.

P2.199   B: Practices with high QOF scores might be making more earlier diagnoses, resulting in greater admission rates for elective treatment

Practices with high QOF scores are more likely to be in areas of low deprivation. Exception reporting will inflate the QOF score but not affect the admission rate. Non-medical staff tend to be very good at rigid, protocol-led work, such as collecting data, but are less capable of managing complex problems.

P2.200   E: Standing blood pressure

This woman has symptoms of postural hypotension and this can be confirmed by checking blood pressure supine and standing. A drop of 20 mmHg is considered significant. Common causes include antihypertensives, L-dopa and anxiolytics. Other common causes include venous pooling after prolonged standing, poor muscle tone, eg bed-bound patients or hypovolaemia (blood loss, diarrhoea). A 24-hour tape is useful for the diagnosis of intermittent arrhythmia whereas a 24-hour blood pressure can differentiate white coat hypertension from sustained hypertension. An ECG is also indicated in this situation but a standing blood pressure should be carried out as part of her baseline observations.

Index

Question numbers beginning with 'P' refer to the practice papers at the end of the book.